Human Psychoneuroimmunology

Edited by

Kavita Vedhara

MRC Health Service Research Collaboration
Department of Social Medicine, University of Bristol, UK

and

Michael R. Irwin

Cousins Center for Psychoneuroimmunology, UCLA Neuropsychiatric
Institute, USA

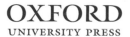

OXFORD
UNIVERSITY PRESS

*This book has been printed digitally and produced in a standard specification
in order to ensure its continuing availability*

OXFORD
UNIVERSITY PRESS

Great Clarendon Street, Oxford OX2 6DP

Oxford University Press is a department of the University of Oxford.
It furthers the University's objective of excellence in research, scholarship,
and education by publishing worldwide in

Oxford New York

Auckland   Cape Town Dar es Salaam Hong Kong Karachi
Kuala Lumpur Madrid Melbourne Mexico City Nairobi
New Delhi Shanghai Taipei Toronto
With offices in
Argentina Austria Brazil Chile Czech Republic France Greece
Guatemala Hungary Italy Japan South Korea Poland Portugal
Singapore Switzerland Thailand Turkey Ukraine Vietnam

Oxford is a registered trade mark of Oxford University Press
in the UK and in certain other countries

Published in the United States
by Oxford University Press Inc., New York

ISBN   978-0-19-856884-1

Printed and bound by CPI Antony Rowe, Eastbourne

Contents

List of Contributors

Robert Ader
Center for Psychoneuroimmunology,
Research Department of Psychiatry,
University of Rochester School of
Medicine and Dentistry,
Rochester, NY, USA

Michael H. Antoni
Department of Psychology,
Coral Gables,
FL 33124, USA

Roger Booth
Department of Molecular Medicine
and Pathology,
The University of Auckland,
New Zealand

Lena Brydon
Department of Epidemiology and
Public Health,
University College London, UK

Sheldon Cohen
Department of Psychology,
Carnegie Mellon University,
Pittsburgh, PA, USA

Jason C. Cole
Cousins Center for
Psychoneuroimmunology,
UCLA Neuropsychiatric Institute,
University of California Los Angeles,
CA, USA

Jason R. Dahn
Miami VA Medical Center,
Miami, FL, USA

Ronald Glaser
Department of Molecular Virology,
Immunology, and Medical Genetics,
Institute of Behavioral Medicine
Research, and Comprehensive
Cancer Center,
Ohio State University,
Columbus, OH, USA

Victoria L. Green
Postgraduate Medical Institute,
University of Hull in Association
with Hull–York Medical School and
Hull and East Yorkshire Hospitals
NHS Trust, Hull, UK

John Greenman
Postgraduate Medical Institute,
University of Hull in Association
with Hull–York Medical School and
Hull and East Yorkshire Hospitals
NHS Trust, Hull, UK

Cobi J. Heijnen
University Medical Center Utrecht,
Laboratory of Psychoneuroimmunology,
Utrecht, The Netherlands

Michael R. Irwin
Cousins Center for
Psychoneuroimmunology,
UCLA Neuropsychiatric Institute,
University of California Los Angeles,
CA, USA

Annemieke Kavelaars
University Medical Center Utrecht,
Laboratory of Psychoneuroimmunology,
Utrecht, The Netherlands

Joey M. Kaye
University of Bristol,
Henry Wellcome Laboratories for
Integrative Neuroscience and
Endocrinology,
Bristol, UK

Stafford L. Lightman
University of Bristol,
Henry Wellcome Laboratories for
Integrative Neuroscience and
Endocrinology,
Bristol, UK

Gregory E. Miller
Department of Psychology,
University of British Columbia,
2136 West Mall,
Vancouver, BC V6T 1Z4,
Canada

Frank J. Penedo
Department of Psychology,
University of Miami,
Coral Gables, FL, USA

Deidre B. Pereira
Department of Clinical and
Health Psychology,
College of Public Health and
Health Professions,
University of Florida,
Gainesville, FL, USA

Bruce S. Rabin
Professor of Pathology and Psychiatry,
Medical Director,
UPMC Healthy Lifestyle Program,
Pittsburgh, PA, USA

Donald M. Sharp
Postgraduate Medical Institute,
University of Hull in Association with
Hull–York Medical School,
Hull, UK

Andrew Steptoe
Department of Epidemiology
and Public Health,
University College London, UK

Kavita Vedhara
MRC HSRC,
University of Bristol, UK

Leslie G. Walker
Postgraduate Medical Institute,
University of Hull in Association
with Hull–York Medical School,
Hull, UK

Andrew A. Walker
Postgraduate Medical Institute,
University of Hull in Association
with Hull–York Medical School,
Hull, UK

E. C. Y. Wang
Section of Infection and Immunity,
University of Wales College of Medicine,
Cardiff, UK

Eric V. Yang
Department of Molecular Virology,
Immunology, and Medical Genetics,
Ohio State University,
Columbus, OH, USA

Chapter 1

Introduction to immunology and immune–endocrine interactions

Bruce S. Rabin

1.1 Introduction

This chapter provides a basic introduction to the 'I' of PsychoNeuroImmunology. An understanding of how the immune system functions to maintain health and sometimes damage tissue will be described. This understanding will be developed by providing information about the cellular and soluble functional components of the immune system, how their interaction with each other produces specific antibody and cell-mediated protection against infectious disease, and how the stressor-induced hormonal response alters immune function. The chapter is not a complete review of immunology. Details of textbooks that the reader can use to obtain a more complete education are given in the References.[1–3]

1.2 The biological context: the immune system

What is referred to as the 'immune system' consists of a variety of interactive cells and soluble molecules. The immune system patrols the blood and the tissues, looking for the presence of substances that are foreign to the body, which are collectively referred to as 'antigens' (usually infectious agents), and whose presence can produce illness. When the immune system identifies the presence of a foreign material it is turned on, directs its attention to the material and helps to kill, inactivate, and remove it from the body. Sometimes the process of removing an infectious agent from the body will damage tissue. Sometimes the reaction of the immune system to an antigen will produce the clinical condition known as 'allergy'.

The process of immune-mediated removal of infectious agents from the body may be relatively benign. For example, bacteria that have penetrated the skin may result in the local accumulation of white blood cells, producing a pimple. Less benign, but tolerable, is immune-mediated removal of the influenza virus from the nose or throat. This may result in increased mucus secretion, a temperature elevation, aching joints, loss of appetite, lethargy, and recovery after a few days.

A more severe response to a virus infection occurs when, for example, the hepatitis virus infects liver cells. The killing of the infected liver cells results in temporarily impaired liver function, resulting in jaundice and extreme lethargy. However, when all the infected liver cells are removed, the damaged liver regrows, leading to normal health.

Finally, an extreme response occurs when, for example, the immune system reacts to a virus that has infected the cells of the pancreas that produce insulin. Efficient removal of the infected cells will produce some damage but leave enough insulin-producing cells to maintain normal glucose control. However, if there is prolonged killing of the infected cells, there may be too few left for normal glucose control and the individual will become diabetic. Unfortunately, unlike the liver, the pancreas does not regrow when damaged.

Good health is associated with an immune system that is functioning well. The hormonal response to the perception of high levels of stress in an individual's life can alter the function of the immune system so that proper elimination of infectious agents is impaired. Thus stress may be a factor leading to altered health through alteration of the function of the immune system.

1.3 Organization of the immune system

Our understanding of how the immune system functions is constantly changing as researchers continue to delve into the intricacies of newly identified populations of lymphocytes and cytokines, as our understanding of the interactions between cells and cytokines are modified, and as our understanding of the importance of the complement system is expanded. In the clinical applications of immunology we are gaining new insights into why autoimmune diseases develop, how resistance to infectious diseases is achieved, and how the immune system resists the spontaneous development of malignancy. However, our detailed understanding of these clinical conditions depends on a more complete knowledge of the development and function of the immune system. The following discussion provides an introduction to components of the immune system and how they function.

1.3.1 Primary lymphoid tissue

Lymphocytes are formed and mature to become functional in the bone marrow and thymus. 'Primary' immune responses are not initiated in these tissues.

1.3.1.1 Bone marrow

The bone marrow is the source of mature oxygen-transporting red blood cells, platelets for blood clotting, and various types of white blood cells. Cells termed 'stem cells' give rise to the various types of blood cells. Under the influence of specific growth factors (proteins that bind to receptors on cell surfaces and activate cell maturation and growth) stem cells for white blood cells will mature into each specific type of white blood cell.

1.3.1.2 **Thymus**

The thymus is a tissue resting on top of the heart. Maturation of immature lymphocytes coming from the bone marrow occurs within the thymus, and the mature cells enter the bloodstream and tissue. They are referred to as T lymphocytes and are involved in reactions called 'cell-mediated immunity'. T lymphocytes that react against the individual's own tissue are eliminated in the thymus. Lymphocytes that are functionally useless are also eliminated.

The thymus increases in size from birth to puberty and then decreases. The epithelial cells of the thymus produce hormones that are associated with maturation of T lymphocytes. The concentration of these thymic hormones in the blood begins to decrease at approximately 60 years of age. The effects of stress on thymus hormone production are uncertain.

1.3.2 **Cells**

1.3.2.1 **White blood cells**

If blood is collected and prevented from clotting and allowed to settle in a tube, the red blood cells will fall to the bottom and a white layer of cells is formed on top of them. The cells which form this white layer are commonly called 'white blood cells' or 'leucocytes'. Some white blood cells have granules in their cytoplasm. These granules contain enzymes that help to digest materials that these cells ingest. The granular cells are called neutrophils, eosinophils, basophils, and monocytes. White blood cells without granules are called lymphocytes and monocytes. White blood cells are also classified on the basis of the shape of the nucleus. Lymphocytes and monocytes have a round nucleus and are sometimes called 'mononuclear' cells. Granulocytes have a lobulated nucleus and therefore are sometimes called 'polymorphonuclear' cells.

1.3.2.2 **Granulocytes (polymorphonuclear) cells**

Neutrophils are involved in the ingestion (phagocytosis) of solid particles such as bacteria. They are attracted to areas where they are needed through a process called 'chemotaxis', and they have the ability to bind foreign particles (such as bacteria) to their surface by a process called 'opsonization' by which particles can be ingested and killed. Antibodies produced by the immune system participate in opsonization by helping neutrophils to ingest bacteria.

Eosinophils help to protect against infections caused by parasites by releasing substances that are toxic to them. They also migrate to sites of allergic reactions where the enzymes released from the eosinophils can damage normal tissue.

Basophils have granules containing histamine which, when released from the cell, will cause some of the symptoms of allergic disease (itching, runny nose, difficulty in breathing). Basophils do not usually enter tissue. A cell with a similar appearance and function is the mast cell. Mast cells are present in tissue and do not circulate.

1.3.2.3 **Mononuclear cells**

Monocytes ingest foreign materials which enter the body. When a monocyte enters tissue it becomes enlarged and is called a macrophage. Infectious agents that are ingested by monocytes and macrophages are often killed when a T lymphocyte activates the monocyte or macrophage.

Lymphocytes: there are several types of lymphocyte, each with a different function. Lymphocytes do not phagocytose.

B **lymphocytes** produce antibody. They are formed in the bone marrow and mature to become capable of recognizing foreign antigen by specific antibody receptors on their surface.

T **lymphocytes** do not produce antibody. They are called T lymphocytes because they mature and become capable of recognizing a foreign antigen in the thymus gland. T lymphocytes are active in the immune reactions termed 'cell-mediated immunity'.

There are several different populations of T lymphocytes that are identified by the presence of unique protein markers on their surface. All T lymphocytes have a surface marker called CD3. In addition, T lymphocytes have either the CD4 or CD8 marker. Thus they are CD3 and CD4 positive or CD3 and CD8 positive.

CD4 T cells are classified as 'helper T cells' because they promote immune reactions. CD8 T cells are capable of killing tissue cells and are referred to as 'cytotoxic T cells'.

CD4 cells can be further subdivided into two classes: CD4-Th1 and CD4-Th2. The Th1 and Th2 cells produce different cytokines and have different functional properties. As a general rule, the CD4-Th1 cells are effective by helping macrophages to kill bacteria that the macrophage has ingested and by helping to activate the CD8 cell (the CD8 cell can kill tissue cells that are infected with a virus). The CD8 T cell is commonly referred to as a 'cytotoxic' lymphocyte. Examples of cytokines produced by Th1 cells are interferon-gamma (INF-γ), interleukin 2 (IL-2), and tumour necrosis factor-beta (TNF-β). As a general rule CD4-Th2 cells are important in inducing B cells to release antibody. Examples of cytokines produced by Th2 cells are IL-4, IL-5 IL-6, IL-10, and IL-13.

Another lymphocyte population is known as the natural killer (NK) lymphocyte. These lymphocytes are not T or B cells. They contain a few granules in their cytoplasm and have the capability of killing tissue cells that have been infected by a virus or which may be malignant. They recognize that a tissue cell has been infected by a virus but, unlike T cells, do not have the capability of recognizing that a particular virus has infected the cell.

1.3.2.4 **Dendritic cells**

Another population of cells that is essential for the function of the immune system is the 'dendritic cells'. These cells are found in all tissues of the body. They have the capability of presenting antigens to T lymphocytes. The antigens are either ingested into the dendritic cells or synthesized within the dendritic cells. Technically, dendritic cells are not white blood cells. They have high concentrations of MHC I and MHC II molecules as well as costimulation molecules on their membranes (MHC is discussed in section 1.5.2). Dendritic cells are very efficient at activating an immune response. Dendritic cells in the spleen or lymph nodes initiate immune responses by interacting with a T cell that has antigen-recognizing receptors for the antigen being displayed in the MHC I or MHC I on the membrane of the dendritic cell.

1.3.3 Secondary lymphoid tissue

Lymphocytes are produced in primary lymphoid tissue (bone marrow) and mature to be capable of recognizing an antigen (B lymphocytes mature in the bone marrow and T lymphocytes mature in the thymus gland). In addition to being found in blood, lymphocytes accumulate in organized tissue called secondary lymphoid tissue (lymph nodes, spleen, mucosal-associated lymphoid tissues).

Lymphocytes that have surface receptors for an antigen, but are naive in the sense that they have not yet been activated to make an immune response to the antigen, become activated to the antigen to which they bear surface-recognition molecules in the secondary lymphoid tissues. The activation requires interaction between (1) antigen-presenting dendritic cells and CD4 T lymphocytes and B lymphocytes for antibody production, (2) antigen-presenting dendritic cells and CD4 T lymphocytes for development of a cellular immune reaction, and (3) antigen-presenting dendritic cells and CD4 T lymphocytes and CD8 T lymphocytes if cytotoxic lymphocytes are to be generated.

1.3.3.1 Lymph nodes

Lymph nodes are organized accumulations of lymphocytes and dendritic cells surrounded by a capsule with a blood supply and connective tissue through which lymph flows. Lymph is fluid that accumulates in tissue and drains back to the bloodstream through small capillary tubes called 'lymphatics'.

Lymphocytes accumulate along the path of the lymphatic vessels forming nodules that are called 'lymph nodes'. Lymph fluid passes through the node on its path back to the bloodstream. There are many lymph nodes located along the lymphatic vessels so that the fluid passes through many nodes as it moves from the periphery to the vasculature. As the lymph fluid passes through the lymph nodes it accumulates lymphocytes from the nodes which eventually pass into the bloodstream.

Another way for lymphocytes to enter a node is by traversing the endothelial cells that line the capillaries carrying blood to the node. The endothelial cells lining the post-capillary venules in the node are large (called 'high endothelial' cells) and have adhesion molecules to which naive lymphocytes bind. The naive lymphocytes pass from the blood through the high endothelial cells and enter the node. Lymphocytes that have been activated in response to an antigen lose the adhesion molecule that binds them to the high endothelial cells and can only enter the node from a lymphatic that drains tissue.

1.3.3.2 Spleen

The spleen is the largest lymphoid organ. It is inserted into the blood circulation and filters blood, removing antigens and old or damaged erythrocytes.

Antigen that is in the bloodstream will pass into the spleen where it is ingested by dendritic cells. Antibody production is initiated by the antibody-producing B lymphocytes upon appropriate interaction with activated antigen-specific T cells.

1.4 Soluble molecules

1.4.1 Antibody

Antibody can affect an infectious agent or a soluble product of the infectious agent. Antibody molecules do not penetrate cells and therefore are effective against antigens that remain in an extracellular location. Such antigens include bacteria, soluble substances released from bacteria, virus that has been shed by a cell, and parasites.

1.4.1.1 Characteristics of antibody

All serum proteins can be classified in one of five large subgroups based on how rapidly they migrate in an electrical field. The five groups are albumin, alpha-1 globulin, alpha-2 globulin, beta globulin and gamma globulin. Antibody molecules belong to the gamma globulin subgroup.

There are five classes of antibody molecules that together comprise gamma globulin. Each class is called an immunoglobulin because it has immune function (Fig. 1.1). The five classes of immunoglobulin (Ig) are IgG, IgA, IgM, IgD, and IgE. Each class of immunoglobulin has its own heavy chain; identification of each class is based on the heavy chain as the light chains are common to all classes.

1.4.1.2 Physiological function of immunoglobulin classes

IgG IgG is effective in neutralizing toxins (such as tetanus or diphtheria toxin) which are produced by microorganisms. There are four subclasses of IgG. The IgG1 and IgG3 subclasses adhere to phagocytic cells and are able to activate the complement system. Therefore IgG1 and IgG3 are effective in providing protection against many microorganisms by participating in the removal of infectious agents. Half of the IgG is in blood and the other half is in tissue. Thus IgG helps protect the entire body from infection. At birth the fetus is protected from infection by IgG which has crossed the placenta.

IgA IgA is found in serum and in the external secretions of the body. In the external secretions (sweat, colostrum, tears, saliva, gastrointestinal tract, bronchi) IgA exists as a dimer of two basic units held together by a joining chain and containing a polypeptide component which is termed the secretory component. The secretory component

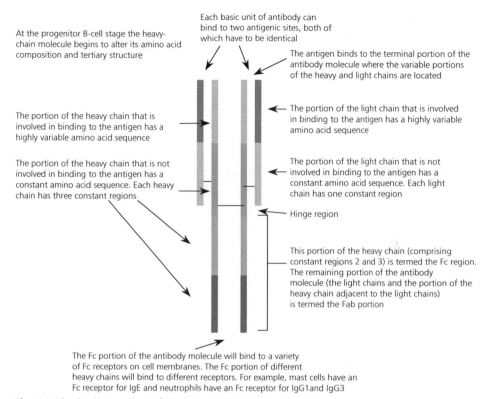

At the progenitor B-cell stage the heavy-chain molecule begins to alter its amino acid composition and tertiary structure

Each basic unit of antibody can bind to two antigenic sites, both of which have to be identical

The antigen binds to the terminal portion of the antibody molecule where the variable portions of the heavy and light chains are located

The portion of the heavy chain that is involved in binding to the antigen has a highly variable amino acid sequence

The portion of the light chain that is involved in binding to the antigen has a highly variable amino acid sequence

The portion of the heavy chain that is not involved in binding to the antigen has a constant amino acid sequence. Each heavy chain has three constant regions

The portion of the light chain that is not involved in binding to the antigen has a constant amino acid sequence. Each light chain has one constant region

Hinge region

This portion of the heavy chain (comprising constant regions 2 and 3) is termed the Fc region. The remaining portion of the antibody molecule (the light chains and the portion of the heavy chain adjacent to the light chains) is termed the Fab portion

The Fc portion of the antibody molecule will bind to a variety of Fc receptors on cell membranes. The Fc portion of different heavy chains will bind to different receptors. For example, mast cells have an Fc receptor for IgE and neutrophils have an Fc receptor for IgG1 and IgG3

Fig. 1.1 The basic structure of the immunoglobulin molecule.

transports IgA onto the external secretions. The function of IgA in serum is not well understood. The major interest in IgA is in its role as a protective substance in the external secretions. Secretory IgA may interfere with the ability of microorganisms to adhere to the mucosal surfaces of the body and to penetrate tissue. The secretory component is synthesized in the epithelial cells which line the mucosal surfaces. The IgA which appears in the external secretions is produced locally by plasma cells underlying the epithelium.

IgM IgM, which consists of five of the basic units, is the largest immunoglobulin. It is efficient as a protective agent against infectious agents because a single molecule bound to a bacterium can activate the complement system. Following stimulation of the immune system by an antigen, the initial antibody response is IgM. Approximately 90% of IgM is in the blood.

IgD Most of the IgD class of immunoglobulin is found on the surface of immature B lymphocytes. The serum concentration of IgD is very low. The role of IgD on the cell surface may be to function as an antigen recognition receptor; however, its clinical significance is unknown.

IgE Small amounts of IgE are found in serum. Most IgE, and the IgE that is responsible for producing the clinical symptoms of allergy, binds to the surface of tissue mast cells or circulating basophils. Degranulation of mast cells occurs when two molecules of IgE that are reactive to the same antigen locate next to each other on the surface of the mast cell, and both interact with the same antigen molecule. The products that are released from the mast cell are responsible for producing the changes in tissue that are referred to as allergy. Histamine is responsible for the immediate allergic reaction and leukotrienes for the sustained reaction.

1.4.2 Complement

Complement is the term applied to a group of sequentially interacting serum proteins that participate in mediating an inflammatory response in tissue. Activated complement attracts polymorphonuclear leucocytes to the site of a bacterium, increases the permeability of blood vessels to allow phagocytic cells into the tissue, and allows cells and fluids to escape from blood vessels and enter tissue. Complement promotes the ingestion of insoluble particles, including bacteria, by phagocytic cells. Fully functional complement can produce holes in cell membranes and cause tissue damage.

1.4.2.1 Properties of complement

Complement is a series of serum proteins that are activated by antigen–antibody complexes or directly by microorganisms. Activation of complement on a cell membrane results in the formation of a membrane-attack complex that produces holes in the membrane. Small biologically active fragments of complement components released during the activation process dilate blood vessels and attract phagocytic cells.

There are two pathways for complement activation. One initiates complement through antibody molecules that bind to an antigen. This is called the 'classical' complement pathway. The other is called the 'alternate' complement pathway and activates complement by the component called C3 adhering to an infectious agent that has entered the body.

The complement components termed C1, C2, and C4 are part of the classic pathway and are activated by C1 binding to antibody that has adhered to an antigen. These complement components then bind and activate C3. The alternate complement pathway initiates activation at C3. Thus C3 is the central aspect of the complement cascade and is where the classic and alternate pathways converge.

As the alternate pathway activates complement in the absence of antibody it is one of the first line defenses against infection. Human cells have a receptor for an inactivator of the bound C3, but bacteria do not. Therefore the alternate complement pathway initiates the components of the complement sequence that are important for mediating an inflammatory response and phagocytosis of bacteria by neutrophils.

The ingestion of infectious agents is enhanced by the C3b component of complement that adheres to the membrane of infectious agents. C3b binds to receptors on macrophages and neutrophils to enhance the ability of the cells to ingest an infectious agent to which complement has attached. Other small molecules split off from C3 and C5, called C3a and C5a, respectively, cause smooth muscle to contract and stimulate mast cells and basophils to secrete histamine. Histamine causes an increased permeability of blood vessels and allows more antibodies, cells, and complement to reach the site of infection. In addition, C3a and C5a attract neutrophils to the site of complement activation.

An example of complement-mediated tissue damage occurs when a patient receives an ABO blood group incompatible transfusion; for example, group A red blood cells are given to a group O recipient. Blood group O individuals have antibody to blood group A. When this occurs, the antibody binds to the red blood cells and activates the complement system, and the red blood cells are lysed (ruptured due to fluid entering the cell through the holes in the membrane created by complement).

1.4.3 Cytokines

Cytokines are soluble proteins released from a cell that can influence the activity of other cells. Cytokines are produced by lymphocytes, monocytes, and macrophages, as well as by tissue cells and cells of the central nervous system. Cytokines bind to receptors on cells. One way in which cells can communicate with each other is by one cell producing a cytokine that binds to a receptor on another cell and activates a cell function.

The nomenclature used to identify cytokines is to call each an 'interleukin' followed by a number. For example, 'interleukin 2' is a cytokine produced by CD4 lymphocytes with the biological property of promoting division of T lymphocytes.

1.4.3.1 Properties of cytokines

Cytokines have the function of mediating and regulating immune responses and inflammatory conditions. Cytokines initiate their function by binding to specific receptors on cell surfaces. Cytokine production is transient and cytokines are not stored in cells. Many cell types, both of the immune system and of other tissue cells, produce cytokines. The targets of cytokines are cells of the immune system and tissue cells. For example, cytokines can produce an elevation of plasma cortisol or body temperature.

1.4.3.2 Examples of cytokines

IL-1

- IL-1 causes an exodus of neutrophils from bone marrow
- IL-1 stimulates collagen release by cells in the skin
- IL-1 is involved with the formation of bone
- IL-1 activates liver cells to release acute phase reactants such as C-reactive protein

- IL-1 has an effect on behaviour and produces sleepiness, loss of appetite, and temperature elevation

IL-2

- IL-2 is a signal for DNA replication and cell division
- IL-2 often acts on the same cells that produce it (autocrine) and on nearby cells (paracrine)
- CD4 cells produce enough IL-2 so that they do not need other sources
- CD8 cells do not produce enough IL-2 on their own and need IL-2 produced by CD4 cells
- the quantity of IL-2 synthesized by CD4 cells influences the magnitude of the immune response
- IL-2 stimulates the growth and function of NK cells
- During a vigorous immune response, shed IL-2 can be detected in serum
- IL-2 is produced by the Th1 subset of CD4 cells

IL-4

- IL-4 is primarily involved in the growth and differentiation of activated B cells
- IL-4 is the only known cytokine that stimulates B lymphocytes to produce IgE for IgE production
- IL-4 is produced by the Th2 subset of CD4 cells

1.4.4 Chemokines

Chemokines are a family of low-molecular-weight chemoattractant molecules that mediate inflammation. Chemokines induce target-cell-specific directional migration of leucocytes (lymphocytes, monocytes, and neutrophils) within tissue sites of inflammation. Chemokines act in conjunction with adhesion molecules to give specificity to the cell composition of inflammatory infiltrates. The leucocyte composition at an inflammatory focus is determined, in large part, by the spectrum of chemokines produced at the site.

1.5 Molecules that are attached to cells

1.5.1 Adhesion molecules

The inflammatory process involves cell movement along adhesion molecules. White blood cells must not only be able to move about in the intravascular space, but they must also be able to adhere to the endothelial cells lining the blood vessels at sites where an inflammatory process is required. Such interactions between lymphocytes and blood vessels are constantly occurring in lymph nodes as part of the mechanism by which lymphocytes migrate from circulation to the lymph nodes.

Leucocyte emigration from the bloodstream into tissue involves a coordinated series of complex events. The presence of an infectious agent or tissue damage sends signals to the adjacent endothelial cells and to leucocytes which cause these cells to become 'activated'. The activation is expressed by the leucocytes adhering to the endothelial cells and then rolling along the endothelial cells as they are pushed by the flow of blood. The rolling leucocytes will eventually stick to a specific location on the endothelium which has expressed increased concentrations of adhesion molecules. Once the leucocytes stick to a point on the endothelial cells, they squeeze between the endothelial cells and migrate to the site within the tissue where they are being attracted.

1.5.2 The major histocompatibility complex

Tissue from one individual transplanted to another is rejected because there are antigens present on the donor tissue that differ from those of the recipient. These antigens stimulate the immune system just as infectious agents do. The antigens that determine whether tissue is compatible between donor and recipient are termed 'histocompatibility antigens'.

The histocompatibility antigens that have an effect on transplant rejection are termed the 'major histocompatibility antigens' and are coded for by a set of clustered genetic loci termed the 'major histocompatibility complex' (MHC).

The primary function of the major histocompatibility antigens is not to elicit destruction of transplanted tissue but rather to present foreign antigens to T lymphocytes. This takes place on the surface of the antigen-presenting cell (dendritic cells, B lymphocytes, macrophages). Thus the foreign antigen (a peptide) is recognized by T lymphocytes in conjunction with a self-antigen (the MHC molecule).

In humans, the MHC molecule is referred to as the human leucocyte antigen (HLA) molecule. This is because the common tissue that is used to detect the presence of these molecules is the 'leucocyte' (white blood cell) and the technique originally used to detect these molecules was to use antibodies that were specific for each of the unique HLA molecules.

There are two classes of histocompatibility antigens, class I and class II. Class I present antigenic peptides that are synthesized within the cytoplasm of the antigen-presenting cell. Class II present antigens that are ingested into and then digested into small peptides by cells. The important cells that present antigen in MHC molecules are the dendritic cells, macrophages, and B lymphocytes.

To be presented in the groove of a MHC II molecule a large protein molecule must be digested into small peptides of approximately 10–14 amino acids. Ingested antigen is degraded into small peptides that are placed into the grooves of MHC II molecules for presentation to T lymphocytes. Peptides synthesized within the antigen-presenting cell are placed into the groove of MHC I molecules. MHC I molecules present antigens to the CD8 class of T lymphocytes (cytotoxic lymphocytes) and MHC II molecules present antigens to the CD4 class of T lymphocytes (helper and mediators of cell-mediated immunity). Every MHC molecule must have a peptide in its groove or it will not move from the cytoplasm to the cell membrane of the antigen-presenting cell.

1.5.3 T-cell receptors

The T-cell receptor (TCR) is the means by which the T cell recognizes an antigen peptide in the MHC molecule. The TCR can only recognize antigen when the antigen

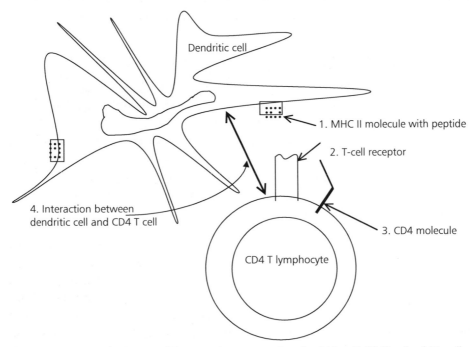

Fig. 1.2 Activation of a CD4 T cell by an antigen-presenting dendritic cell. (1) The dendritic cell ingests a foreign antigen, digests it into small peptides, and places the peptides into the groove of the MHC II molecule. This occurs within the cytoplasm of the dendritic cell. The MHC molecule is then placed onto the membrane of the dendritic cell with the peptide accessible to a CD4 T cell. (2) A naive CD4 T cell that, by chance, has a TCR with specificity for the peptide in the MHC molecule can form an interaction between the TCR and the peptide. In the lymph node this occurs in the paracortical area. (3) When the TCR fits into a MHC groove and binds to the peptide, the CD4 molecule will be able to approach and bind to its receptor on the external portion of the MHC molecule. (4) Once the T cell has bound to the MHC molecule, there are additional interactions that take place to strengthen the binding and activate the T cell. There are costimulatory molecules on the T cell and dendritic cell that interact with each other, the dendritic cell releases cytokines that help the T cell to become activated, and the T cell releases cytokines that increase its activation. The T cell is converted from a naive to an activated T cell. The activated T cell can provide help to a B cell to release antibody to the antigen that activated the T cell or it may go to the blood and tissue where it looks at MHC molecules that may be presenting the same peptide that activated the T cell. If it finds the peptide, the T cell will initiate a cell-mediated immune reaction to kill the cell presenting the peptide.

is bound to MHC molecules and the complex of MHC and antigen is associated with accessory molecules (CD3 and CD4 or CD8). Unlike the antibody molecule, the TCR is not secreted.

The purpose of the TCR is to locate either T helper cells (CD4) or T cytotoxic cells (CD8) at the site of a foreign pathogen (Fig. 1.2). The CD4 cells will mediate an inflammatory response by attracting other cells (such as polymorphonuclear leucocytes, macrophages, and monocytes) to the tissue where the foreign microorganism is located, and the CD8 cells will kill tissue cells which are infected with a virus.

1.5.4 Costimulatory molecules

Accessory membrane molecules, termed 'costimulatory molecules' strengthen the interaction between the T cell and antigen-presenting cell, and between T-helper cells and B lymphocytes. They do not have antigenic specificity so that, regardless of the antigenic peptide to which the TCR is binding, the same costimulatory molecule functions to hold the T cell to the antigen-presenting cell or B cell. In addition to strengthening the binding between cells, the costimulatory molecules send messages to the T-cell cytoplasm indicating that the cell has reacted with another cell.

1.6 The inflammatory response

Inflammation is a response that occurs to rid the body of an infectious agent or to remove and repair damaged tissue. It is localized to the site in the body where the infectious agent or tissue damage is found. Inflammation is characterized by pain, heat, redness, and swelling at the site where it occurs. It may be acute (occurring without activation of the immune system) or chronic (involving activation of the immune system). Redness (caused by a dilation of blood vessels) and pus (pus is an accumulation of white blood cells in tissue) at the site of a splinter is an example of inflammation.

The white blood cells that move out of the bloodstream into tissue where they are needed are the inflammatory cells. These primarily consist of neutrophils with fewer monocytes that become macrophages when they locate in tissue. Acute inflammation is the rapid accumulation (often within minutes) of neutrophils and monocytes in tissue in response to the presence of an infectious agent or damaged tissue.

White blood cells circulate in the blood, but when an infectious agent is present in tissue they must leave the blood and enter the tissue. The attraction of inflammatory cells to the site of an infectious agent in tissue is mediated by chemokines which are released by macrophages and tissue cells that are present at the site of invasion by the infectious agent. Chemokines are a family of low-molecular-weight molecules that contribute to the development of tissue inflammation.

In a healthy person the response to infectious agents or tissue injury is rapid and efficient and will frequently lead to resolution (resolution means that the eliciting agent is removed) before the immune system is activated (this is called 'acute inflammation')

(Fig. 1.3). In an individual with an overwhelming infection or who is chronically ill or who may be experiencing a high level of stress, the acute inflammatory response does not work efficiently and the immune system becomes activated and participates in the inflammatory response (when the immune system participates it is called 'chronic inflammation').

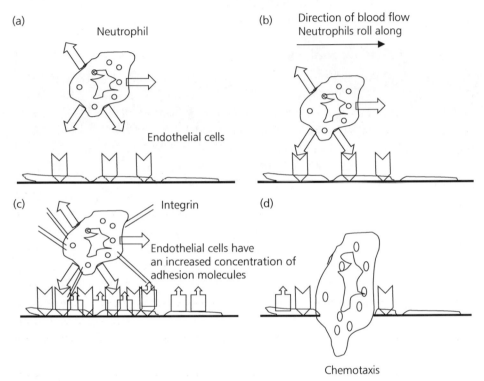

Fig. 1.3 Schematic diagram of the acute inflammatory response. (a) A neutrophil with L-selectin adhesion molecules is loosely adherent to the endothelial cells that express adhesion molecule receptors to which the neutrophils bind. (b) The blood flow rolls the loosely adherent neutrophil along the walls of the blood vessel. (c) A bacterium entering the tissue activates the macrophages adjacent to the blood vessels to release cytokines. The cytokines cause the endothelial cells to increase the production of selectin adhesion molecules and the neutrophils to increase their concentration of an adhesion molecule called an integrin. The increased concentration of adhesion molecules causes the neutrophil to stop rolling and stick at the site of increased adhesion molecules. (d) After becoming adherent, the neutrophil follows a chemotactic gradient towards the macrophages that are responding to the presence of the bacterium. When the neutrophils reach the bacterium they ingest it. Ingestion is enhanced by the process of opsonization. In this case, opsonization is caused by the deposition of the C3b component of complement through the alternate complement pathway. The components of the alternate complement pathway are C3a which causes increased vascular permeability and chemotaxis, C5a which causes chemotaxis, and C3b which causes opsonization.

1.7 **Host defense**

Dividing the functional aspects of the body's defense against infectious disease into two broad categories helps us to understand that some defense mechanisms do not have to be activated by the presence of an infectious agent, while others require activation by the infectious agent. Innate immunity is always active, while adaptive immunity must be turned on by the infectious agent.

1.7.1 **Innate immunity**

The innate immunity system, which protects the body from infection, is always active and continuously patrols the body for the presence of infectious agents. It does not attack the body itself because of regulatory mechanisms that prevent this from occurring. This defense mechanism works rapidly the first time that the body encounters the infectious agent. Regardless of how many times the host experiences the foreign material, the magnitude of the response does not increase, indicating that innate immunity has no memory. If we relied on the adaptive immune system alone for protection from infection, we would probably die from infections because it can take 4–5 days for the immune response to be activated. The innate immunity system which protects against infectious organisms is activated very quickly, often within minutes. Both white blood cells and soluble substances in plasma are involved in this process.

1.7.1.1 Some components of the innate protective system

- Physical barriers: skin and mucous membranes.
- Phagocytic cells: these are white blood cells that engulf infectious agents, and kill them. The phagocytic cells do not have specific immunity to the infectious agent. Phagocytic cells are the polymorphonuclear leucocytes, monocytes, and macrophages.
- NK cells: a class of lymphocytes that react to malignant cells and cells infected with virus and kill the cells.
- Blood-borne molecules: enzymes that interfere with growth of infectious agents.
- Complement: a group of interactive serum proteins that participate in mediating an inflammatory response in tissue. Activated complement attracts polymorphonuclear leucocytes and allows cells and fluids to escape from blood vessels and enter tissue. Fully functional complement can produce holes in cell membranes.

1.7.2 **Adaptive immunity**

This immune defense reaction occurs after exposure to an antigen and involves lymphocytes that become specifically reactive to the antigen that activated the immune response. It shows specificity (meaning that the immune reaction will be directed to the substance which elicited the immune response and not to other substances).

Specific immunity has the characteristic of memory, i.e. exposure to a substance that the immune system has reacted to previously will stimulate a more rapid response than the first response.

Antigen is the activator of the immune system. The immune system reacts to the presence of an antigen. An antigen is usually something that is foreign to the body such as an infectious agent. When immunized against tetanus, tetanus is the antigen. When immunized against polio, polio virus is the antigen. When the immune system reacts against an antigen, it may neutralize its ability to damage the body or the immune system may actually cause the antigen (e.g. a bacterium) to be killed.

1.7.2.1 Some components of the acquired or specific protective system

- ◆ Antigen: a substance which enters the body and stimulates a specific response by the immune system that results in the production of antibody or activation of an antibody-independent cell-mediated reaction.
- ◆ Specificity of an immune response: the immune response (whether antibody or cell-mediated) reacts only with the specific antigen which activated the immune system to produce the antibody or cell-mediated response. Another antigen will stimulate or evoke another specific immune response. The immune response is specific to the antigen that stimulated that particular immune response.
- ◆ Memory: when the immune system encounters an antigen to which it has already reacted (been sensitized to) it will respond much more rapidly than it did to the first encounter. The reaction time (the time between the immune reactive cells encountering the antigen and the immune cells acting) is decreased and the magnitude of the immune response is increased.

1.8 The antibody response

The components and course of a normal antibody response developing in the lymph node are discussed. Similar events occur in the spleen. The lymph nodes are responsible for producing antibody to antigens that enter tissue and the spleen is responsible for producing antibody to antigens that are present in the bloodstream.

The mechanisms of activation of antibody production in the primary antibody response (the response that occurs the first time that the immune system encounters the antigen) and in the secondary antibody response (the response that occurs during re-exposure to an antigen that has previously activated the immune system) are different. The primary response requires conversion of naive T lymphocytes (T lymphocytes that are capable of reacting to an antigen but has not yet done so) to activated T lymphocytes (T lymphocytes that have responded to the presence of an antigen and can respond more quickly than naive T lymphocytes).

The antibody-producing B lymphocytes are also converted from naive to activated cells. In the secondary response, the necessary T and B lymphocytes are present and reintroduction of antigen rapidly increases their function. The earliest detection of antibody during a primary response is usually 4 days after the injection of antigen, while antibody elevation is detected within 24 h in a secondary response. This suggests that stress hormones may have different effects on altering the primary and secondary antibody responses. When studying the effect of stress on altering antibody production, it is necessary to establish whether a primary or secondary response is being studied.

1.8.1 Producing the primary antibody response

If antigen is introduced into tissue (e.g. by injection into the skin), dendritic cells in skin and muscle are involved. If the antigen is introduced across a mucosal membrane (e.g. the nasal mucosal), dendritic cells in mucosal sites are involved.

Dendritic cells ingest and degrade protein antigens into small peptides of approximately 8–12 amino acids. The peptides are then inserted into MHC class I and MHC class II molecules and displayed on the membrane of the dendritic cells. If the dendritic cells are located in the spleen, they can initiate the next step of immune activation. If they are located in the skin, muscle, or mucosa, they lose their adhesiveness at the site where they are located and go to the lymph node draining the local site. On the way they are altered, becoming less capable of phagocytosis, and become antigen-presenting cells. When they reach the node they bind to a CD4 T cell that can recognize the antigen in the MHC molecule. The dendritic cell converts naive cells to activated CD4 T cells in paracortical areas of secondary lymphoid organs.

The naive B cells follow the same circulation pattern, as do the naive T cells. A naive B cell in the paracortical region of the lymph node has the opportunity to encounter antigen that has been injected into the subject. It binds the antigen to antigen-specific antibody molecules on its surface, ingests the antigen, digests it, and presents it in MHC molecules. The activated T cell (activated by a dendritic cell) binds to the same antigenic peptide on the B cell that activated it on the dendritic cell. The T cell releases cytokines that provide the help that the B cell requires to release antibody and produce a specific class of antibody (IgG, IgA, IgE).

Once the B lymphocyte has begun to release antibody, the antibody will combine with free antigen that will still be present in the lymph node. The combination of antigen and antibody will stick to the surface of a cell in a part of the lymph node called the follicle. This cell is called a 'follicular dendritic cell'. The B lymphocyte that is producing antibody to the antigen actually has some of the antibody stuck in the cell membrane. The antibody-producing B lymphocyte will move into the follicle and stick to the antigen bound to the follicular dendritic cell. This has two important implications: (1) the B lymphocyte will die unless it is attached to the antigen on the follicular dendritic cell, and (2) over time the antibody produced by the B cell will increase the tightness of its binding to the antigen.

1.9 **Cell-mediated immunity**

A local delayed hypersensitivity reaction is the delayed hypersensitivity skin test reaction. The test determines whether an individual has been infected with, for example, the organism that causes tuberculosis. A small amount of antigen from the organism is injected into the skin and, if there are memory lymphocytes for the antigen, a reaction will occur in 48–72 h.

Intradermal injection of the antigen that an individual has previously been sensitized to produce redness and a firm swelling (due to the accumulation of cells at the injection site) of the skin. Histologically, when the reaction is at its peak the infiltrate is predominantly mononuclear cells, of which about 80–90% are monocytes. Monocytes are not known to have immunological specificity. Therefore they are probably brought to the reaction site by cytokines released from the antigen-specific lymphocytes that react with the antigen.

Delayed hypersensitivity involves antigen-processing cells (dendritic cells), CD4-Th1 lymphocytes that are activated by antigen presented in the MHC II molecules of dendritic cells, and cells associated with inflammation (phagocytic cells).

Another reaction that does not involve antibody is the response mediated by cytotoxic lymphocytes. This reaction involves antigen-presenting cells and CD8 lymphocytes. In the reaction of cytotoxic T lymphocytes, the antigen-presenting cell presents antigen with the class I MHC complex. The cytotoxic reactions are involved in resistance to viral infections, rejection of transplanted tissue, and reactions to malignant tissue.

Cytotoxic T lymphocytes kill target cells by lysis (punching holes or 'pores' in the target cell membrane). The pores are formed by a protein called perforin (pore forming protein) or cytolysin and several enzymes.

Although the cytotoxic T-cell mechanism of resistance to infectious agents is not a true delayed hypersensitivity response (as it lacks an inflammatory cell component), it is an important host defense mechanism and therefore is included as a cell-mediated reaction.

Cell-mediated reactions provide protection against infectious agents that are located within cells. The presentation of a peptide of the antigen in an MHC molecule indicates that the antigen-presenting cell has been infected. The T cell can then target that particular cell for destruction.

1.10 **Immunopathological mechanisms of disease**

The primary purpose of the immune system is to protect the body from invasive microorganisms. However, at times the immune system, using the same mechanisms that protect from disease, may produce reactions that damage host tissue. The reactions are frequently referred to as hypersensitivity reactions, as an indicator of the heightened immune reactivity associated with these reactions. There is clear evidence for at least four types of hypersensitivity reactions:

1.10.1 Type 1 reactions

Type 1 reactions are induced by antigens known as allergens which result in the production of the IgE class of immunoglobulin. IgE mediates the release of a variety of pharmacological active substances from tissue mast cells and circulating basophils. The released mediators have an effect on tissue that leads to an increase in vascular permeability (so that fluids escape into the extravascular tissue), constriction of airways (with resultant difficulty in exhaling air from the lungs), an increase in mucus production, and the activation of sensory nerve endings (with a resultant itching sensation).

1.10.2 Type 2 reactions

Type 2 reactions primarily involve the combination of IgG or IgM antibodies with accessible antigens on cell surfaces. The antigen may be a natural constituent of the cell surface or may be adsorbed onto the cell surface. The interaction of antigen and antibody may have the following effects.

1 They may activate the complement system and cause death or lysis of the target cell

2 They may result in adherence of antibody-coated cells to phagocytic cells and phagocytosis of the antibody-coated cell.

3 They may alter the function of the cell without causing the cell to be killed. All antibodies reacting with membrane antigens are not necessarily cytotoxic. For example, antibody to the acetylcholine receptor is part of the pathogenesis of myasthenia gravis.

Similarly, in autoimmune anaemia an individual synthesizes IgG antibodies against his or her own red cells. Binding of the antibodies activates the complement system and the cells are either removed by phagocytosis or destroyed by lysis. To achieve activation of complement there have to be two IgG antibodies located adjacent to each other on the red cell membrane. This requires as many as 800–1000 molecules of IgG to be present on the surface of the red cell. Smaller amounts of IgG antibody will promote removal of the antibody-coated erythrocytes by the phagocytic cells of the spleen and liver. Antibodies directed to cell surface antigens do not necessarily destroy the cell. Sometimes antibodies to cell surface receptors may alter the physiology of the cell. Again in myasthenia gravis, an antibody to the acetylcholine receptor at the neuromuscular junction of striated muscle causes removal of the receptor and interferes with transmission of a signal to initiate contraction of striated muscle. Similarly, in Graves' disease an antibody to the thyroid-stimulating hormone receptor produces activation of the receptor with a resultant increase in the production of thyroid hormone.

1.10.3 **Type 3 reactions**

Antigen–antibody (immune) complexes form when circulating antibody binds to the soluble (not part of a cell) specific antigen for which the antibody has specificity. The phagocytic cells of the spleen, liver, and lung normally remove immune complexes from the circulation. If more complexes are formed than can be removed by mononuclear phagocytes, the complexes will be deposited in tissue. In tissue the complexes will activate the complement system.

The amount of immune complex formed and the location of the complex determines the type of reaction. When the complexes are deposited in tissue near the site of an injected antigen, the reaction is called an Arthus reaction. Complexes formed in the bloodstream may deposit in blood vessel walls, the kidneys, the synovium, and the choroid plexus of the brain. Thus systemic deposition of immune complexes is associated with vasculitis, nephritis, and arthritis. This reaction is called serum sickness.

1.10.4 **Type 4 reactions**

This is cell-mediated immunity which was described in section 1.9.

1.11 **Autoimmunity**

An immune response to an individual's own tissue is an autoimmune response. This can usually be determined by detecting the presence of antibodies to the tissue which are known as 'autoantibodies'. If the autoimmune response produces tissue damage, an autoimmune disease results. Many people, especially those aged over 60 years, will have autoantibody without the presence of disease. However, the antibody may be an indicator of slowly evolving tissue damage.

Normally, immune reactions to self-antigens do not occur because of a phenomenon called 'tolerance'. When tolerance is broken, autoimmune reactions and disease result. Immune tolerance is the inability to make an immune response to one's own antigens (self-antigens). Lymphocytes capable of reacting with self-antigens must be removed from the repertoire of immune cells so that the immune system does not attack the self.

B-cell tolerance occurs in the bone marrow where B lymphocytes are maturing. As soon as the specific antibody molecule appears on the membrane of the B lymphocyte, binding to antigen will render the B cell tolerant through either cell death or functional impairment. As the only antigens that should be present in the marrow are self-antigens, tolerance to self should develop while immune responses to other antigens remain. This process requires that the antigen binds tightly to the antibody molecule. However, this does not usually occur and autoreactive B lymphocytes commonly occur in most individuals.

T-lymphocyte tolerance occurs in the thymus gland. Immature T cells leave the bone marrow and pass through the blood to the thymus. They mature in the thymus and develop receptors on their membranes (TCRs) that can bind to specific antigen. If the

TCR reacts with a self-antigen that is present in the thymus and is being presented in an MHC molecule, the self-reactive T cell either dies or is rendered inactive.

The mechanism of removing self-reactive T cells is more efficient than that of removing self-reactive B cells. Thus, although B lymphocytes may be present that can release antibody to self-antigen, the inability of these cells to receive help from a T cell precludes the formation of these autoantibodies.

However, as autoimmune diseases are not uncommon, there must be ways in which self-tolerance is broken. Indeed, there are several mechanisms for this. In some individuals a response to an infectious agent can initiate the autoimmune response. Thus, if stress decreases the ability of the immune system to resist infectious agents and the infectious agent carries an antigen that is identical or similar to a self-antigen, tolerance may be broken. In individuals who have an autoimmune disease, stress is often associated with exacerbation of the disease. This is probably due to stress hormones altering the balance between the CD4 Th1 and CD4 Th2 cells with a resultant increased reactivity of the Th1 cells.

In identical twins, there is a concordance of approximately 50% for autoimmune disease. Thus, in 50% of identical twins, where one twin has an autoimmune disease, the other twin does not. This suggests that genetic factors are important for the development of autoimmune diseases, but the environment is also important. Thus genetic factors may predispose to disease development, but disease does not occur unless combined with the proper environment. The genetic factors may involve having a major histocompatibility locus that is capable of presenting the self-antigen to T cells.

1.12 Stressor-induced immune alteration

1.12.1 Hormonal changes

As has been discussed above, components of the immune system are found in the bone marrow, blood, lymph nodes, and spleen, and are dispersed throughout tissue. The cells of the immune system are bathed in plasma, the liquid component of blood. The chemical composition of plasma has a regulatory effect on the function of immune cells. There is assumed to be an optimal concentration of vitamins, minerals, protein, and hormones that allow immune components to function at their maximum capability. Elevation of a single component may alter the function of the immune system. For example, stress will elevate the concentration of hormones such as glucocorticoids (cortisol or corticosterone) and catecholamines (epinephrine or norepinephrine).[4-6] As lymphocytes have receptors for these hormones,[7] binding of hormones to their receptors may alter immune function.

One way that hormonal alteration may alter immune function is related to a changed function of multiple immune components. For example, decreased function of T and B cells with a lowered amount of antibody production following immunization may occur. Another pathway of lowered antibody production following immunization could occur if a single cell type is functionally altered. For example, a reduction of CD4 function, a reduction of B-cell function, or decreased presentation capability of dendritic cells may each contribute to lowered antibody production. Thus a change in antibody-producing capability may be due to stressor-induced changes of dendritic, T, and B cells, or to a change in just one of these components. Obviously, measuring antibody production following immunization provides a summative effect but does not allow determination of whether a single immune component is responsible for the change.

Another concern relates to the actual hormone that is responsible for altered immune function. Does stress alter the concentration of one, two, three, or more hormones, each of which can alter immune function. Of course, we only know what we measure. Therefore the use of specific hormonal antagonists is important to help clarify which hormones have functional effects on the immune system.[8]

1.12.2 Can stress alter cytokine production?

There are numerous studies showing that an elevation of stress hormones alters production of cytokines.[9] As cytokines are important for activation of many components of the immune response (activation of T cells, promoting antibody production by B cells, and activating the acute inflammatory response), this may be one of the most important ways that stress alters the defense against infectious disease.

1.12.3 Can stress alter the acute inflammatory response?

The hormonal response to stress can alter the acute inflammatory response by altering the production of proinflammatory cytokines that mediate the inflammatory response.[10,11] It is possible that each phase, from generation of IL-1 that increases adhesion molecules to ingestion and killing of bacteria, is altered. Thus stress may decrease the ability of the innate defense system to develop a localized inflammatory response, which will remove bacteria from tissue that they have invaded.

For a normal inflammatory response to occur, neutrophils must migrate from their point of adherence on endothelial cells to the tissue site where they are needed. Studies have shown that adhesion molecule expression is also modified by stress hormones.[12]

1.12.4 Can stress alter the chronic inflammatory response?

The chronic inflammatory response requires the immune system to become activated. An impaired activation of the immune system will decrease the efficiency of elimination of the infectious agent that first initiated the acute inflammatory response and then the chronic inflammatory response.

We now give an example of the course of a disease that differs depending on the efficacy of the immune system in eliminating an infectious agent. Infection of liver cells with the hepatitis B virus does not damage the liver cells. Destruction of liver cells with resultant jaundice is due to the immune system killing the infected cells. Most infected individuals recover fully after the immune system kills all the infected liver cells. However, there are some individuals who become infected with hepatitis B and are then incapable of completely eliminating the infected cells, resulting in a continuous infection with liver cells being destroyed as new ones are formed (the liver has the unique capability of being able to regenerate itself after it is damaged). This condition is called 'chronic active hepatitis' and is associated with an impaired ability of the immune system to kill all the infected hepatocytes. Although this example is dramatic, it should serve to highlight the importance of having an effective immune system and the possibility that stress can reduce the ability of the immune system to eliminate infected tissue cells.

1.12.5 Can stress alter the antibody response?

Ingestion, degradation, placing into MHC molecules, and presentation of MHC molecules on the dendritic cell membrane are all essential aspects of initiating the antibody response. Not all of these have been studied to determine their susceptibility to stress, but studies of MHC presentation have shown that it is reduced.[13] Activation of the appropriate T-lymphocyte and cytokine production by the T lymphocyte is altered by stress. Whether stress hormones specifically alter B-cell function is not clear.[14]

1.12.6 If stress suppresses immune function, how does stress predispose to the development of autoimmune disease?

A logical concern relates to how stress, which is usually associated with a decrease in the function of the immune system, can be associated with diseases that are thought to be caused by increased immune activity. This can occur through alteration of the regulatory components of the immune system[15] or through an increased susceptibility to infectious diseases with a subsequent increased risk of an autoimmune response.

Obviously, the relationship between the effects of stress on altering the function of the immune system and the development of an autoimmune disease is complex. Further complications are related to different patients with the same disease having different aetiologies to their disease. Eventually, clarification of the factors that contributed to the development of an autoimmune disease in a particular patient will depend upon identifying the immune pathway that was responsible for the disease in that patient. This, in turn, will allow a more precise characterization of the role of stress in the pathogenesis of autoimmune disease to be identified.

1.13 Conclusion

Each month brings new understanding of how the immune system is capable of recognizing an antigen and producing either antibody or a cell-mediated reaction to the antigen. As basic and clinical immunologists further clarify how the immune system functions to maintain health, understanding the mechanisms of stressor-induced immune alteration will become increasingly relevant. The eventual goal of psycho-neuroimmunologists is to develop interventions that will contribute to the maintenance of the function of the immune system and resultant achievable high quality of health and of life. This begins with an understanding of how the immune system functions.

References

1 Abbas AK, Lichtman AH (2001). *Basic Immunology*. Philadelphia, PA: W.B. Saunders.

2 Janeway C Jr, Travers P (2001). *Immunobiology—The Immune System in Health Disease*, 5th edn. New York: Garland.

3 Roitt I, Brostoff J, Male D (2001). *Immunology*, 6th edn. London: Mosby.

4 Negao AB, Deuster PA, Gold PW, Singh A, Chrousos GP (2000). Individual reactivity and physiology of the stress response. *Biomed Pharmacother* **54**: 122–8.

5 Nagatomi R, Kaifu T, Okutsu M, Zhang X, Kanemi O, Ohmori H (2000). Modulation of the immune system by the autonomic nervous system and its implication in immunological changes after training. *Exerc Immunol Rev* **6**: 54–74.

6 Sanders VM, Straub RH (2002). Norepinephrine, the beta-adrenergic receptor, and immunity. *Brain Behav Immun* **16**: 290–332.

7 Glaser R, Lafuse WP, Bonneau RH, Atkinson C, Kiecolt-Glaser JK (1993). Stress-associated modulation of proto-oncogene expression in human peripheral blood leukocytes. *Behav Neurosci* **107**: 525–9.

8 Bachen EA, Manuck SB, Cohen S, *et al.* (1995). Adrenergic blockade ameliorates cellular immune responses to mental stress in humans. *Psychosom Med* **57**: 366–72.

9 Rabin BS (1999). *Stress, Immune Function, and Health: The Connection*. New York: John Wiley.

10 Kunz-Ebrecht SR, Mohamed-Ali V, Feldman PJ, Kirschbaum C, Steptoe A (2003). Cortisol responses to mild psychological stress are inversely associated with proinflammatory cytokines. *Brain Behav Immun* **17**: 373–83.

11 Glaser R, Kiecolt-Glaser JK, Marucha PT, MacCallum RC, Laskowski BF, Malarkey WB (1999). Stress-related changes in proinflammatory cytokine production in wounds. *Arch Gen Psychiatry* **56**: 450–6.

12 Goebel MU, Mills PJ (2000). Acute psychological stress and exercise and changes in peripheral leukocyte adhesion molecule expression and density. *Psychosom Med* **65**: 664–70.

13 Sonnenfeld G, Cunnick JE, Armfield AV, Wood PG, Rabin BS (1992). Stress-induced alterations in interferon production and class II histocompatibility antigen expression. *Brain Behav Immun* **6**: 170 8.

14 Cohen S, Miller GE, Rabin BS (2001). Psychological stress and antibody response to immunization: a critical review of the human literature. *Psychosom Med* **63**: 7–18.

15 Sanders VM (1998). The role of norepinephrine and beta-2-adrenergic receptor stimulation in the modulation of Th1, Th2, and B lymphocyte function. *Adv Exp Med Biol* **437**: 269–78.

Chapter 2

Psychological stress and endocrine axes

Joey M. Kaye and Stafford L. Lightman

2.1 Introduction

Throughout the history of medicine, reference has been made to the influence of negative emotions and psychological distress on physical health.[1] However, it has only been in the last few decades that clear scientific evidence supporting such a notion has been provided. In a number of recent large epidemiological surveys[2–6] impaired psychological functioning has been shown to be associated with an increased prevalence of serious medical conditions such as coronary heart disease, osteoporosis, diabetes, dementia, and premature death. Thanks to advances in scientific research techniques the specific biological processes and pathways that are responsible for the adverse consequences of psychological stress can now be studied in detail. Most of this research has focused on the neural, endocrine, and immune systems as these provide the principal multidirectional paths of communication between the brain and peripheral organs. This chapter will concentrate on the individual components that comprise the endocrine response to psychological stress.

2.2 Principles of endocrinology

The endocrine system is comprised of a series of specialized cells that release chemical messengers or **hormones** into the bloodstream. These hormones are carried to all parts of the body where, by binding to specific receptors, they influence the activity and function of target cells and organs. The fundamental roles of these hormones include reproduction, growth and development, energy storage and utilization, and the maintenance of a physiological equilibrium or homeostasis. Physiological homeostasis refers to all those processes necessary to sustain cell survival and function, including autonomic cardiovascular activity such as heart rate and blood pressure control, breathing and temperature regulation, and the maintenance of salt, water and acid–base balance. These systems are continually active, both when the organism is at rest (a time when growth, feeding and reproduction predominate) and when it is under stress (where survival responses become active and the former behaviours are suppressed).[7]

2.2.1 **Anatomical organization of endocrine systems**

All endocrine systems are regulated to some extent by the central nervous system and many brain sites are involved in interpreting, integrating, and organizing the stress response. The hypothalamic–pituitary–adrenocortical (HPA) axis and the sympatho-adrenomedullary (SAM) axis are the principal endocrine stress-response systems.[8,9]

2.2.1.1 Hypothalamic–pituitary unit

The hypothalamus acts as an integration centre regulating numerous essential functions including appetite, thirst, temperature regulation, sleep, the reproductive cycle, stress, and some aspects of arousal and behaviour.[7] It receives and integrates many neural and endocrine messages and responds by either sending neural messages to other parts of the brain or releasing a variety of specific regulatory hormones. The hypothalamus sits at the base of the brain around the third ventricle and is connected to the pituitary gland via the pituitary stalk. Within the hypothalamus, specific neurosecretory cells are located in functionally discrete groups or **nuclei**. Hormones produced by these nuclei gain access to the pituitary by being either transported down axons of the pituitary stalk to the posterior lobe of the pituitary or released into a network of small blood vessels that surround the pituitary stalk which are then carried in the bloodstream to the anterior lobe of the pituitary.

In response to appropriate stimuli, the hypothalamic-derived releasing hormones corticotrophin-releasing hormone (CRH), growth-hormone-releasing hormone (GHRH), thyrotropin-releasing hormone (TRH), and gonadotropin-releasing hormone (GnRH) stimulate the synthesis and release of anterior pituitary adrenocor-ticotropic hormone (ACTH), growth hormone (GH), thyroid-stimulating hormone (TSH), leutinizing hormone (LH), and follicle-stimulating hormone (FSH) respect-ively. When released into the general circulation, these hormones act on specific target tissues to stimulate the release of further hormones, each with its own unique function. ACTH stimulates cortisol production from the cortex of the adrenal gland. Cortisol in humans (corticosterone in animals) is the main effector hormone of the HPA axis, gaining access to every cell in the body and influencing many essential stress-related cellular processes.[10,11] GH acts on the liver to release insulin-like growth factor 1 (IGF-1) which promotes energy provision for protein and collagen synthesis.[7] TSH acts on the thyroid gland to release thyroid hormone which regulates the rate of metabolic processes within all cells, and LH and FSH are important in regulating fertility and sex hormone production (testosterone in males and oestrogen in females).[7,8,12,13]

Arginine vasopressin (AVP), prolactin and oxytocin all reach the posterior pituitary by being transported down axons from neurons originating in the hypothalamus.[7] All three have been shown to play a role in anxiety behaviour and the neuroendocrine response to stress,[13] although they all have important additional roles. AVP derived from the posterior pituitary, for example, is responsible for the maintenance of salt and water balance,[7] whereas AVP produced by the same hypothalamic nuclei as CRH acts synergistically with CRH to modify the HPA response to stress.[14]

The effect that a hormone has on a particular target cell depends on its interaction with specific receptors located on or within that cell. Differences in the tissue distribution, binding affinity, and functional characteristics of receptors may produce specific differences in the action of a particular hormone at different sites. The effect of cortisol within the brain, for example, is determined by two receptors with different distributions and affinities for glucocorticoids.[15] High-affinity, type I, or mineralocorticoid (MR) receptors have a limited distribution within the brain, and are mostly found in the hippocampus where they are involved in feedback processes that are important for the normal day-to-day variation in cortisol levels. In contrast, low-affinity, type II, or glucocorticoid (GR) receptors have a more widespread distribution,[15] and are important regulators of the glucocorticoid response to stress.[9,10,16,17] Different receptor subtypes similarly determine the various actions of AVP. Within the kidneys, V2 receptors are responsible for the osmotic regulatory function of AVP. V1a receptors are located within the brain, vascular smooth muscle, and the liver, whereas V1b receptors within the pituitary gland determine its role in modifying the HPA response to stress.[18]

2.2.1.2 Brainstem autonomic unit

The autonomic nervous system is regulated by a group of interconnected brainstem neurons and can be broadly separated into two divisions, the sympathetic nervous system (SNS) and the parasympathetic nervous system (PNS).[19] These brainstem nuclei have extensive connections with other parts of the brain, including the frontal lobes, the limbic and paralimbic areas, the hypothalamus, and the cerebellum.

The SNS originates from nuclei in the lower brainstem that use norepinephrine as their principal neurotransmitter. These noradrenergic nuclei, centred on the **locus coeruleus**, project downward to the intermediolateral columns of the spinal cord. Cell bodies from here send **preganglionic** fibres into a chain of ganglia that run along both sides of the spinal column. **Postganglionic** fibres give rise to sympathetic nerves that supply the heart, blood vessels, lungs, gut, kidneys, and other organ systems. These nerves principally release norepinephrine from their terminals close to the site of action. Other preganglionic fibres also innervate the adrenal medulla and regulate the release of epinephrine into the general circulation.[19,20]

Catecholamines, the effector hormones of the SNS, are initially derived from the amino acid tyrosine that is converted sequentially to dopamine, norepinephrine, and then epinephrine. These hormones act through specific cell-surface receptors of which several subtypes exist, including α, β_1 and β_2 receptors. Epinephrine acts through both α and β receptors, whilst norepinephrine acts principally on α receptors. These receptors are all widely distributed and account for the rapid effects that these hormones have on many physiological processes.[9,12,20]

The PNS originates from several brainstem nuclei that give rise to the vagus nerve and to a plexus of nerves at the base of the spinal cord. In general, the PNS has effects opposite to those of the SNS, although the two systems may augment each other through the positive action of one and the active withdrawal of the other.[9,19]

2.2.2 Physiology of endocrine function

2.2.2.1 Hormone and receptor function

When hormones arrive at their target cell, they can influence the activity of that cell by binding to specific receptors located either on the cell surface or within the cell body or nucleus. Binding to a cell-surface receptor triggers a cascade of signals within the cell that can rapidly lead to changes in cell function. These **second-messenger** cascades may result in the release of preformed products that have been stored within the cell or, alternatively, changes in cell function can occur more slowly through the interaction with the genetic material of the cell.[21]

For example, cortisol binds to receptors located within the cell itself. These hormone–receptor complexes are then transported into the nucleus of the cell where they interact with specific binding sites on DNA termed glucocorticoid-response elements. These sites regulate the rate at which gene transcription and subsequent protein synthesis occurs, and binding can either promote or inhibit these processes. Within the cell, these hormone–receptor complexes can also have more rapid non-genomic effects through interaction with other intracellular pathways.

2.2.2.2 Feedback

A high degree of precision over the release of specific hormones is maintained by the hierarchical structure of endocrine systems and the concept of **feedback**. Once released, a hormone will act on specific receptors located on target cells, and will also act on receptors located at the site where its own releasing hormones were originally produced. These receptors respond to the presence of a biologically active hormone by suppressing the amount of further releasing hormone produced or released.[21] For example, cortisol acts at the level of both the hypothalamus and anterior pituitary, reducing the amount of releasing hormone (CRH and ACTH, respectively) produced and consequently limiting the amount of further cortisol released into the circulation. Similarly, low cortisol levels will have the effect of removing CRH and ACTH suppression, thereby allowing cortisol levels to rise appropriately. In this way, cortisol release is carefully regulated according to metabolic need.[7,8] In addition to this direct form of feedback control, some hormone systems, including cortisol, also have indirect feedback control. Cortisol acts on the hippocampus, a site important in memory formation which is also vulnerable to the negative effects of excessive cortisol exposure. As part of the protective mechanism to limit excessive cortisol exposure, a subset of hippocampal neurons that release the neurotransmitter γ-aminobenzoic acid (GABA) project to the hypothalamus where GABA inhibits CRH release, thus contributing to the negative feedback effect on cortisol.[22] A further feedback loop occurs between the HPA axis and the immune system involving the action of cytokines. These polypeptides regulate the growth and function of immune cells and are released predominantly in response to immune or infectious stimuli, but also in response to other forms of physical or psychological stress.[23] Cytokines have been shown to stimulate hypothalamic CRH release with subsequent ACTH and cortisol production. Cortisol itself then acts to dampen and restrain the activity of stimulated immune cells, thereby ensuring that the inflammatory response is kept appropriate to the body's needs.[24]

2.2.2.3 Patterns and rhythms

Hormone release can be either continuous (e.g. thyroid hormone) or pulsatile (e.g cortisol, LH, and GH). The amount of hormone produced will depend on the frequency and amplitude of each pulse and results in hormone levels that can vary over hours, days, or even weeks.[7] For example, cortisol release varies over a 24 h period with a peak in the early morning, corresponding to an increased CRH pulse amplitude, and a trough in the late afternoon. This day-to-day variation is referred to as a **circadian rhythm**.[25] Within this circadian rhythm, the absolute amount of cortisol released will vary between individuals depending on the frequency of pulse generation, and is referred to as an **ultradian rhythm**.[10] Several hormones show a daily circadian rhythm, whilst others vary over different time periods. For example, female reproductive hormones vary over weeks, determining the menstrual cycle.[7]

2.3 Theoretical basis for endocrine activation following psychological stress

2.3.1 Overview

In the face of any threat or challenge, either real or perceived, an organism must mount a series of coordinated and specific hormonal, autonomic, immune, and behavioural responses that allow it to escape or adapt to this threat.[2,9,12] In order to cope success fully with a particular stressor, the characteristics and intensity of the response must match that posed by the threat itself. Further, the duration of the response should be no longer than is otherwise necessary for a successful outcome.[26] The consequences of a response that is inadequate or excessive in terms of its specificity, intensity, or dura tion may be one or more of a number of psychological or physical pathologies.[2,12,27]

In the early 1900s, Walter Cannon introduced the concept of homeostasis—an ideal steady state for all physiological processes, disruption of which initiated an emergency 'fight or flight' response typical of sympatho-adrenomedullary activation where coordinated body processes would work together to restore this ideal balance.[28] Hans Selye[29,30] also emphasized the importance of multiple integrated systems that respond in a coordinated fashion to a particular stressor.[8] He highlighted the importance of the HPA axis in the stress response when he described the **general alarm reaction** which is an early response to a noxious stimulus characterized by non-specific activation of the principal endocrine response systems, the HPA and SAM axes. Continued stress exposure to the same noxious agent had lasting effects on the endocrine, immune, and other systems characterized by adrenal gland enlargement, gastric ulceration, and lymphatic atrophy.[2,31] Seyle termed this the **general adaptation syndrome,** and he noted that recovery from this state was possible provided that the stress was terminated. However, continued or repeated exposure usually resulted in exhaustion and ultimately death.[30,31]

In the 1950s followers of Freudian theory suggested that psychological stress could produce similar responses. Freud held that maternal influences and early childhood trauma had profound and long-lasting effects on the psychological and physical health of the individual.[30] Animal studies by Levine,[30] and subsequently many others,[32] have demonstrated long-term endocrine changes as a consequence of stress, especially psychological stress, experienced in early development. Further work by Mason[33] has shown that psychological stressors are some of the most potent stimuli of the endocrine stress response, particularly when they involve elements of novelty, uncertainty, and unpredictability.[34] This was highlighted by the observation that anticipating an event can be as potent an activator of the stress response as the event itself.[30]

The idea that all stress is damaging and that this damage occurs as a consequence of excessive hormone production was initially implied by the observation that various endocrine diseases were often associated with overt psychopathology and that this corrected itself once the endocrine condition resolved.[35] This led several authors to postulate that single-hormone abnormalities (either excesses or deficiencies) where responsible for specific behavioural consequences such as depression or schizophrenia.[35] Although this notion is no longer accepted, it did lead on to the idea that abnormalities of neurotransmitters and neurotransmitter systems are more likely to be responsible for certain psychopathologies, and that pharmaceutical agents that target these systems could produce successful treatments.[35] More recently, it has become apparent that the stress response is beneficial in protecting an individual from a harmful situation and that the brain can learn, adapt, and adjust its future response to be more efficient and effective.[2] Problems arise when the stress is sustained or becomes repetitive. The principal stress-responsive systems are energy expensive, and our ability to continually adapt to and recover from stress (a process termed **allostasis**[22]) is diminished when we choose a lifestyle consisting of a poor diet, little exercise, disturbed sleep, the consumption of cigarettes and alcohol, etc. The consequences of failing to recover adequately from each stressful episode (or **allostatic load**) is the promotion of ill-health through high blood pressure, hypercortisolism, suppressed immune function, and poor growth and reproduction.[2,9,22,26] Ultimately, the consequences for long-term physical and mental health are significant.

2.3.2 Hypothetical coordinated time-dependent response

The stress-response system has evolved as both an early warning system capable of recognizing potential or existing threats and a response system that can initiate and drive the necessary processes required to escape or confront the threat. By its very nature, the response must be dynamic, beginning rapidly with brain and behavioural activation, followed quickly by physiological activation.[36] These processes are characterized by positive feedback and feedforward loops that enhance and reinforce themselves as well as recruiting other arms of the stress response. Slower-acting hormone systems are recruited into the cascade, providing checks and balances to the already active but energy-expensive systems, putting a brake on the whole response to ensure that it is kept appropriate to the type of stress faced and to its intensity and duration, and ensuring that the response is switched off when the threat has been adequately dealt with.[17,37]

Changes in the internal or external environment that represent either real or potential threats are recognized with the parts of the brain responsible for receiving, integrating, interpreting, and then relaying this information to those areas responsible for coordinating the necessary response. This brain activation can be detected within milliseconds and proceeds over seconds to minutes as the response continues to unfold. Stereotypical orienting behaviour, initiated within seconds, gradually gives way to more goal-directed behaviour that is specific to the stressor being faced and the environment in which it is occurring.[37]

Activation of the autonomic nervous system occurs within seconds, mediated by the release of catecholamines from sympathetic nerves and the adrenal medulla, and enhanced by a withdrawal of parasympathetic activity.[20,28] These systems promote the immediate physiological, motor, and behavioural responses needed in the face of acute physical or psychological stress. Within minutes of the onset of this cascade of events, hypothalamic releasing hormones stimulate the release of pituitary hormones, with the appearance of ACTH signalling the recruitment of the HPA axis into the process.[7,9,10] The cortisol response is much slower, with peak levels not seen for 15–20 min after the onset of the stress. Early actions of the HPA system provide additional energy resources for the stress response, whilst slower gene-related effects over the next few minutes to hours serve to restrain ongoing actions of the stress response which, if left unchecked, may prove to be unsustainable for the individual.[9,12]

2.3.3 Specific components of the stress system (Fig. 2.1)

2.3.3.1 The HPA axis

Hormone action Corticotropin-releasing hormone, identified by Vale *et al.*[38] in 1981 as the 41 amino acid peptide responsible for promoting the synthesis and release of ACTH, is also widely distributed throughout the central nervous system. It is found within the cortex where it has important effects on behaviour and cognitive processing, within the

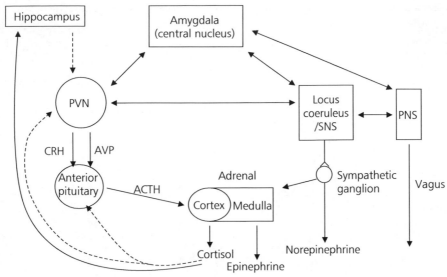

Fig. 2.1 Principle components and interactions of the endocrine stress-response system. Solid lines indicate activation; broken lines indicate inhibition.

brainstem where interactions with sympathetic and parasympathetic centres influence autonomic functioning, and within limbic and paralimbic regions such as the amygdala where it influences the expression of mood and anxiety-type behaviours.[7,8,10,39]

CRH-stimulated activation of the HPA axis cascade results in the release of large amounts of adrenal glucocorticoids into the circulation.[9,10,12] Glucocorticoids, in general, have two fundamental roles in the stress response.[17] First, during stress-free periods basal levels have a role in **preparing** the organism for future stress exposure. This involves energy storage and conservation by promoting glucose and fat uptake and opposing energy utilization. They also prime the immune system for future activation and promote memory formation of previous stressors so that future exposure to the same or a similar stressor may facilitate a more rapid and efficient response. The second role is that of a **modulating** effect at the time of stress exposure itself. Initially, glucocorticoids enhance the cardiovascular effects of catecholamines and vasopressin, promote energy provision and utilization, influence and enhance appropriate stress-related behaviours, and stimulate certain aspects of the immune response.[17,40,41] However, most of these responses would occur even in the absence of any circulating glucocorticoids. It is perhaps even more important that, once the stress response has been initiated, some of the principal actions of glucocorticoids are to suppress and restrain the activity of these systems, in particular the SAM and immune systems. In doing so, glucocorticoids provide an essential regulatory balance to ensure that the stress response is appropriate in terms of both its intensity and duration, and that all these responses are 'switched off' when the stress has been successfully dealt with.[2,42,43]

Animal studies The functional role of CRH and its receptors within the brain has been extensively investigated in animals and has included anatomical lesion studies, CRH-receptor knockout mice, and antibodies or CRH-like compounds with either inhibitory or stimulatory effects on CRH receptors.[13,14,31,44,45] Overall, the addition of CRH seems to promote anxiety-like behaviour and increases the physiological effects of stress, whilst inhibiting CRH suppresses both stress-related behaviour and physiological changes. In several studies the administration of CRH directly into the brains of rodents decreased exploratory behaviour, increased fear and conflict behaviour, and suppressed feeding and sexual activity.[45,46] CRH also stimulated stress-related physiological changes, including increases in heart rate and blood pressure.[47] At least two CRH receptors have been identified within the brain. $CRH-R_1$ is widely distributed in the pituitary, brainstem, cerebellum, and amygdala, and appears to mediate stress-induced HPA axis activation as well as stress-related (and possibly spontaneous) anxiety behaviour. Some evidence for this includes the demonstration that $CRH-R_1$ knockout mice display increased behavioural activity consistent with reduced anxiety in situations where normal mice display increased anxiety. Additionally, following acute stress, these animals show a blunted ACTH and glucocorticoid response.[39] Similarly, studies of compounds that block $CRH-R_1$ suggest that treated animals display reduced anxiety to some, but not all, anxiety-provoking situations as well as displaying a reduced HPA hormone response to high-intensity stressors.[45]

$CRH-R_2$ has a more restricted distribution and a much higher affinity for CRH-like peptides, particularly urocortin II, than for CRH. Studies of $CRH-R_2$ knockout mice as well as $CRH-R_2$ inhibitors have yielded less consistent results, with animals displaying a mix of both increased and decreased anxiety behaviour and mixed hormonal responses to stress that were dependent on such factors as the gender of the animal and the type of provoking stimulus.[45]

In addition to driving both HPA and behavioural responses to stress, CRH also modulates the autonomic immune responses and other endocrine responses to stress. CRH activity in the brain activates central sympathetic systems with subsequent increases in epinephrine and norepinephrine release, decreased parasympathetic outflow, and an overall increased sympathetic tone with increased heart rate, blood pressure, and cardiac output.[12,47,48] Bidirectional influences between CRH and the immune system result in stimulation of the HPA axis by cytokines (interleukins 1 and 6, and tumour necrosis factor-α) with increased cortisol release. Cortisol itself has widespread anti-inflammatory actions, although there is evidence that locally produced CRH and autonomic–immune interactions stimulated by CRH can have pro-inflammatory effects.[12,41]

Human studies Whilst much of the understanding of the biology of CRH is derived from studies in rodents, human studies have indicated that dysregulation of CRH function contributes to the pathophysiology of several disorders including depression, post-traumatic stress disorder, disorders of sleep, stress-related menstrual irregularity and infertility, manifestations of the metabolic syndrome, and functional gastrointestinal disorders.[9,31,48] Further, targeting CRH peptides and their receptors is increasingly seen as an effective means of managing these various conditions, and a number of CRH agonists and antagonists are currently under evaluation in clinical and preclinical studies. Oral CRH-R$_1$ receptor antagonists have been shown to decrease anxiety-related endocrine, autonomic, and behavioural responses in rat and primate models.[41,49] They have also been safely trialled in a human phase II clinical study of patients with major depression[50] who showed an improvement in depression and anxiety symptoms on treatment and a significant worsening following discontinuation of treatment.

The specific response of glucocorticoids and the HPA axis to psychological stress in humans has been evaluated in numerous experiments in recent years.[51] Experimental laboratory protocols, including mental arithmetic tasks, speech and public speaking tasks, and video game playing, have been developed to try and examine the response to a standardized and consistent challenge. The relevance of the biological response has also been examined in individuals facing real life stressors such as bereavement, academic examinations, anticipation of surgery, and parachute jumping.[51]

Laboratory studies that have included mental arithmetic, the Stroop colour word test, and video game playing are not associated with a consistent elevation in cortisol.[51,52] In contrast, public speaking, either alone or in combination with some of the former stressors, is associated with a significant rise in cortisol, albeit with a wide inter-individual variation.[51–53] Repeated exposure to both physical and psychological stressors typically results in a gradual decline in cortisol responses, a phenomenon termed **habituation**.[54] However, a proportion of individuals fail to habituate[51] and may be at greater risk of the adverse consequences of chronic overexposure to stress hormones.[55]

Activation of the HPA axis during real life stress, particularly bereavement, occurs in some but not all individuals.[51,56] Notably, it appears to be a feature of bereavement that is associated with significant anxiety[57] and/or symptoms of depression.[51]

Anticipation of a significant stress, such as surgery or an academic examination, is also associated with HPA axis activation. Although surgery itself (which is a physical stress) is associated with further cortisol release, this is not a consistent feature during examinations.[51,58,59] Further, both anxiety levels before an examination and expected performance are poorly correlated with changes in cortisol levels during the examination itself.[51]

Everyday work stress, job strain, and intensity of perceived job-related stressors are in general associated with HPA axis activation, with the greatest activation seen with more intense pressure.[51,60] However, within an individual, cortisol levels are a poor predictor of job strain at the time they are measured.[51,61]

Patterns of secretion and feedback Cortisol secretion is precisely controlled by the complex feedback system that regulates the HPA axis. Whilst significant variability exists between individuals, within an individual both the circadian and ultradian rhythms of cortisol are tightly controlled and highly stable. Repeated or chronic stress with consequent CRH hyperactivity and excessive or unrestrained cortisol exposure has been shown to result in hippocampal neuronal damage and impaired hipppocampal function.[2] The hippocampus is involved with contextual memory formation and is also an essential part of the cortisol negative feedback system. Impaired memory formation, particularly for emotional events, may exacerbate future stress responses under similar circumstances, whilst impaired negative feedback further exacerbates the hypercortisolism. Rosmond et al.[62] were able to demonstrate that the HPA axis in non-stressed individuals is characterized by a wide circadian rhythm (with distant morning zeniths and evening nadirs), a discrete but small response to an acute stress, and appropriate suppression of cortisol levels following the administration of an exogenous glucocorticoid, indicating a normal pattern of secretion with an intact feedback mechanism. In contrast, chronically stressed individuals displayed a decreased circadian variability (due to decreased morning zeniths and increased evening nadirs), a large acute stress response, and inadequate cortisol suppression, indicating an altered pattern of secretion and impaired negative feedback with resultant cortisol hypersecretion. The effect of this hypercortisolism in the brain includes depression and anxiety,[3] whilst in the periphery it is associated with bone loss, obesity, hypertension, insulin resistance, and other features of the metabolic syndrome.[3] Further, some patients with cancer have been shown to have alterations to their neuroendocrine and immune axes which may have implications for their disease progression and outcome. Several studies have indicated that major stressful life events are more likely to be associated with cancer relapse,[63] whilst a supportive social network and positive psychosocial interventions had a protective effect. The probable mechanisms for this include HPA axis dysregulation and immune dysfunction. For example, Sephton et al.[64] have demonstrated poorer survival from breast cancer in women with an abnormally flattened cortisol diurnal rhythm that was also associated with low natural killer (NK) cell number and activity.

2.3.3.2 Arginine vasopressin

Hormone action AVP released from magnocellular cells of the paraventricular nucleus (PVN) and the supraoptic nucleus in response to osmotic and haemodynamic stimuli promotes water and electrolyte retention in the kidneys,[8] whilst AVP derived from parvocellular cells of the PVN acts synergistically with CRH to stimulate the release of ACTH.[11,65]

Animal studies Acute psychological stress paradigms in animals have suggested that AVP levels are not altered during these forms of stress.[66,67] Rather, AVP appears to be more important as a mediator of ACTH release during chronic stress. Chronic stress increases AVP expression within the PVN,[65,68] whilst inhibitors of AVP impair the HPA response to various stressors including insulin-induced hypoglycaemia and restraint stress.[69] As mentioned earlier, glucocorticoid levels are initially high during chronic or repeated stress, with negative feedback downregulating CRH receptors and subsequently suppressing CRH and ACTH responses. As a result, CRH responses often decline with time in the face of high cortisol levels (habituation). However, exposure to a novel stress during this time restores the original HPA response, and this is mediated by AVP whose receptors do not show the same downregulation (in some circumstances they may be upregulated).[68,70]

Human studies There is limited information documenting AVP responses to psychological stress. However, Scott and Dinan[71] have recently suggested that the impaired HPA axis regulation that commonly accompanies major depression in humans reflects AVP activity rather than CRH. Therefore AVP may be an important target in the design of therapeutic agents for this condition.

AVP appears to sensitize the pituitary to the effects of a superimposed novel stressor, suggesting that AVP and CRH are regulated independently and that against a background of chronic stress, where continued excessive cortisol release would have an overall detrimental effect, AVP may help to maintain an adequate HPA response to a novel stressor.[68]

2.3.3.3 The sympatho-neural and sympatho-adrenomedullary axis

Hormone action The hallmark sympathetic 'fight or flight' response, as described by Cannon[28], is characterized by global activation of the SAM system and features typical physiological and behavioural activation including increase of heart rate, increased blood pressure, and rapid breathing. Fear, vigilance, sensory arousal, and motor activation, often with trembling, goose bumps, and piloerection (hair standing on end), also occur. Release of glucose stores, immune activation, and increased blood flow to essential organs such as the brain, whilst inhibiting non-essential activity like digestion, together produce a 'state of emergency' which can rapidly attend to a sudden change in physiological balance.[12,20] This response is characterized by its speed of onset, its ability to begin in anticipation of an event being stressful, and its interaction with other stress-responsive systems.[20] This interaction can occur through either neural connections or increased blood flow that transports other messengers (such as hormones and cytokines) more rapidly to their respective sites of action.[20]

Human studies Whilst the 'fight or flight' reaction is a useful way of describing the global SAM response to various stressors, it is clear from several studies that the adrenomedullary and sympathetic nervous responses to stress are regulated independently and the components of each vary in their response to different stressors.[72] For example, in humans the physical stress of cold or exercise is associated with both epinephrine and norepinephrine responses, whereas the response to insulin-induced hypoglycaemia is mediated predominantly by epinephrine alone.[20]

Psychological stress is also a potent stimulus of the SAM axis, with activation occurring at generally lower levels of stress than that required to generate an HPA response.[49,54,73] Several laboratory-based stress paradigms, including mental arithmetic and public speaking tasks either alone or in combination,[54,74] are associated with significant catecholamine release and an increase in heart rate and blood pressure.

Catecholamine responses to real life stressors have been more difficult to measure.[51,59] Several authors have demonstrated significant responses in anticipation of academic examinations or surgical stress, or immediately prior to a first-time parachute jump.[36,51] Additionally, significant increases in epinephrine have been noted during examinations, and both epinephrine and norepinephrine increase during the parachute jump.

There are few studies documenting the catecholamine response during other real life stressors such as bereavement or work-related stress.[51] However, recent studies examining the role of specific events that may trigger an acute myocardial infarction have implicated activation of the SAM axis as the mechanism by which acute cardiac ischaemia is produced following physical exertion or negative emotions such as anger, tension, or sadness.[75] A similar mechanism is postulated as the cause of increased cardiac deaths seen to occur in spectators of important and dramatic sporting events that have a negative outcome[76] and the decrease in deaths following similar events in which there is a positive outcome.[77]

Unlike cortisol and the HPA axis, SAM (catecholamine, heart rate, and blood pressure) responses to either exercise or psychological stress do not show the same continuum, although differences between individuals are apparent when anticipating a stress or in response to cold stress.[53,55,78] Concordance between high anticipatory or cold-induced heart rate responses and high-stress-induced cortisol responses has allowed the classification of individuals as high or low responders, with the hypothesis that either hypo- or hyper-reactivity of the stress response will influence an individual's susceptibility to developing various psychological, metabolic, or immune-related disorders.[56]

Patterns of secretion and feedback Concordance between SAM responses and the HPA axis has its foundation in a large number of neuroanatomical and behavioural studies indicating the importance of strong bidirectional neuronal influences of the brainstem catecholamine centres and CRH-mediated pathways including the PVN.[31,74] This translates into a powerful feedforward system where stress-induced activation of catecholaminergic systems activates and in turn is further activated by stress-responsive CRH neurons.[31] Such an interaction would serve to appropriately reinforce the principal early stress-response systems following an acute threat, but altered sensitivity of one or the other may significantly contribute to the disordered activity of the endocrine stress response that underlies many psychological conditions. For example, hyperactivity of the locus coeruleus–catecholamine system with subsequent CRH hyperactivity and reduced feedback sensitivity has been postulated as a likely mechanism for the endocrine changes seen in depression and anxiety states.[31,79,80]

Neuropeptide Y (NPY), a 36 amino acid peptide, is an additional important component of the sympathetic nervous system. It is found within sympathetic brain centres where it has important regulatory effects on both the HPA and SAM axes, influences appetite and feeding behaviour, and may also have anxiolytic properties.[12] In the periphery, it is found within sympathetic nerve fibres associated with blood vessels and immune cells. Released with norepinephrine, neuropeptide Y contributes to the control of blood pressure, blood flow, and lymphocyte traffic.[81]

2.3.3.4 Prolactin

Hormone action Prolactin, which is predominantly required for milk production during lactation, has been shown in both animal and human experiments to be released in response to acute stress, although its role is yet to be fully determined.[9,12,51]

Animal studies High prolactin levels in rodents, such as those occurring during lactation, are associated with reduced expression of anxiety behaviour and HPA axis suppression.[82] Further, intracerebroventricular administration of prolactin in rats reduced both behavioural anxiety and corticosterone responses to a superimposed stress, whilst a prolactin receptor antagonist given by the same route enhanced anxiety behaviour.[83]

Human studies A few studies of both laboratory and real life psychological stress have measured prolactin responses, but little consistency between responses has been shown.[36,51] In some studies of academic examination stress and parachute jumping, prolactin levels have been shown to increase, whilst other forms of psychological stress have shown either no change or even decreases in prolactin levels.[36,51]

2.3.3.5 The growth, thyroid, and reproductive axes

Hormone action Anterior pituitary GH release is stimulated following some acute stressors.[9] GH itself stimulates the release from the liver of IGF-I which acts on many different tissues, but whose main role in acute stress is the release of energy stores from the liver.[7] Laboratory psychological stressors are generally not associated with a change in GH levels,[51] although some studies of parachute jumping or bereavement recall have shown a GH response.[36,84] During chronic emotional disorders such as anxiety or depression, GH levels are suppressed through the combined influence of CRH, which stimulates GH inhibitory peptides such as somatostatin, and direct action of glucocorticoids on the GH gene.[12]

Similarly, the thyroid axis is also suppressed in response to chronic stress-induced HPA axis activation, and thyroid hormone levels seem to follow a similar pattern to GH levels in response to both laboratory and real life psychological stressors.[12,51]

Hypothalamic TRH is inhibited by CRH and somatostatin, whilst glucocorticoids inhibit both TSH release from the pituitary and thyroid hormone (T_4) release from the thyroid gland.[7,9] Further, they also reduce the conversion of T4 to its more active form, tri-iodothyronine (T_3), in peripheral tissues.[7]

The reproductive axis is also very sensitive to the inhibitory influences of CRH, glucocorticoids, and components of other stress-responsive pathways such as inflammatory cytokines and endorphins.[12] Chronic HPA axis activation from physical or psychological stress, as in highly trained athletes or people with anorexia nervosa, is commonly associated with suppression of reproductive hormone release, and particularly with menstrual cycle inhibition in women.[9,51,85]

2.3.3.6 Other neurohormonal systems

Oxytocin, a posterior pituitary hormone required for the induction of labour, is also released during stress.[66] Currently, its precise function during stress is unclear, but some recent evidence suggests that it acts to oppose or modulate the action of AVP.[66]

The **renin–angiotensin** system is an important hormonal system that regulates circulating blood volume and blood pressure. It is activated in response to haemodynamic stressors such as blood loss, but renin is also released during acute psychological stress as part of the activation of the sympathetic nervous system and may have a role in the anticipatory phase of the stress response.[66]

Substance P is activated during pain and chronic inflammatory stress and appears to add to the inhibitory influence some inflammatory mediators have on CRH and the HPA axis. In addition, substance P increases sympathetic activation in response to pain.[12]

2.3.4 Sources of intra- and inter-individual variation

The cascade of hormone release described above will vary depending on the nature of the stressor itself and the individual within whom the stress is occurring. Even major physical stressors, which themselves produce fairly stereotypical responses, will show differences in the magnitude of responses between individuals dependent on the psychological factors that characterize the individual and the context in which the stressor is occurring. Further, purely psychological stressors show significant inter-individual variability in both the magnitude and quality of the response.[43] Several potential mechanisms underlie this variation, including activation of different neuroanatomical pathways, genetic influences, the role of early life experiences and development, specific characteristics of the individual concerned, such as personality, coping style, and comorbid illness, and numerous situational and environmental differences such as social status and the extent of personal support networks.[55,74,78,86]

2.3.4.1 Stressor-dependent factors

A few discrete brain circuits are the first to be activated in response to stress, and it is these that initiate the cascade of events that follow. In reference to the HPA axis, Herman and Cullinan[87] highlight two discrete pathways responsible for activating this axis: first, catecholamine-mediated pathways, termed 'limbic-insensitive' pathways, that project directly from the brainstem to the PVN, and, secondly, 'limbic-sensitive' pathways that originate from the amygdala. Crucially, the activation of these pathways is dependent on the characteristics of the particular stressor being faced. Limbic-insensitive stressors, such as hypoxia, haemorrhage, and inflammation, represent an immediate threat to survival and require a rapid, directed, and automatic response. Other stressors, such as novelty or restraint in animals or the various forms of psychological stress in humans, are not an immediate threat to survival and are only considered stressful when compared with previous or similar experiences. These limbic-sensitive stressors require a degree of cognitive processing and interpretation before they are recognized as constituting a threat or a stress. This is not to say that the response is any less dramatic. In fact, psychological stressors are often perceived far more intensely, with a much greater negative impact on the individual, than are physical stressors.[88]

Animal studies that have examined hormonal, cardiovascular, and immune responses, as well as specific brain activation following different stressors, have clearly shown different profiles of neuroendocrine activation. Differences occurred with both changes in the intensity of a specific stress and when one type of stress was compared with another,[89,90] suggesting that each stressor has its own neurochemical 'signature' producing a unique pattern of central and peripheral neuroendocrine activation which, in concert with similar behavioural, physiological, and immune responses, produces a response that is appropriately matched to the particular threat being faced.[89]

2.3.4.2 Genetic influences

The activity of several different components of the stress response are to some degree inherited, such that differences in genetic make-up confer structural and functional variations in these components. Advances in molecular techniques have allowed the development of knockout and transgenic animal models that either over- or under-express specific components of the stress system. These models can be used to analyse the relevant contribution of each component of these systems and the importance of the genetic variations realized. We have already mentioned the CRH receptor knockout studies, where under-expression leads to reduced anxiety, impaired HPA and SAM activity, and altered immune responsiveness. In contrast, over-expression is associated with increased anxiety and features of glucocorticoid excess.[45,48] Similar studies have examined the role of other components of the stress-response system and have included pituitary hormones and their receptors, steroid hormones, biosynthetic enzymes, regulatory proteins, enzymes involved in the synthesis of catecholamines, transport proteins, and different hormone receptors.[91] Another example is the neurotransmitter serotonin which exerts considerable influence over the HPA and SAM axes and contributes significantly to mood and anxiety behaviours.[92,93] Genetic polymorphisms of the numerous serotonin receptors are one of many factors known to influence the expression of psychiatric illness, particularly depression, and the hormonal changes often seen in association with such psychopathology.[94]

Few studies have been performed in humans. However, as one example, Kirschbaum et al.[95] have shown that monozygotic twins have a stronger correlation between baseline and stimulated cortisol levels following three separate psychological challenges than is observed in dizygotic twins.

2.3.4.3 Developmental factors

Early life experience, including prenatal, but particularly postnatal and early infancy experience, has been shown in animal models to have lifelong effects on the endocrine stress-response system.[43,96] At birth, an intact stress-response system exists that is responsive to stimuli pertinent to the young individual such as cold, pain, and separation. However, the first few years of life are a period of rapid and intense learning with the brain recording and processing new experiences every day. Unlike the adult brain, the developing brain displays 'plasticity', with new nerve branches and connections being formed continuously. Stress that occurs during this time can have profound effects on the developing brain and can permanently alter the function of these systems.[43,96,97] The effect of early life stress on CRH gene expression, glucocorticoid feedback sensitivity, and the subsequent activity of the HPA axis in adulthood is particularly well documented.[96] In rodents, mild stress, such as brief periods of immobilization or maternal separation during the first few weeks of life, decreases CRH responsiveness and HPA axis activation to other acute stressors during adulthood. In the long term, this translates into an improved resilience to stress as adults. In contrast, more severe stress, such as prolonged maternal separation, alters factors such as CRH gene expression and sensitizes the HPA axis to the effects of additional stress exposure. This effect persists into adulthood, manifesting itself as a lowered resistance to stress and an increased vulnerability to the negative impact of physical, psychological, and immune stressors with an increased susceptibility to anxiety.[98,99]

A similar effect of adverse early life experience on endocrine function and psychological illness in humans has been more difficult to demonstrate. However, recent epidemiological surveys have clearly shown that children who have suffered psychological neglect, physical or sexual abuse, or parental loss are much more likely to display mood or anxiety disorders during adulthood than are those who have not been exposed to such trauma.[100,101] Further, adult survivors of childhood sexual abuse are more likely to display altered HPA axis activity even in the absence of overt clinical depression or psychopathology.[101]

2.3.4.4 Individual/host characteristics

As mentioned, the principal factor that distinguishes psychological from physical stressors is that psychological stress requires some form of cognitive processing to occur first. Comparisons are made between prior experience and the current situation, and if differences exist between what was expected and what is actually happening, arousal or stress increases.[30] Modifying this are such factors as the level of control that the individual perceives him- or herself to have over the threat, the extent to which the threat and its consequences are predictable, and the degree of feedback received concerning how well the individual is coping with the threat.[30,43] Thus the less control a person feels they have over a challenging situation, the more unpredictable it is, and the less they know about how well they are coping with it, the greater will be the stress response. These concepts of controllability, predictability, and feedback are important in human research, as the degree to which an individual perceives they either have or lack control and predictability depends on their personality and coping style as well as their prior experience with the same or similar stress.[88]

A number of studies in animals have examined factors such as social isolation, status within social groups, and the importance of the mother–child relationship, and they have highlighted profound and long-term effects on the HPA axis and other stress-response systems.[88] These studies suggest that individuals with poorly formed social networks or who have experienced significant disruptions to these relationships have an impaired ability to cope with additional stress and that this is associated with chronic disruption to their neurohormonal stress-response systems. Further, studies in humans have shown that individuals who anticipate more adversity from a particular threat are more likely to experience a negative outcome, and that these individuals are typified by high levels of neuroticism, high anticipatory anxiety, social isolation, and poor psychological defences.[52,53,55,102] Following certain stressors, these individuals usually demonstrate larger and longer-lasting cortisol and SAM stress responses and a lower rate of habituation.[26,102] In addition, these so-called high responders also display impaired immune responses (such as NK and T-lymphocyte cell number and function) to a variety of stressors. The authors imply that these individuals are more susceptible to the negative health consequences of neuroendocrine and immune dysfunction.[52,53,55,102] In support of this, several epidemiological studies in humans have indicated that the presence of positive social relationships in the form of familiar social partners and/or close salient and supportive social relationships is an important influence on an individual's ability to cope with stress. On the other hand, social disadvantage, low socio-economic status, and loss of important interpersonal relationships (e.g. through divorce or death of a spouse) are associated with an increased risk of significant psychological and physical morbidity including an increased risk of depression and anxiety, breast cancer, cardiovascular disease, and inflammatory bowel disease.[2–5,41,64]

2.4 Practical considerations

Endocrine systems are dynamic, with a number of factors influencing the accuracy and relevance of hormone measurement and interpretation.

2.4.1 Hormone distribution and site of action

It is important to remember that a particular hormone may be differentially distributed and the presence of hormone in one compartment (e.g. in the bloodstream) does not necessarily reflect its activity or content in another compartment (e.g. the brain). For example, CRH is an important neurotransmitter that is found throughout the brain, but is not normally found in significant quantities in the peripheral blood. CRH can be measured in spinal fluid, but routine sampling of this in humans is impractical and can be dangerous. However, during pregnancy CRH derived from the placenta can be found in large quantities in the peripheral blood, although this bears no relationship to CRH activity in the brain.[7]

Another example is norepinephrine which is principally released at its local site of action, the sympathetic nerve terminal. Plasma norepinephrine levels reflect the combined effects of spillover from local production, adrenomedullary release into the bloodstream, metabolism, and renal clearance. Thus plasma norepinephrine levels represent only an approximation of local sympathetic activity, but despite this they remain a valid means of measuring sympathetic responses.[51]

2.4.1.1 Peripheral blood

Sampling of hormones from the peripheral bloodstream is relatively easy. However, blood sampling is often painful and can provoke anxiety in some individuals, which may result in significant changes in stress hormone release. It is usually necessary to place an indwelling catheter first and allow the subject to rest for at least 20–30 min before sampling commences.

Most hormones are also carried in the bloodstream bound to various transport proteins, with only a fraction of the free hormone being present. It is this free hormone that is available for binding to cell receptors. However, many routine hormone assays do not discriminate between bound and unbound hormone, and a change in binding protein levels may appear to alter the total amount of hormone present without actually affecting the amount of free hormone available. Therefore in some cases it is necessary to measure binding protein levels as well as specific hormone levels.[21]

2.4.1.2 Saliva

Salivary samples are non-invasive, easy to collect, and particularly useful when it is necessary to obtain samples from a large number of subjects in their natural environment. They can also be used with children or other vulnerable groups where repeated blood sampling is impractical or unethical. Salivary samples have been most widely used for cortisol, with the additional advantage that salivary cortisol is present in its free unbound state, thus avoiding the potential confounding effects of binding proteins. The main disadvantage is that several hormones are either not detected in saliva or salivary levels do not accurately reflect peripheral blood levels. For example, prolactin, growth hormone, and the catecholamines cannot be reliably measured from saliva.

2.4.1.3 Urine

Urine samples are also simple to collect non-invasively, and several hormones including cortisol, growth hormone, and the catecholamines can be measured from urinary samples. However, urine measures reflect hormone exposure over relative long periods (hours) and are more useful in evaluating total hormone exposure or changes in the pattern of daily hormone release (e.g. changes in the diurnal rhythm of cortisol production) rather than rapid changes following acute stressors.[51] In addition, factors affecting renal clearance will also affect the amount of hormone present in the urine. Vasoconstriction, for example from increased sympathetic activity, may decrease the renal clearance of catecholamines.[20]

2.4.2 Patterns and rhythms

Differences in the profiles of hormone release are important to consider when interpreting hormone measurements, especially single-hormone measurements performed at rest. The time of day the measurement is taken is relevant to hormones that have a diurnal variation, whilst the ultradian rhythm of some hormones results in a large variation in hormone levels between individuals at any one time of the day. For example, GH is released in a pulsatile fashion approximately every 90 min, with most release occurring overnight (particularly in males). Differences could thus be expected depending on the time of day as well as where within the 90 min pulse (peak versus trough) the sample is taken.

2.4.3 Feedback

The activity of both direct and indirect pathways of feedback regulation on the various hormonal systems needs to be considered when measuring and interpreting hormone levels. For example, female reproductive hormones influence a number of feedback systems, and hormone measurements in women need to be interpreted in relation to the timing of the menstrual cycle or to the use of exogenous hormones such as those in the oral contraceptive pill.[7]

2.4.4 The example of the HPA axis

The complexity surrounding the patterns of cortisol release and feedback illustrates the importance of considering all these issues when attempting to measure the activity of the HPA axis, as it is necessary to decide first whether one is interested in the activity of the axis in the basal or resting state, or the normal pattern of hormone release during a diurnal cycle, or the integrity of feedback systems to respond appropriately, or the ability of the axis as a whole to mount a response to a specific challenge.

First morning plasma or salivary cortisol levels reflect the state of the axis under resting conditions, but provide little other information regarding the dynamic responsiveness of the axis. A 24 h urine cortisol collection provides a total estimate of cortisol exposure for that time period which may predict cortisol over-exposure. Not infrequently, however, an abnormal circadian pattern can occur (e.g. a flattened rhythm with loss of the evening nadir) without an absolute increase in 24 h cortisol output. Intermittent plasma or salivary cortisol measures may better predict changes in circadian rhythms.

The integrity of feedback pathways can be determined by the administration of exogenous glucocorticoid, such as dexamethasone, in the evening, followed by an early morning cortisol measurement. Failure to suppress the morning cortisol peak adequately indicates an abnormality in normal feedback pathways, as is commonly seen in patients with depression.[80]

Dynamic testing of the HPA axis, i.e. measuring its ability to respond or react to a specific challenge, has been more difficult to perform and interpret. Several approaches have been described including psychological stimuli such as public speaking and mental arithmetic tasks, physical stimuli including pain or cold exposure, and pharmacological challenges such as insulin-induced hypoglycaemia.[54,74] Whilst dynamic testing is probably the best means of assessing the role of the HPA axis, many of the stimuli used are limited by ethical, practical, and reliability issues, and a single optimal test for use in humans is still lacking.

2.4.5 Laboratory considerations

As described earlier, the timing of hormone release following stress will vary depending on the particular hormone of interest and its specific function. It is important to consider the number and frequency of samples that need to be taken in order to determine both the change in hormone levels over time and the peak change. Peak increases in catecholamines, ACTH, and AVP occur rapidly, usually within minutes of exposure to acute stress, whilst cortisol responds more slowly, with peak increases typically seen 15–20 min after exposure.[51]

Once a sample has been collected, the stability of the hormones of interest needs to be considered as some hormones degrade rapidly. For example, cortisol is quite stable in both plasma and saliva and it is quite appropriate for subjects to collect and store salivary samples at home over a few days before they are processed. However, other hormones are much less stable and strict sampling and processing procedures need to be followed to avoid samples being lost. Epinephrine and norepinephrine are rapidly oxidized at room temperature and collection requires pre-chilled collection tubes, the addition of anti-oxidants, and rapid separation and freezing of the collected plasma. This can significantly restrict the collection of catecholamines from subjects outside the laboratory setting.

Finally, the use of exogenous hormones, medications, or other drugs such as glucocorticoids, oestrogen, or opiates can interfere with specific hormone measurements through either direct effects on the activity of the relevant axis or cross-reactions with biochemical assays.

2.5 **Conclusions and future directions**

It is clear that psychological stress is a fundamental stimulus for the principal endocrine stress-response pathways and that an individual's psychological characteristics are important modifiers of these responses. Moreover, it is also well established that impaired functioning of these stress-response systems is central to the pathophysiological pathways that underlie many psychiatric, immune, and physical disorders. The challenge for the future is the need to develop tools that can accurately and consistently measure the reactivity of these systems and the consequences of their activation. It is essential to be able to do this in individuals, in order to predict their vulnerability to illness, and in large populations, in order to measure the impact of stress and the efficacy of any therapeutic intervention. Further, there is a need to expand our current understanding of the mechanisms that produce stress-related pathophysiology in order to design more effective therapies.

2.5.1 **Measures of stress reactivity**

As already discussed, the ability of an individual to mount a neurohormonal response and the characteristics of that response to a specific stressor provide a much more useful means of assessing the integrity of the stress response than static tests of individual neuroendocrine axes. Currently, an optimal test of the stress-response system is lacking. The present challenge is to develop a means of accurately, safely, and reliably activating the stress response in order to predict disease susceptibility within both individuals and larger population groups.

2.5.2 **Measures of stress consequences**

As well as being able to measure the reactivity of stress systems, it is essential to develop ways of consistently recording the consequences of exposure to both acute and chronic stress. Probably the greatest challenge is to produce a universally accepted definition of stress. Whilst we all understand the concept, an accepted scientific definition still eludes us, making our ability to define and measure the consequences of stress, be they psychological, physiological, immune, or endocrine, that much more difficult.

2.5.3 **Mechanisms of disease**

Much more progress is being made in understanding the mechanisms by which activation and dysregulation of stress-response systems leads to overt psychological and physical disease, particularly in the field of molecular biology. The use of new molecular techniques, such as knockout and transgenic animal models and genetic profiling of individuals and population groups, has allowed the study of the role of specific hormones, neurotransmitters, receptors, transport proteins, enzymes, and second-messenger pathways in the development of stress related disease. For example, CRH-hyper-responsive Fischer rats demonstrate an exaggerated HPA response to stress and are more prone to infections and tumours but more resistant to inflammatory and autoimmune disorders. Lewis rats, on the other hand, are genetically CRH-hypo-responsive with relative hypocortisolaemia and show a reduced incidence of infections and tumours but an enhanced risk of inflammatory and autoimmune disorders.[1,41]

2.5.4 Therapeutic intervention

Ultimately, the goal behind understanding these processes is to be able to identify individuals at risk and to provide effective therapeutic options to minimize or prevent the negative impact of stress on health. Understanding the pathways that intertwine stress, health, and disease will allow the development of new treatments for conditions that cause severe and long-term ill health in many members of the community. For example, melancholic depression is characterized by CRH hypersecretion, impaired cortisol feedback, and hypercortisolaemia.[103] Post-traumatic stress disorder, on the other hand, is also characterized by central CRH hyperactivity but a relative hypocortisolaemia.[86] In both conditions, there is increasing evidence that targeting the CRH system has the potential to produce new and effective treatments.[86]

References

1 Sternberg EM (1997). Emotions and disease: from balance of humors to balance of molecules. *Nat Med* **3**: 264–67.

2 McEwan BS (1998). Protective and damaging effects of stress mediators. *N Engl J Med* **338**: 171–9.

3 Chrousos GP, Gold PW (1998). A healthy body in a healthy mind—and *vice versa*—the damaging power of 'uncontrollable' stress. *J Clin Endocrinol Metab* **83**: 1842–5.

4 Chrousos GP (2000). The role of stress and the hypothalamic–pituitary–adrenal axis in the pathogenesis of the metabolic syndrome: neuro-endocrine and target tissue-related causes. *Int J Obes Relat Metab Disord* **24**(Suppl 2): S50–5.

5 Krantz DS, McCeney MK (2002). Effects of psychological and social factors on organic disease: a critical assessment of research on coronary heart disease. *Annu Rev Psychol* **53**: 341–69.

6 Rozanski A, Blumenthal JA, Kaplan J (1999). Impact of psychological factors on the pathogenesis of cardiovascular disease and implications for therapy. *Circulation* **99**: 2192–2217.

7 Thorner MO, Vance ML, Laws ER Jr, Horvath E, Kovacs K (1998). The anterior pituitary. In Wilson JD *et al.* (eds), *Williams Textbook of Endocrinology* (9th edn) Philadelphia: W.B. Saunders, 249–340.

8 Carrasco GA, van der Kar LD (2003). Neuroendocrine pharmacology of stress. *Eur J Pharmacol* **463**: 235–72.

9 Chrousos GP (1998). Stressors, stress, and neuroendocrine integration of the adaptive response. The 1997 Hans Seyle Memorial Lecture. *Ann NY Acad Sci* **851**: 311–35.

10 Harbuz MS, Lightman SL (1992). Stress and the the hypothalamo-pituitary-adrenal axis: acute, chronic and immunological activation. *J Endocrinol* **134**: 327–39.

11 Lightman SLL (1994). How does the hypothalamus respond to stress. *Semin Neurosci* **6**: 215–19.

12 Habib KE, Gold PW, Chrousos GP (2001). Neuroendocrinology of stress. *Endocrinol Metab Clin North Am* **30**: 695–728.

13 Reichlin S (1998). Neuroendocrinology. In Wilson JD *et al.* (eds), *Williams Textbook of Endocrinology* (9th edn) Philadelphia: W.B. Saunders, 165–248.

14 Ma XM, Lightman SL (1998). The arginine vasopressin and corticotrophin-releasing hormone gene transcription responses to varied frequencies of repeated stress in rats. *J Physiol* **510**: 605–14.

15 de Kloet RE (1991). Brain corticosteroid receptor balance and homeostatic control. *Front Neuroendocrinol* **12**: 95–164.

16 Young EA, Lopez JF, Murphey-Weinberg V, Watson SJ, Akil H (1998). The role of mineralocorticoid receptors in hypothalamic-pituitary-adrenal axis regulation in humans. *J Clin Endocrinol Metab* **83**: 3339–45.

17 Sapolsky RM, Romero LM, Munck AU (2000). How do glucocorticoids influence stress responses? Integrating permissive, suppressive, stimulatory, and preparative actions. *Endocr Rev* **21**: 55–89.

18 Scott LV, Dinan TG (1998). Vasopressin and the regulation of hypothalamo–pituitary–adrenal axis function: implications for the pathophysiology of depression. *Life Sci* **62**: 1985–98.

19 Gilbey P, Spyer P (1993). Essential organization of the sympathetic nervous system. *Bailliere's Clin Endocrinol Metab* **319**: 413–20.

20 Young JB, Landsberg L (1998). Catecholamines and the adrenal medulla. In Wilson JD *et al.* (eds), *Williams Textbook of Endocrinology* (9th edn) Philadelphia: W.B. Saunders, 665–728.

21 Wilson JD, Foster DW, Kronenberg H, Larsen PR (1998). Principals of endocrinology. In Wilson JD *et al.* (eds), *Williams Textbook of Endocrinology* (9th edn) Philadelphia: W.B. Saunders, 1–10.

22 McKewan BS (2000). The neurobiology of stress: from serendipity to clinical relevance. *Brain Res* **886**: 172–89.

23 Turnbull AV, Rivier CL (1999). Regulation of the hypothalamic-pituitary-adrenal axis by cytokines: actions and mechanisms of action. *Physiol Rev* **79**: 1–71.

24 John CD, Buckingham JC (2003). Cytokines: regulation of the hypothalamic–pituitary–adrenal axis. *Curr Opin Pharmacol* **3**: 78–84.

25 Horrocks PM, Jones AF, Ratcliffe WA, *et al.* (1990). Patterns of ACTH and cortisol pulsatility over twenty-four hours in normal males and females. *Clin Endocrinol* **32**: 127–34.

26 Kiecolt-Glaser JK, McGuire L, Robles TF, Glaser R (2002). Emotions, morbidity and mortality. New perspectives from psychoneuroimmunology. *Annu Rev Psychol* **53**: 83–107.

27 Vanltallie TB (2002). Stress: A risk factor for serious illness. *Metabolism* **51**: 40–5.

28 McCarty R (1994). Regulation of plasma catecholamine response to stress. *Semin Neurosci* **6**: 197–204.

29 Selye H (1956). *The Stress of Life*. New York: McGraw-Hill.

30 Levine S (2000). Influence of psychological variables on the activity of the hypothalamic–pituitary–adrenal axis. *Eur J Pharmacol* **405**: 149–60.

31 Koob GF (1999). Corticotropin releasing factor, norepinephrine and stress. *Biol Psychiatry* **46**: 1167–80.

32 Brunson KL, Avishai-Eliner S, Hatalski CG, Baram TZ (2001). Neurobiology of the stress response in early life: evolution of a concept and the role of corticotropin releasing hormone. *Mol Psychiatry* **6**: 647–56.

33 Mason JW (1968). A review of psychoneuroendocrine research on the pituitary–adrenal cortical system. *Psychosom Med* **30**: 576–607.

34 Ursin H (1998). The psychology in psychneuroendocrinology. *Psychoneuroendocrinology* **23**: 555–70.

35 Brambilla F (2000). Psychoneuroendocrinology: a science of the past or a new pathway for the future? *Eur J Pharmacol* **405**: 341–9.

36 Richer SD, Schurmeyer TH, Schedlowski M, *et al.* (1996). Time kinetics of the endocrine response to psychological stress. *J Clin Endocrin Metab* **81**: 1956–60.

37 Eriksen HR, Olff M, Murison R, Urin H (1999). The time dimension in stress responses: relevance for survival and health. *Psychol Res* **85**: 39–50.

38 Vale WW, Spiess S, Rivier C, Rivier J (1981). Characterization of a 41-residue ovine hypothalamic peptide that stimulates secretion of corticotropin and beta-endorphin. *Science* **213**: 1394–7.

39 Owens MJ, Nemeroff CB (1991). Physiology and pharmacology of corticotropin releasing factor. *Pharmacol Rev* **43**: 425–73.

40 Tsigos C, Chrousos GP (2002). Hypothalamic–pituitary–adrenal axis, neuroendocrine factors and stress. *J Psychosom Res* **53**: 865–71.

41 O'Connor TM, O'Halloran DJ, Shanahan F (2000). The stress response and the hypothalamic–pituitary–adrenal axis: from molecule to melancholia. *Q J Med* **93**: 323–33.

42 Goldstein DS, McEwan B (2002). Allostasis, homeostasis and the nature of stress. *Stress* **5**: 55–8.

43 Sapolsky RM (1994). Individual differences and the stress response. *Semin Neurosci* **6**: 261–9.

44 Jessop DJ, Harbuz MS, Lightman SL (2001). CRH in chronic inflammatory stress. *Peptides* **22**: 803–7.

45 Bakshi VP, Kalin NH (2000). Corticotropin releasing hormone and animal models of anxiety: gene–environment interactions. *Biol Psychiatry* **48**: 1175–98.

46 Jones DNC, Kortekaas R, Slade PD, Middlemiss DN, Hagan JJ (1998). The behavioural effects of corticotropin releasing factor-related peptides in rats. *Psychopharmacology* **138**: 124–32.

47 Jezova D, Ochedalski M, Glickman M, Kiss A, Aguilera G (1999). Central corticotropin-releasing hormone receptors modulate hypothalamic–pituitary–adrenocortical and sympathoadrenal activity during stress. *Neuroscience* **94**: 797–802.

48 Gammatopoulos DK, Chrousos GP (2002). Functional characteristics of CRH receptors and potential clinical applications of CRH–receptor antagonists. *Trends Endocrinol Metab* **13**: 436–44.

49 Habib KE, Weld KP, Rice KC, *et al.* (2000). Oral administration of a corticotropin releasing hormone receptor antagonist significantly attenuates behavioural, neuroendocrine, and autonomic responses to stress in primates. *Proc Natl Acad Sci USA* **97**: 6079–84.

50 Zobel AW, Nickel T, Kunzel HE, *et al.* (2000). Effects of the high-affinity corticotropin-releasing hormone receptor 1 antagonist R121919 in major depression: the first 20 patients treated. *Psychiatry Res* **34**: 171–81.

51 Biondi M, Picardi A (1999). Psychological stress and neuroendocrine function in humans: the last two decades of research. *Psychother Psychosom* **68**: 114–50.

52 Sgoutas-Emch SA, Cacioppo JT, Uchino BN, *et al.* (1994). The effects of an acute psychological stressor on cardiovascular, endocrine and cellular immune response: a prospective study of individuals high and low in heart rate reactivity. *Psychophysiology* **31**: 264–71.

53 Kirschbaum C, Prussner JC, Federenko I, *et al.* (1995). Persistent high cortisol responses to related psychological stress in a subpopulation of healthy men. *Psychosom Med* **57**: 468–74.

54 Singh A, Petrides JS, Gold PW, Chrousos GP, Deuster PA (1999). Differential hypothalamic–pituitary–adrenal axis reactivity to psychological and physical stress. *J Clin Endocrinol Metab* **84**: 1944–8.

55 Cacioppo JT, Malarkey WB, Kiecolt-Glaser JK, *et al.* (1995). Heterogeneity in neuroendocrine and immune responses to brief psychological stressors as a function of autonomic cardiac activation. *Psychosom Med* **57**: 154–64.

56 Biondi M, Picardi A (1996). Clinical and biological aspects of bereavement and loss-induced depression: a reappraisal. *Psychother Psychosom* **65**: 229–45.

57 Jacobs SC, Mason J, Kosten TR, Kasl SZ, Ostfeld AM, Whaby V (1987). Urinary free cortisol and separation anxiety early in the course of bereavement and threatened loss. *Biol Psychiatry* **22**: 148–52.

58 Brooks JE, Herbert M, Walder CP, Selby C, Jeffcoate WJ (1986). Prolactin and stress: some endocrine correlates of preoperative anxiety. *Clin Endocrinol* **24**: 653–6.

59 Semple CG, Gray CE, Borland W, Espie CA, Beastall GH (1988). Endocrine effects of examination stress. *Clin Sci* **74**: 255–9.

60 Cummins SE, Gervitz RN (1993). The relationship between daily stress and urinary cortisol in a normal population: an emphasis on individual differences. *Behav Med* **19**: 129–34.

61 Harenstam A, Theorell T (1990). Cortisol elevation and serum gamma-glutamyl transpeptidase in response to adverse job conditions. How are they interrelated? *Biol Psychol* **31**: 157–71.

62 Rosmond R, Dallman M, Björntorp P (1998). Stress related cortisol secretion in men: Relationship with abdominal obesity, endocrine, metabolic and hemodynamic abnormalities. *J Clin Endocrinol Metab* **83**: 1853–9.

63 Speigel D, Sephton SE, Terr AI, Stites DP (1998). Effects of psychosocial treatment in prolonging cancer survival may be mediated by neuroimmune pathways. *Ann NY Acad Sci* **840**: 674–83.

64 Sephton SE, Sapolsky RA, Kraemer HC, Spiegel D (2000). Diurnal cortisol rhythm as a predictor of breast cancer survival. *J Natl Cancer Inst* **92**: 994–1000.

65 Ma X, Levy A, Lightman SL (1997). Emergence of an isolated arginine vasopressin (AVP) response to stress after repeated restraint: a study of both AVP and corticotropin-releasing hormone messenger ribonucleic acid (RNA) and heteronuclear RNA. *Endocrinology* **138**: 4351–7.

66 van de Kar LD, Blair ML (1999). Forebrain pathways mediating stress-induced hormone secretion. *Front Neuroendocrinol.* **20**: 1–48.

67 Hashiguchi H, Ye SH, Morris M, Alexander N (1996). Single and repeated environmental stress: Effect on plasma oxytocin, corticosterone, catecholamines and behaviour. *Physiol Behav* **61**: 731–6.

68 Aguilera G, Rabadan-Diehl (2000). Vasopressinergic regulation of the hypothalamic–pituitary–adrenal axis: implications for stress adaptation. *Regul Pept* **96**: 23–9.

69 Linton EA, Tilders FJ, Hodgkinson S, Berkenbosch F, Vermes I, Lowry PJ (1985). Stress-induced secretion of adrenocorticotropin in rats is inhibited by administration of antisera to ovine corticotropin-releasing factor and vasopressin. *Endocrinology* **116**: 966–70.

70 Ma XM, Lightman SL, Aguilera G (1999). Vasopressin and corticotrophin-releasing hormone gene responses to novel stress in rats adapted to repeated restraint. *Endocrinology* **140**: 3623–32.

71 Scott LV, Dinan TG (2002). Vasopressin as a target for antidepressant development: an assessment of the available evidence. *J Affect Disord* **72**: 113–24.

72 Bornstein SR, Chrousos GP (1999). Adrenocorticotropin (ACTH)- and non-ACTH-mediated regulation of the adrenal cortex: neural and immune inputs. *J Clin Endocrinol Metab* **84**: 1729–36.

73 Malarkey WB, Pearl DK, Demers LM, Kiecolt-Glaser JK, Glaser R (1995). Influence of academic stress and season on 24-hour mean concentrations of ACTH, cortisol, and beta-endorphin. *Psychoneuroendocrinology* **20**: 499–508.

74 Gerra G, Zaimovic A, Mascetti CG, *et al.* (2001). Neuroendocrine responses to experimentally-induced psychological stress in healthy humans. *Psychoneuroendocrinology* **26**: 91–107.

75 Chi JS, Kloner RA (2003). Stress and myocardial infarction. *Heart* **89**: 475–6.

76 Carroll CD, Ebrahim S, Tilling K, Macleod J, Davey Smith G (2002). Admissions for myocardial infarction and World Cup football: database survey. *BMJ* **325**: 1439–42.

77 Berthier F, Boulay F (2003). Lower myocardial infarction mortality in French men the day France won the 1998 World Cup of football. *Heart* **89**: 555–6.

78 Negrao AB, Deuster PA, Gold PW, Singh A, Chrousos GP (2000). Individual reactivity and physiology of the stress response. *Biomed Pharmacother* **54**: 122–8.

79 Ressler KJ, Nemeroff CB (1999). Role of norepinephrine in the pathophysiology and treatment of mood disorders. *Biol Psychiatry* **46**: 1219–33.

80 Gold PW, Goodwin F, Chrousos GP (1988). Clinical and biochemical manifestations of depression: relationship to the neurobiology of stress. Part 2. *N Engl J Med* **319**: 413–20.

81 Elenkov IJ, Wilder RL, Chrousos GP, Sylvester V (2000). The sympathetic nerve—an intergrative interface between two supersystems: the brain and the immune system. *Pharm Rev* **52**: 595–638.

82 Torner L, Toschi N, Pohlinger A, Landgraf R, Neumann ID (2001). Anxiolytic and anti-stress effects of brain prolactin: Improved efficacy of antisense targeting of the prolactin receptor by molecular modelling. *J Neurosci* **21**: 3207–14.

83 Torner L, Toschi N, Nava G, Clapp C, Neumann ID (2002). Increased hypothalamic expression of prolactin in lactation: involvement in behavioural and neuroendocrine stress responses. *Eur J Neurosci* **15**: 1381–9.

84 Kosten TR, Jacobs S, Mason J, Wahby V, Atkins S (1984). Psychological correlates of growth hormone response to stress. *Psychosom Med* **46**: 49–57.

85 Knol BW (1991). Stress and the hypothalamus–pituitary–testis system: a review. *Vet Q* **13**: 104–14.

86 Ehlert U, Gaab J, Heinrichs M (2001). Psychoneuroendocrinological contributions to the etiology of depression, posttraumatic stress disorder and stress-related bodily disorders: the role of the hypothalamus–pituitary–adrenal axis. *Biol Psychiatry* **57**: 141–52.

87 Herman JP, Cullinan WE (1997). Neurocircuitry of stress: central control of the hypothalamo–pituitary–adrenocortical axis. *Trends Neurosci* **20**: 78–84.

88 Levine S, Ursin H (1991). What is stress? In Brown MR, Koob GF, Rivier C (eds), *Stress: Neurobiology and Neuroendocrinology*. New York: Marcel Dekker.

89 Pacak K, Miklos P, Yadid G, Kvetnansky R, Kopin I, Goldstein D (1998). Heterogenous neurochemical responses to different stressors: a test of Selye's doctrine of nonspecificity. *Am J Physiol* **275**: R1247–55.

90 Pacak K, Miklos P (2001). Stressor specificity of central neuroendocrine responses: implications for stress-related disorders. *Endocrin Rev* **22**: 502–48.

91 Bornstein SR, Böttner A, Chrousos GP (1999). Knocking out the stress response. *Mol Psychiatry* **4**: 403–7.

92 Dinan T (1996). Serotonin and the regulation of hypothalamic–pituitary–adrenal axis function. *Life Sci* **58**: 1683–94.

93 Lowry CA (2002). Functional subsets of serotonergic neurones: implications for control of the hypothalamic–pituitary–adrenal axis. *J Neuroendocrinol* **14**: 911–23.

94 Veenstra-VanderWeele J, Anderson GM, Cook EH Jr, (2000). Pharmacogenetics and the serotonin system: initial studies and future directions. *Eur J Pharmacol* **410**: 165–81.

95 Kirschbaum C, Wust S, Faig HG, Hellhammer DH (1992). Heritability of cortisol responses to human corticotropin-releasing hormone, ergometry, and psychological stress in humans. *J Clin Endocrinol Metab* **75(6)**: 1526–30.

96 Brunson KL, Avishai-Eliner S, Hatalski CG, Baram TZ (2001). Neurobiology of the stress response in early life: evolution of a concept and the role of corticotropin releasing hormone. *Mol Psychiatry* **6**: 647–56.

97 Lopez JF, Akil H, Watson SJ (1999). Role of biological and psychological factors in early life development and their impact on adult life. Neural circuits mediating stress. *Biol Psychiatry* **46**: 1461–71.

98 Bremner JD, Vermetten E (2001). Stress and development: biological and psychological consequences. *Dev Psychopathol* **13**: 473–89.

99 Sapolsky RM (1997). The importance of a well groomed child. *Science* **277**: 1620.

100 Mullen PE, Martin JL, Anderson JC, Romans SE, Herbison GP (1996). The long-term impact of the physical, emotional and sexual abuse of children: a community study. *Child Abuse Negl* **20**: 7–21.

101 Heim C, Newport DJ, Bonsall R, Miller AH, Nemeroff CB (2001). Altered pituitary–adrenal axis responses to provocative challenge tests in adult survivors of childhood abuse. *Am J Psychiatry* **158**: 575–81.

102 McCleery JM, Goodwin GM (2001). High and low neuroticism predict different cortisol responses to the combined dexamethasone–CRH test. *Biol Psychiatry* **49**: 410–15.

103 Gold PW, Chrousos GP (1999). The endocrinology of melancholic and atypical depression: relation to neurocircuitry and somatic consequences. *Proc Assoc Am Physicians* **111**: 22–34.

Chapter 3

Assessment of the immune system in human psychoneuroimmunology

K. Vedhara and E. C. Y. Wang

3.1 Introduction

Since the pioneering observations of Ader and Cohen[1] concerning the susceptibility of the immune system to behavioural conditioning, there has been a dramatic increase in research dedicated to stress–neuroendocrine–immune interactions and their consequences for immunomodulation, i.e. the field of psychoneuroimmunology (PNI). One area within this field that has attracted considerable attention has been the phenomenon of stress-related immune impairment in humans. Many immunological changes have been reported, however, one of the major challenges facing human PNI research concerns the clinical significance of these immune alterations in people who experience psychological stress.

In this chapter, we review and evaluate some of the more frequently used *in vitro* and *in vivo* immunological techniques in the hope that a clearer understanding of what these assays can tell us will inform the discussion of the significance of stress-related immune impairment in humans. We commence with a brief description of the immune system (for a more detailed description see Chapter 1), followed by a review of the assays typically used in PNI. The review of each assay includes a description of the rationale behind its use, a technical account, a commentary on the advantages and limitations of the assay, and a consideration of their clinical relevance. The empirical work considered in this chapter has been conducted primarily with humans and, with the exception of the section on delayed hypersensitivity skin tests (DTh), focuses on sampling from peripheral blood.

3.2 The biological context: the immune system

Our immune systems are confronted with a wide variety of infectious agents on a daily basis. However, for the most part, these are eradicated or contained long before they have an opportunity to result in symptoms. The processes by which the immune system is believed to achieve this have been described earlier in this text and elsewhere;[2–4] however, a brief summary follows. Skin and mucosal secretions act as the first, physical barriers to infection. If these are breached, the immune system comes into play. The immune system can be divided into 'innate' and 'acquired' components. The innate immune system acts immediately and consists of mediators that recruit cells to the site of infection, aid in triggering pathways of repair, and kill pathogens outright (e.g. the complement cascade). In addition, there are defined subsets of white blood cells that potentiate these effects, whilst also ingesting and killing pathogens themselves [e.g. neutrophils, natural killer (NK) cells, and macrophages]. If the pathogen survives or evades these assaults, the acquired immune system comes into action. Acquired immunity is highly specific (see below) and slower to act, but it has the advantages of developing both increased specificity as it matures and 'memory' of prior exposure. Thus it is able to mount a faster and more intense response when re-exposed to the same pathogen.

A diagrammatic summary of the principal features of acquired immunity and some parts of innate immunity are presented in Figure 3.1 which shows the cascade of immune events which occur in response to a pathogenic challenge (the numbers in parentheses in the following description refer to Fig. 3.1). Following contact with an antigen-presenting cell (APC), the pathogen is taken up either by infection (as is the case for a virus) or by being 'swallowed' by the APC. The proteins that make up the pathogen are then 'processed', during which they are broken down into small fragments called peptides (1). Because these peptides are derived from the pathogen

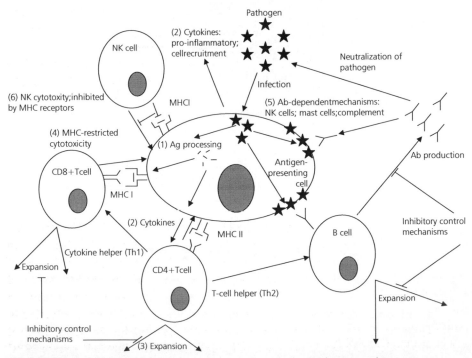

Fig. 3.1 Principal features of immune system activity: Ab, antibody; Ag, antigen.

and nothing else, they create a pathogen-specific 'footprint' that can then be recognized by the acquired immune system as being different from the host and thus, worthy of an immune response. This is achieved by binding of the peptides to a family of molecules called the major histocompatibility complex (MHC) and presentation to defined populations of white blood cells (T cells) that make up the specific arm of the immune response. T cells express a cell surface protein called the T-cell receptor (TCR) which recognizes MHC with the pathogenic peptides attached, resulting in activation. T cells can be broadly divided into two subsets with distinct functions and different MHC recognition patterns. CD4+ T cells recognize peptides bound to MHC class II and release soluble factors that aid the development of the immune response (cytokines) (2). CD8+ T cells recognize peptides bound to MHC class I and 'kill the messenger' (4). The cytokines from CD4+ T cells (2) trigger activation, differentiation, and expansion (3) of the cytotoxic CD8+ T cells (4) and antibody-producing B cells. Antibodies form the soluble arm of the immune system and have a range of different functions including direct inactivation of the pathogen, complexing with antigen to allow removal of the pathogen, activation of complement, and acting as a recognition 'bridge' for cell types which express antibody receptors (e.g. mast cells, NK cells, and eosinophils) (5). NK cells are another cytotoxic cell subset. They kill cells that do not express MHC I (6), and so counteract T-cell evasion mechanisms that reduce expression of MHC I.

It is evident from this brief description that the immune system is made up of several diverse yet interconnected components, and that the successful eradication of pathogens is dependent upon harmonious communication between these components. It is also clear that immune dysfunction could occur at any level; thus the nature of the immune impairment is necessarily related to the location of the dysfunction. In the remainder of the chapter we discuss the assays that have been used to assess the competence of the human immune system in PNI research.

3.3 The empirical evidence

3.3.1 *In vitro* measures of the immune system

3.3.1.1 Lymphocyte subsets

Rationale The successful eradication of pathogens is dependent, in part, upon the existence of adequate numbers of immune cells and appropriate cell ratios. This is evident in diseases such as human immunodeficiency virus (HIV) infection in which the loss of CD4+ cells disables the rest of the immune system, thus making the HIV-infected patient vulnerable to a multitude of infections.[5] Similarly, immunity to herpes simplex virus I (HSVI) is known to be dependent upon NK cell activity.[6] Thus a reduction in these cells leaves the host vulnerable to increased viral activity. The clinical relevance of cell counts has led to the widespread use of total white blood cell (WBC) counts, WBC differentials[7–9], and lymphocyte subset counts as indices of immune system efficacy.[10–12]

Technical description The estimation of numbers and proportions of immune cell subsets is conducted by flow cytometric (FACS) analysis. Individual cells in suspension (normally taken from samples of peripheral blood) pass through a laser in a stream of isotonic solution. Gross cell subsets, such as granulocytes, lymphocytes, and macrophages, are differentiated by their physical properties, which cause light to scatter in definitive patterns. The degree of forward scatter indicates cell size, while side scatter reveals the extent of cell granularity. The differentiation of lymphocyte subsets is achieved by the staining of cells with fluorochrome-bound monoclonal antibodies (mAbs) which bind to antigens on the cell surface. The laser excites the fluorochromes present on the mAbs, resulting in the emission of different wavelengths of light. These emissions are detected by the flow cytometer and allow relative quantification of the amount of these antigens on the surface or within the cell. The systematic nomenclature of these immune cell antigens has led to the identification of over 230 cluster designation (CD) markers and this number continues to increase. The CD nomenclature is related to phenotype and not necessarily function, although in some cases there is an overlap. An overview of some of the most frequently measured cell subsets and markers is presented in Table 3.1.

Advantages A cursory glance at the literature reveals that the enumerative assessment of cellular immunity in PNI research has traditionally focused on major cell subsets[10,12,13] and, more recently, on markers of T-cell activation.[14–16] Several key advantages are gained by such assessments. First, several investigators have demonstrated that significant and selective changes occur in leucocyte subpopulations in response to acute stress.[10,17] Thus it is clear that the measurement of cell counts is an effective way of assessing the effects of acute stress. Secondly, the measurement of cell activation markers offers insight into the extent and nature of cellular activation and therefore may be more closely aligned with assessments of cell function. Indeed, the assessment of these markers can inform the debate on the ways in which stress may affect the immune system. This is demonstrated in the results of a study which reported that caregivers of demented patients displayed an increase in CD8 cells but poorer T-cell proliferation.[15] However, an assessment of the numbers of cells exhibiting the CD38 activation marker revealed that both CD4 and CD8 cell subpopulations contained reduced percentages of CD38 cells. Thus the poorer proliferation could be attributed to the reduction in activated T cells, as evidenced by CD38 percentages. Therefore the potential for activation markers to elucidate the stress–immune system relationship further would appear to be considerable. Finally, when combined with functional assays, enumerative assessments of lymphocyte subpopulations allow one to ascertain whether observed alterations in cell numbers are of functional relevance and, conversely, whether apparent alterations in immune function are due to changes in the functional efficacy of the cells or simply to changes in cell numbers.

Table 3.1 The identity/function of some of the most frequently assessed lymphocyte sub-populations

Antigen	Identity/Function
CD3	Present on all T cells. Molecular complex associated with the TCR and responsible for TCR-mediated transduction
CD4	Present on T helper cells which direct the nature (i.e. cellular or humoral) of an immune response
CD8	Present on suppressor and cytotoxic T cells
CD16/CD56	Combined expression of CD16 and CD56, but lack of CD3, is a marker for NK cells
CD19 and CD20	Two primary B-cell markers
CD57	Found on a proportion of T and NK cells; present as a carbohydrate moiety on a variety of as yet unnamed glycoproteins on lymphocytes. Identifies very late stage differentiated effector cells in the CD8+ T-cell population
Chemokine receptors (e.g. CCR7)	Four families of chemokine receptors responsible for chemotaxis and migration of cells. Different cell types (ranging from neutrophils and basophils to T cells and macrophages) express different C, CC, CXC, or CX3C receptors at different stages of development depending on their function and tissue migration patterns. Some, such as CCR7, are used to differentiate between naive, central memory, and effector memory T-cell subsets
Markers of T-cell activation	
HLA-DR	This antigen is expressed on T cells, B cells, and monocytes following activation.
CD25	The induction of CD25 on T cells occurs approximately 48 h after T-cell activation, serving to increase the sensitivity of T cells to IL-2 (a T-cell growth factor necessary for T-cell proliferation). Therefore CD25 induction can be used as a T-cell activation marker. Recent research has indicated that it also identifies a subset of CD4+ T cells that are immunoregulatory
CD27	A lymphocyte-specific TNFR family member, expression of which is highly induced by activation. TNFR family members are involved in immune organ development, immune cell differentiation, and immune response regulation
CD28	T-cell activation is dependent on TCR signalling and co-stimulatory molecules. CD28 is one such molecule. It is found on a proportion of T and B cells (terminally differentiated), but is downregulated on T cells following antigenic exposure. Mutually exclusive expression with CD57
CD38	Present on activated T cells and terminally differentiated B cells as well as onepithelial cells and cells of the monocyte lineage, although its function is unknown
CD45RA and CD45RO	The CD45RA antigen is believed to indicate T-cell 'resting' status, i.e. the cell has not yet been activated, although recent research has indicated that it also identifies 'effector memory' T cells. In contrast, CD45RO antigen is believed to indicate recent cell activation and a marker for 'central memory'. The expression of these antigens is reversible
CD69	This antigen is expressed on all lymphocytes (T, B, and NK cells) and neutrophils following activation
CD71	This antigen is induced following T-cell activation. However, it is expressed before CD25 and thus can be used as an earlier activation marker for T cells

Limitations Several limitations also exist with the measurement of cell subsets. The first of these concerns the observation that cell numbers do not necessarily correlate well with cell function.[18–20] For example, Anesi et al.[20] reported evidence of poorer T-cell responses to a mitogen in subjects with major depressive disorder, but found no evidence of a significant alteration in T-cell numbers. Similarly, Kang et al.[19] reported that an examination period was associated with a reduction in NK cell activity, although NK cell counts during the same period actually increased. Thus one cannot draw conclusions regarding the functional efficacy of cells from the measurement of cell numbers. A second concern is that cell numbers fluctuate according to a number of factors, such as cell migration, circadian rhythms, etc.,[21] none of which have implications for the effectiveness of the immune system. For example, Marsland et al.[10] speculated that the effects of stress on lymphocyte subsets may be mediated by changes in haemoconcentration (i.e. plasma volume), as periods of acute psychological stress are known to affect haemoconcentration. This proposal was examined by reanalysing data from four previous studies on the effects of acute stress on lymphocyte subsets. The initial findings had shown evidence of stress-related increases in NK and CD8 cells, but no effects on CD4 and CD19 cells. However, after adjusting for haemoconcentration, the increases in NK and CD8 cells were augmented, and decreases in CD4 and CD19 cells became apparent. These results provide strong support for plasma volume being an important mediator of stress effects on circulating cell counts; and further suggest that researchers should be cognizant of the fact that any alterations in lymphocyte subpopulations may, in part, reflect physiological events rather than stress-induced variations. Finally, there is often some overlap in lymphocyte subsets, many of which have different functions. For example, CD8+ cells can be divided into several subpopulations (e.g. CD8+CD28+, CD8+CD28−, CD8+CD57+, CD8+CD57−). Thus, unless the populations are defined precisely, the interpretation of lymphocyte counts can be problematic.

Recommendations The above considerations would appear to advocate a reassessment of the way in which lymphocyte counts are used in PNI research. For example, we propose that the quantification of cell numbers is most informative when combined with functional assessments. In addition, the study of cell ratios may offer a more cogent index of immune system activity. For example, the normal ratio of CD4 to CD8 cells is 2 : 1, and this ratio is altered in the presence of some infections.[22] Therefore it would be appropriate to adopt the ratio of CD4 to CD8 ratio as an outcome measure in investigations designed to explore issues such as the relationship between stress and infections. We also contend that activation markers, used in conjunction with or in isolation from lymphocyte counts, may offer a more efficacious index of immune system activity for two main reasons. Firstly, they are closely related to markers of cell function and/or differentiation. For example, the markers CD45RA, CD45RO and CCR7 identify three subsets of T cells: (i) naive (have not previously met their specific antigen), (2) central memory (have met antigen, but cannot perform their functions immediately), and (3) effector memory (have met antigen and are capable of immediate effector function).[23] Secondly, they can inform the debate on the ways in which stress may affect the immune system. For example, the assessment of both CD25 and CD71 would offer insight into the stage at which T-cell activation may be affected (see Table 3.1). One final area of worthy of attention concerns the measurement of cell adhesion molecules and chemokine receptors. Both identify the differentiation/activation state of lymphocytes and their ability to circulate and home to different tissue,[23,24] and their measurement is becoming more common in PNI.

Clinical implications Immune cells travel through the bloodstream and between tissues, and therefore there is little doubt that the numbers and proportions of cells in circulation provide an indication of the state of leukocyte distribution and redistribution in the body.[17] Thus the enumerative assessment of cells informs us of the ability of the immune system to respond to potential or ongoing immune challenges.

3.3.1.2 Cytotoxicity assays

Rationale One of the major functions of the immune system is to remove foreign or 'non-self' cells such as those infected with virus, cells which are immortalized (i.e. cells which have lost the normal controls that inhibit perpetual cell division), and cells that are tumorigenic. Active killing (i.e. cytotoxicity) of such cells can be carried out by both T cells and NK cells and is measured by cytotoxicity assays. It is believed that the body regularly produces non-self cells, and so the ability of the immune system to identify and destroy these cells is an important feature of its activity and therefore a highly relevant immune outcome measure.

Technical description Standard cytotoxicity assays are based on the principle that cells capable of cytotoxic action, i.e. T or NK cells (also referred to as effectors), release cytolitic molecules (e.g. perforin) which create holes within the membrane of the target cell, and that this action results in the eventual destruction of the target. As a consequence, the assay involves incubating non-self targets with a radiolabelled substance which they absorb. The non-self targets are then incubated with either NK or T cells. If the selected effector cell type is efficient and viable, the non-self targets will be destroyed and the previously absorbed radiolabelled substance will be released. The amount of radiolabel in a standard volume of supernatant is then measured and compared with a negative control (i.e. no effector cells present and therefore no cell lysis) and a positive control (i.e. 100% lysis of targets caused by detergent). Hence, cytotoxicity is a measure of the release of radiolabelled substances from the targets after their outer membranes have been breached. However, it should be noted that this is not the only form of killing used by effectors. Advances in our understanding of apoptosis (also known as programmed cell death) have shown that T and NK cells are capable of inducing 'suicide' in non-self targets through the disintegration of DNA and cell structure without destroying the membrane of the target cell.[25] Furthermore, these two killing mechanisms are not mutually exclusive. Current models suggest that cytotoxic cells use perforin to create holes in the cell's membrane and that this, in turn, facilitates the introduction of factors (granzymes) that induce apoptosis.[26] This model explains the ability of cytotoxic cells to kill different targets irrespective of their differential resistance to pore-forming molecules. Assays exist which measure apoptosis, but these will not be considered here.

The two subsets of effectors recognize their targets in different ways and different conclusions can be drawn from each assay. Thus NK and T-cell assays will be considered separately. With regard to NK cell cytotoxicity, the typical assay involves the incubation of NK cells with a specific target known to be susceptible to NK cell killing. These targets are generally tumour cell lines such as K 562 or Molt 4, and cytokines such as interferon are often used to activate the NK cells beforehand. The ratio of effector to target is determined by cell counting, and in this way a more accurate calculation of the number of NK cells needed to destroy a predetermined number of targets is possible. In contrast, T-cell cytotoxicity assays involve taking a cell line of targets which are not susceptible to NK cells (usually a mouse B lymphoblastoid cell line such as JY) and which express a receptor for antibodies and coating them with a mouse anti-human CD3 monoclonal antibody.[27] CD3 is a T-cell-specific marker; thus anti-CD3 antibodies serve to activate all T cells and hold the targets in close proximity, allowing cytotoxic mechanisms to take place. This assay is considered to measure 'total T-cell cytotoxic capability'. An additional assay worthy of consideration is lymphokine activated killer (LAK) activity. This assay measures non-specific cytotoxicity against a wide range of targets following activation by high concentrations of IL-2. This assay is used most widely in studies relating to tumour cells. Finally, antigen-specific cytotoxic assays also exist.[28] In their purest form, these assays involve targets (e.g. a B-cell line) which express an appropriate MHC I, i.e. an MHC which is restricted to the TCR expressed by the effector. The target cells are coated with the peptide that is recognized by the TCR. In this way, targets which do not express the correct MHC I, or which are coated with an inappropriate peptide, are not recognized by the effector cells.

Advantages Cytotoxicity assays inform us about the cytotoxic potential of the subsets in question, i.e. T or NK cells. Therefore a reduction in cytotoxicity would indicate a defect in the response, although it would not identify the mechanisms underlying this defect. Cytotoxicity assays confer many advantages, and this is evidenced by the number of PNI investigations in which NK cell and T-cell cytotoxity assays have been employed.[29–32] First, the assays themselves are robust and relatively easy to perform. In particular, NK cytotoxic assays use effectors that are easy to stimulate in short-term culture against transformed cell line targets that are also easy to grow. This also applies to the anti-CD3 directed 'total' T-cell cytotoxicity assay mentioned above. In contrast, antigen-specific cytotoxic T-cell lines and clones require long-term culture and are more difficult to grow. However, once established they are very sensitive, with significant killing at effector-to-target ratios <1. This allows the investigation of other cellular or cytokine-derived influences on cytotoxicity. Furthermore, the targets (normally virally infected, peptide-loaded, or transformed cell lines) are generally well defined and therefore can be clinically enlightening. For example, malignant melanoma cell lines can be used in assays using samples from patients with the disease. Finally, because the mechanisms of cytotoxicity are fairly well understood, relatively precise delineation of any observed defect is possible.

Limitations

NK cells Most investigations of NK cell cytotoxicity have several methodological difficulties which make it difficult to conclude that the target destruction witnessed has been caused exclusively by NK cells. First, some investigators use whole peripheral blood mononuclear cells (PBMCs) as effectors,[29,33] and NK cells constitute only a small and variable part of such samples. Secondly, PBMC samples clearly contain other cell subsets, some of which are capable of non-specific tumour line killing (e.g. CD3+ and CD57+ T cells[27]). Thirdly, some groups have examined NK cytotoxicity using only non-adherent cells (i.e. adherent cells are removed before the assay). However, adherent populations produce some cytotoxic activity and their removal can also result in alterations in cytokine release. Together, these factors could result in erroneous conclusions regarding the extent of NK cytotoxic activity. Finally, cytotoxicity assays define NK cell activity according to the cell's ability to kill particular tumour lines. However, the extent to which responses to these lines (which have been transformed in culture for long periods) are indicative of physiologically active cytotoxic responses is not clear.

T cells With regard to T-cell cytotoxicity, it should be noted that anti-CD3 directed cellular cytotoxicity is known to generate false positives. This is believed to be due to the tendency of the anti-CD3 antibody to produce strong signals, which result in non-physiological T-cell activation.[34] In addition, the target cell line traditionally associated with such assays (P815) is known to be highly susceptible to destruction by a broad range of cell types including macrophages, T cells, and NK cells.[35] Hence this assay involves the use of a non-physiological stimulus against non-physiological targets. Similar physiological criticisms can be directed against LAK assays. It can be argued that effector cells encounter exceedingly high concentrations of IL-2 in local microenvironments (e.g. lymph nodes) during an immune response. However, the concentrations used to generate LAK cells are often 100 times greater than those capable of inducing a proliferative response. In addition, the constitution of LAK cells is not uniform, consisting of varying proportions of NK and T cells (depending on the subject) and a related absence of specificity (LAK cells kill both tumour and normal cells). Together, these limitations highlight the non-physiological nature of LAK assays.

Recommendations It is clear from Figure 3.1 that an end-stage event such as cytotoxicity can be affected in a number of ways. For example, a reduction in cytotoxicity could be caused by defects in antigen presentation, cytokine help, active suppression, defects in perforin release, or just decreased proliferation of effector cells. Thus, if an assay demonstrates reduced cytotoxicity and the assay has been conducted in isolation, information on the mechanisms that may be involved cannot be obtained. The use of additional assays, such as cytokine or proliferation assays, would enable conclusions to be drawn regarding possible mechanisms.

With regard to NK cytotoxicity assays specifically, the methodological limitations described above suggest that future work with this assay would benefit from the use of either purified NK cells (using CD16 and CD56) or the depletion of NK cells from PBMCs. Either approach would ensure that only NK cells were responsible for any cytotoxicity witnessed in the assay. Furthermore, NK cytotoxicity assays should be combined with lymphocyte counts which identify the proportion of NK cells within a given sample. This would, in turn, allow conclusions to be drawn about the efficiency of cytotoxic activity within this subset.

Clinical implications Cellular cytotoxicity is the primary mechanism for removing virally and bacterially infected cells or non-self (i.e. tumorigenic) cells. However, a general defect in cytotoxicity is not necessarily lethal, as demonstrated by studies on perforin knockout mice.[36,37] Rather, the clinical importance of cytotoxicity is dependent on the pathogen. Thus, while no human disease identified to date is totally dependent on cytotoxicity for its clearance, the absence of cytotoxic T lymphocytes is clearly associated with the progression of a number of diseases including HIV[38] and cervical carcinoma.[39] Such findings provide indirect evidence for their role in controlling such diseases.

3.3.1.3 Lymphocyte proliferation

Rationale Lymphocyte proliferation assays are perhaps the most widespread functional *in vitro* assessments of the cellular arm of the immune system.[29,30,39,40] These assays involve the measurement of lymphocyte division (i.e. proliferation) in response to any stimulus. Implicit in the performance of these assays is the assumption that the greater the proliferation, the more effective is the immune response, although it should be acknowledged that it has not yet been determined whether or not such a linear relationship exists. Two main assays of proliferation have been reported: proliferation in response to non-specific stimuli, and proliferation in response to specific stimuli.

Technical description Proliferating cells actively take up thymidine and incorporate it into their DNA. Thus the standard proliferation assay consists of quantitating the uptake of radioactively labelled thymidine (usually tritiated, i.e. labelled with ^{3}H), thereby estimating the amount of cell division that has taken place. Recent years have seen the advent of non-radioactive flow-cytometer-based proliferation assays. Some are very similar to the ^{3}H assays; thus the uptake of the thymidine analogue 5-bromo-2′-deoxyuridine (BrdU) can be measured instead of ^{3}H by using antibodies to BrdU and a flow cytometer as a readout. Another flow-cytometer-based assay uses the fluorescent stable protein dye carboxyfluorescein succinimidyl ester (CFSE) which is incorporated into cells before stimulation. After activation, the dye is evenly divided to daughter cells as the cells divide and therefore the decrease in fluorescence in any particular cell is a measure of the number of cell divisions it has undergone.

The stimuli used to elicit cell division can be both 'specific' and 'non-specific'. The latter are polyclonal stimuli and thus activate most if not all lymphocytes. Typical examples are the lectins PHA, CON A (mainly T cells), and PWM (T and B cells), the anti-CD3 monoclonal antibodies OKT3 and UCHT-1 (only stimulate T cells), and non-specific activators such as phorbol esters (e.g. phorbol myristate acetate). In contrast, T-cell proliferation in response to specific stimuli is dependent upon antigen recognition by TCRs. This is achieved by the presentation of specific peptides, derived from processing foreign protein antigens, in the grooves of MHC I or MHC II molecules (MHC I molecules present antigens to CD8+ cytotoxic T cells, while MHC II molecules present to CD4+ helper T cells). These peptides are then recognized by the TCRs as foreign, and T-cell activation and proliferation ensue.

Advantages Proliferative responses to non-specific stimuli inform the researcher as to whether there is a difference in the general responsiveness of lymphocytes. In addition, the use of different non-specific stimuli, or mitogens, can offer some insight into where in the proliferation process the impairment has occurred. For example, OKT3 antibodies specifically stimulate T cells in culture via the TCR, so that reduced responses would imply a fault in T-cell responsiveness via TCR signalling. In combination, these assays can identify immune defects. Thus lack of responsiveness to CON A (a monocyte-dependent polyclonal lymphocyte activator) but responsiveness to OKT3 would suggest that the reduced proliferation was due to a monocyte defect.

In contrast, the advantage of using specific stimuli is that an examination of the immune response to a specific pathogen is possible. Any foreign antigen which has previously been met by the host's immune response can be tested. Furthermore, because one is examining a highly specific immune response (i.e. only those T cells which recognize the antigen in question), it is possible to undertake a more detailed analysis of specific T-cell responses. Thus any differences between individuals are more clearly defined.

Limitations The principal limitation of proliferation assays using non-specific stimuli is their polyclonal nature. Many investigations have employed this immune index as their outcome measure. However, the results from such investigations do not allow us to identify which subsets of lymphocytes are responding, nor do they inform us on the potential mechanisms involved. In addition, in studies where data on cell counts are not available, it is not possible to discount the possibility that differences in proliferation may simply be caused by alterations in the numbers and ratios of the different lymphocyte subsets in the peripheral blood sample being tested. Furthermore, the synthetic nature of the stimuli used in such assays necessarily limits the scope of the conclusions that can be drawn regarding the efficacy of the immune system in the face of naturalistic pathogens. Finally, the reliability of proliferation assays has also been called into question. Fillion *et al.*[41] explored the reliability of proliferative responses to CON A and PHA in healthy males. Blood samples were taken and assays conducted at baseline and 14, 28, and 42 days later. Their results revealed evidence of significant variability in proliferative responses to both mitogens, particularly between days 14 and 28, and that different dilutions also exhibited different patterns of stability.

Difficulties also exist with proliferation assays which use specific stimuli. Although specific stimuli provide data on the nature of the immune response to a naturalistic pathogen, they are essentially *in vitro* assays from which conclusions regarding *in vivo* processes must be drawn with caution. In particular, it should be noted that the specific stimuli used in such assays tend to come in the form of soluble antigens derived from the pathogen under investigation. CD8+ cells typically have poor responses to such antigens, and thus the proliferative responses that are witnessed are usually derived from CD4+ cells.[42] CD8+ proliferative responses are only observed when intact cells (e.g. virus-infected cells) are used as stimulators. A further difficulty with such assays is that the responses are strongly influenced by how recently the last *in vivo* exposure to the antigen occurred. As it is difficult to control for previous exposure, results from such assays can be confounded by this factor.

Recommendations Proliferation assays involving non-specific stimuli are most informative when the stimulus is chosen with a view to identifying where in the proliferation process the immune dysfunction is occurring. In this regard, the use of multiple mitogens could help to delineate the causes of immune dysfunction.

Clinical implications Proliferation is an intrinsic part of immune responses, occurring in B and T lymphocytes following recognition of antigen by their respective antigen receptors and in the presence of the correct cytokines. The clinical implications are dependent on the magnitude of the defects. While a 50% reduction in proliferative responses may have little clinical effect, total abrogation would result in no immune response to an antigenic challenge and immunodeficiency, as seen in AIDS.[43] A less extreme example comes from reports of decreased specific proliferative responses to varicella zoster virus (VZV) in the elderly.[44] This downregulation of the cellular immune response has been proposed as one of the mechanisms which may explain the increased risk of herpes zoster with advancing age. Together, these data suggest a correlation between reduced T-cell proliferation to a virus and clinical disease.

3.3.1.4 Cytokine and soluble cytokine receptor levels

Rationale Cytokines are soluble factors released by immune cells which control and direct the function of other immune effectors. They act by binding specific receptors on the cell surface, cross-linking of which results in cell stimulation. There are often soluble versions of the cytokine receptors (e.g. sIL-6R, sTNFR) that buffer the effects of the cytokine. Alterations in the concentration of cytokines or their soluble receptors mediate the down- and upregulation of the immune system and thus offer insight into several aspects of immune system activity. Indeed, these molecules represent a major target for clinical treatment (e.g. the anti-TNF antibody infliximab and the soluble TNFR molecule etanercept are now used in the treatment of inflammatory diseases such as rheumatoid arthritis).[45,46] The range of cytokines is extensive and is continually increasing, with several subpopulations also in existence (e.g. interferons, colony-stimulating factors, transforming growth factors, and tumour necrosis factors). Therefore in Table 3.2 we describe the functions of only some of the cytokines which have featured in investigations into the effects of stress on the immune system.

In Table 3.2, we distinguish between type 1 (Th1) and type 2 (Th2) cytokines. Th1 cytokines (e.g. γ-interferon, IL2, etc.) are often referred to as pro-inflammatory cytokines and promote cellular immunity. In contrast, Th2 cytokines (e.g. IL-4, IL-10, etc.) are known as anti-inflammatory cytokines and promote humoral immunity. Further details can be found in the reviews by Cohen and Cohen[47] and Wardle.[48] These two classes of cytokine are mutually inhibitory. Thus the ratio or balance between Th1 and Th2 cytokines is of interest as it informs us as to whether a cellular (Th1) or humoral (Th2) immune response is predominant. In recent years there has been considerable interest in the Th1/Th2 ratio in PNI, with evidence suggesting that periods of both acute and chronic stress can result in a suppression of Th1 immunity, resulting in a shift towards Th2.[49-51]

A number of different systems are used to investigate cytokine levels, namely poly-clonal mitogen stimulation, antigen-specific activation, or broad measurements of

Table 3.2 Functions of the five classes of antibody found in the immune system

Antibody type	Function/description
Immunoglobulin A (IgA)	Secreted in body fluids like tears and therefore protects the mucosal surfaces
Immunoglobulin E (IgE)	Attaches to antigens and then to basophils and mast cells, triggering the release of histamines
Immunoglobulin M (IgM)	Multiple functions including the triggering of complement-mediated lysis and the formation of antibody–antigen complexes which can be cleared by phagocytic cells of the liver
Immunoglobulin G (IgG)	Coats microorganisms making it possible for macrophages and neutrophils to recognize, engulf, and destroy pathogens such as bacteria. This is the most abundant immunoglobulin consisting of multiple isotypes with different functions
Immunoglobulin D (IgD)	Little is known about the function of this antibody

cytokines in circulating plasma or serum. However, cytokines tend to act in the lymph node microenvironment where antigen-presenting cells meet T and B cells.[48] Therefore *in vitro* systems, such as mitogen stimulation or antigen-specific stimulation, are just attempts to imitate a much more complex and subtle set of cellular interactions. Measurement of cytokine levels following mitogen stimulation is the least physiological investigation, as multiple cell subsets of different antigen specificities are activated. It is more a measure of the general ability of a group of cells, as a whole, to produce cytokines. Antigen-specific activation is a better defined system, as the stimulating antigen will only be presented to highly specific effectors. This is a closer representation of *in vivo* events, although it is important to acknowledge that the organization and milieu of cells in peripheral blood are very different from those of cells in lymph nodes. While *in vitro* measurements of cytokines in circulation are the least contrived, such measurements are unlikely to reflect the events in lymph node microenvironments unless systemic infections are taking place.

Technical description One of the most common techniques used for measuring cytokine levels is the enzyme-linked immunosorbent assay (ELISA). Cytokine ELISAs function in the same way as those used to measure antibody titres, apart from the fact that both the antibody used to coat the plate and the enzyme-conjugated antibody are cytokine specific. In brief, plastic plates are coated with the appropriate antigen (i.e. the one which binds to the antibody of interest). The test sample is then introduced onto the plates. At this stage, antibodies specific to the antigen (i.e. the target antibody) are bound to the plate and all non-specific antibodies are washed off. This is followed by the addition of another antibody, specific to the target antibody, which is conjugated with an enzyme. An enzyme substrate is then introduced which, following action of the enzyme, results in a colour change which can be measured quantitatively with a spectrometer. The degree of colour change is related to the amount of enzyme, which in turn is related to the initial concentration of the target antibody. These tests are called 'sandwich ELISAs' because the target antibody is sandwiched between an antigen and another antibody-specific antibody.

An adaptation of the ELISA is the ELISPOT assay. This uses the principle of ELISA but instead of a supernatant, activated cells (normally T cells activated with peptide) are added to plates coated with cytokine-specific antibody. The localized production of the target cytokine results in a footprint around the cytokine-producing cell, which is then visualized after the cell is washed away. By counting the number of spots, the number of cytokine-producing cells in any particular cell mix can be estimated.

Another antibody-based assay is intracellular cytokine staining (ICS). This is a flow-cytometry-based assay that allows the identification of the cell types producing a particular cytokine. Like ELISPOT, this system is not quantitative with respect to the amount of cytokine produced in a culture, but it does define the number and type of cells producing any particular cytokine (e.g. CD4+ T cell versus CD8+ T cell) and therefore gives an idea of the underlying mechanisms taking place within any system.

Two further techniques have been used to measure cytokines: biological assays and the reverse transcriptase polymerase chain reaction (RT-PCR). Biological assays use the particular role of a specific cytokine as a measure of its concentration. An example would be the use of IL-2-dependent T-cell lines (CTLL-2)[52] to measure IL-2 concentration. This involves starving the cell line of IL-2 before introducing a set number of cells to a test supernatant and measuring their proliferation to the IL-2 in that sample. A standard curve is generated using varying concentrations of recombinant IL-2, from which the concentration of IL-2 in the test supernatant can be read. Cell line proliferation assays exist for most of the interleukins.

In contrast, RT-PCR is a molecular biological technique involving the extraction of RNA from a cell sample, its conversion to complementary DNA by reverse transcriptase (RT), and then the polymerase chain reaction (PCR) to amplify the DNA message using oligonucleotide primers so that it can be visualized on an agarose gel.[53]

Finally, a number of technologies that can measure concentrations of multiple cytokines from single samples have recently flooded the market. There are technologies that can measure both DNA and protein, but all of them tend to be expensive. With respect to DNA, there are now a number of 'DNA array' systems (e.g. Affymetrix gene chips) which compare the levels of thousands of genes in two or more different test samples. It should be noted that not only cytokine gene expression but potentially the expression of every gene expressed by the cell in question is measured in such an assay. With respect to measurement of cytokine protein levels, most of the technologies are antibody based. In their simplest form, these include the cytometric bead arrays (CBAs), which measure six cytokines in a single sample and represent multiple ELISAs in a test tube with a readout on a flow cytometer. However, there are also cytokine protein arrays (e.g. the Biocarta system) which measure tens to hundreds of different cytokines from a single sample. These may well represent the future of clinical cytokine research.

Advantages and limitations Cytokine levels are able to inform us about several features of the immune system. First, the lack of certain cytokines suggests potential mechanisms for any functional abnormalities recorded. For example, Kiecolt-Glaser et al.[54] reported that stress in elderly caregivers was associated with a poorer antibody response to influenza vaccine. However, unlike previous investigations, they measured several cytokines (IL-2, IL-1β, and IL-6) and thus were able to speculate on the possible mechanisms involved. Secondly, the level of Th1 and Th2 cytokines inform the researcher about the type of immune response being made to an antigen (i.e. cellular or humoral) and indicate what is probably the most active cell type involved. This is clinically relevant, because different diseases require different immune responses (e.g. asthma is characterized by dominant Th2 responses, while rheumatoid arthritis is characterized by a dominance of Th1). Thus a stress-related shift towards one or other immune process is likely to have important implications for populations with such conditions.

Specific advantages are also conferred by each of the assays used to measure cytokines. For example, ELISAs provide information on the immunoreactivity of cytokines. Furthermore, because monoclonal anticytokine antibodies are used in ELISAs, the investigator can be sure that the quantitative result is an accurate measure of the cytokine concentration. However, ELISAs do not provide information about the actual activity of the cytokine because, even if a cytokine is inactive, it may still be recognized by an antibody. In contrast, biological assays confer the advantage of informing the investigator about the bioactivity of the cytokines being measured, although it should be noted that, because cytokines are pleiotropic and can have very similar functions (e.g. IL-2 and IL-4 both induce T-cell proliferation), biological assays should be carefully controlled. For example, the cell line CT.4R, can be used to estimate concentrations of both IL-2 and IL-4, but for definitive conclusions such assays should be carried out in the presence of inhibitory antibodies to just one of these cytokines.[55] ELISAs also provide little information on the number and type of cells producing the cytokine. However, this information can be obtained from ELISPOT and ICS. The advantage of the RT-PCR method is its incredible sensitivity: RT-PCR can now detect mRNA from a single cell. Unlike biological assays or ELISAs, the results from RT-PCRs are not confounded by the turnover of cytokines. Upon release, there is an active uptake of cytokines such that measures of cytokines in supernatant only reveal a proportion of the total cytokine released. Similarly, cytokines can bind to antagonists which may also interfere with their detection. Cytokine detection by RT-PCRs is not affected by physiological activity of this kind. However, intrinsic to RT-PCR is that it detects the level of messenger RNA and not of protein itself. Many intracellular processes take place between the expression of mRNA and final release of a protein, any of which may be blocked or impaired. Similarly, lack of mRNA does not mean that there is not a stable active cytokine present. Thus RT-PCR is not in itself a measure of actual cytokine levels, but rather a measure that a cell's machinery is ready to generate the cytokine. It is also, at best, semiquantitative (unlike ELISAs), measuring levels of mRNA relative to those of a control gene.

Limitations Perhaps the most significant limitation impeding the widespread use of cytokine determination in PNI is the fact that only a very limited number of cytokines can be detected in the plasma of healthy individuals. Thus the measurement of plasma cytokines is ultimately of greatest utility in 'diseased' populations.

Recommendations Despite some of the considerations outlined above, the measurement of cytokine concentrations offers an exciting opportunity to explore the potential mechanisms underlying stress-related immune dysfunction. It is for this reason that we would advocate the more widespread assessment of multiple cytokines in PNI. In this respect, the future is likely to lie in the use of 'arrays' that measure changes in multitudes of genes and proteins. The only limiting factor of these technologies is expense, but they are already in use in basic science with systems such as the Affymetrix DNA array being used to measure changes in expression of over 10 000 genes in a single assay.

Clinical implications As with many biological systems, and a recurring theme in this chapter, the clinical implications of changes in cytokine levels are dependent on their magnitude. Complete loss of a cytokine is often not immediately lethal, but the resultant immunodeficiency is likely to kill once a pathogen can take advantage of the defect (e.g. IL-7 knockout mice[56]). Where the main role of the cytokine is immunoregulatory, removal can result in autoimmunity as seen in IL-2 knockout mice.[57] However, partial loss often has no clinical significance, as many cytokines are partly redundant.

Changes in groups of cytokines, such as Th1 or Th2, give an indication of the type of immune response occurring (cellular versus humoral). However, dominance of Th1 or Th2 cytokines cannot, in itself, be interpreted as being adaptive or maladaptive. Both cytokine subsets are essential features of the immune response, and only in specific contexts is one or other dangerous to the host. For example, Decker *et al.*[58] reported that surgical stress was associated with a shift in the Th1–Th2 balance in the favour of Th2, as shown by an increase in IL-4 production. However, the significance of this shift is unclear. This study clearly demonstrates that the immunological significance of cytokine concentrations should be interpreted in the context of the pathogen under investigation. For example, Th1 responses (cellular) are vital for the control of leprosy lesions,[59] while a Th2 response (antibody) is much more effective in controlling influenza infection.[60]

3.3.1.5 Antibody assays

Rationale Another popular assay in PNI is the measurement of antibody levels.[61–63] Antibodies are proteins constructed from four polypeptide chains,[64] and are produced by B cells following exposure to antigens. They bind to the antigen which stimulated their development and, via a variety of mechanisms, counteract the pathogenic potential of the antigen. Hence levels of circulating antibody offer some insight into the efficacy of the humoral arm of the immune system.

Five major classes of antibody (known as isotypes) have been identified and defined by their different heavy chains: IgA, IgG, IgM, IgD, and IgE. IgG and IgA can be split further into four subclasses and two subclasses, respectively. The functions of the major isotypes are described in Table 3.3. The different functions are conferred by the non-antigen-binding carboxy-terminal half of the heavy chain.[65] Structurally, the heavy chains differ in the number and location of the disulphide bonds which link the chains and the distribution of their N-linked carbohydrate groups. Further isotype-specific differences are the lack of a hinge region (which increases the flexibility of the antibody) in IgM and IgE, and the polymeric qualities of IgM (which forms

Table 3.3 Cytokines and their functions

Cytokine	Cell expression	Function (Th1 versus Th2)
IL-1	Wide—nearly all immune cells	Wide—*in vivo* causes hypotension, fever, weight loss, acute phase responses
IL-2	T cells	Stimulates growth and differentiation of T, B, NK, LAK cells, monocytes, macrophages (Th1 cytokine)
IL-3	Activated T cells, mast cells, eosinophils	B-cell growth factor; expands haematopoietic precursors; activates monocytes (Th1 cytokine)
IL-4	T cells, mast cells	Multiple biological effects on B and T cells; stimulates IgG4/IgE secretion from B cells (Th2 cytokine)
IL-5	T cells, mast cells, eosinophils	Eosinophil growth and B-cell differentiation factor (Th2 cytokine)
IL-6	Wide—including non-lymphoid cells	Regulates B- and T-cell function, haematopoiesis, and acute phase reactions (Th2 cytokine)
IL-7	Bone marrow, thymic stromal, and spleen	Proliferation and differentiation of B and T cells
IL-8	Activated Th2 T cells	Neutrophil chemoattractant and activator; also attracts basophils and some lymphocytes
IL-9	Wide—including non-lymphoid cells	Enhances proliferation of T cells, mast cells, erythroid precursors (Th2 cytokine)
IL-10	Activated T cells, monocytes	Stimulates proliferation of B, thymocytes, and mast cells; inhibits Th1 cytokine production (Th2 cytokine)
IL-11	Bone marrow, stimulated fibroblasts	Growth factor for multipotential haemopoietic progenitors
IL-12	B cells, monocytes/macrophages	Induces proliferation and differentiation of Th1 cells; enhances NK cells (Th1 cytokine)
IL-13	Activated T cells	Promotes B-cell proliferation and IgM/IgE/IgG4 production (Th2 cytokine)
IL-14	T cells	Enhances proliferation of activated B cells; inhibits Ig synthesis
IL-15	Wide—more by monocytes/epithelial cells	Stimulates growth and differentiation of T, B, and NK cells
IL-18	Keratinocytes, monocyte lineage cells	Enhances IL-12 and IFN-γ production from lymphocytes and boosts NK cytotoxicity (probable Th1 cytokine)
IL-21	Activated CD4+ T cells	Stimulates growth and differentiation of T, B, and NK cells
IFN-γ	T and NK cells	Activates most immune cell types; potentiates antiviral effect of IFN-α and IFN-β (Th1 cytokine)
TNF-α	Wide	General pro-inflammatory cytokine—increases immune cell migration, activates macrophages and neutrophils, potentiates lysis of virus-infected cells
TNF-β	Wide	Important in development of certain lymphoid organs and maturation of the antibody response (Th1 cytokine)

tetramers) and IgA (which forms dimers). Each of these antibodies is ubiquitous, although certain classes tend to predominate in particular fluids. For example, IgA is found primarily in mucous secretions, while IgG predominates in serum. IgE is the antibody recognized by mast cells and basophils, and is the main pathogenic antibody in patients suffering severe allergies. The fluid in which the antibody predominates dictates the nature of the sample collected, and the isotype of the antibody dictates the type of immunity it confers.

Technical description One of the most common techniques used for the quantification of antibodies is ELISA (see above). This assay relies on the highly specific nature of the antigen–antibody interaction. The basic assay can be adapted to measure concentrations of total Ig, different Ig isotypes, or even antigen-specific antibodies.

Advantages ELISAs are straightforward, robust, and extremely sensitive. The assessment of total levels of antibody[61,63] enables the investigator to detect gross immunodeficiency. Furthermore, the measurement of IgA in particular is especially attractive as its production in saliva makes it readily available for measurement. However, the quantification of antibody titres to a specific antigen[66,67] is inherently superior. This approach is based on the premise that once antibodies are made in response to an antigen, the host retains a small proportion of them in the circulation. Therefore it is possible to assess the efficacy of humoral immunity to a specific pathogen with such assays, and these data clearly have great clinical relevance. Much of the work that has been conducted with antigen-specific antibody assays has involved the measurement of antibody titres to latent herpes viruses, such as herpes simplex virus 1 (HSV-1) and Epstein–Barr virus (EBV). These viruses are known to be persistent and reactivating infections in humans.[66–68] Hence, unlike other antigens for which antibody presence is affected by how recently the host has been exposed to the antigen, moderate levels of antibody to the virus are always present in the host. Furthermore, these levels fluctuate in response to viral activity, with an increase in viral replication being associated with an increase in antibody titres. Thus the assessment of antibody titres to latent viruses would appear to be ideally suited to investigations of the effects of stress on one virus-specific aspect of humoral immunity.

Limitations Of all the antibody assays used in PNI, the measurement of total antibody levels is perhaps the most limited. The antigen specificity of antibodies means that only a certain proportion of circulating antibody will respond to any particular antigen. Thus total antibody is a poor index of the specific antibody response and can provide only an imprecise measure of immune system activation. This is perhaps most clearly seen in the literature on secretory IgA (S-IgA), which demonstrates that the relationship between stress and S-IgA is, at best, equivocal.[63,69,70] In their comprehensive review of this literature, Bosch et al.[71] concluded that the equivocal nature of the evidence is, in part, attributable to methodological issues such as variability in the definition of stress, timing of sample collection, effects of salivary flow, etc. However, notwithstanding the possible effects of methodological inadequacy, the clinical relevance of total S-IgA remains questionable. Individuals who are S-IgA deficient are able to maintain good health. Thus the importance of transient changes in S-IgA in response to stress should be interpreted with caution. Indeed, this has led some investigators to examine the effects of stress on other features of secretory immunity, such as lysozyme and bacterial aggregration.[71–73]

In contrast, the quantification of antibody titres to a specific antigen[66–68] is clearly more precise and clinically relevant. However, the antibody response can and does wane in the absence of the stimulating antigen. In addition, antibodies have a limited half-life. Thus the assessment of antigen-specific antibodies is dependent, in part, upon ensuring recent exposure to the antigen. It is for this reason that several investigators have focused on antibody titres to latent viruses where moderate levels of antibody to the virus are always present in the host. Indeed, this approach is likely to grow in popularity in view of new techniques which enable the measurement of latent virus, in particular EBV, in saliva[74] and dried blood spots.[75]

Recommendations It is evident that, in isolation, differences in antibody titres can only inform us that there may be an impairment or increase in the production of antibodies *per se*. However, further information can be obtained on the processes involved by assessing antibody titres in conjunction with functional *in vitro* assays. For example, stimulation with pokeweed mitogen (a lectin which induces T-cell-dependent antibody production by B cells) can inform us whether T or B cells are involved in the altered process. In addition, the selection of different classes of antibody can help to determine which particular immune responses are altered. For example, IgM production is indicative of a 'primary' immune response, i.e. a response to an antigen that has not previously been presented or a response that has waned. Conversely, IgG is indicative of a more specific 'memory' response, i.e. prior exposure to the antigen has occurred.

The process by which B cells change the isotype of the antibody they secrete is called 'isotype switching'.[76] It is regulated by cytokines released from T cells[77] and is accompanied by changes in the region which binds antigen (termed 'somatic hypermutation'[78]), resulting in increased binding efficiency. This maturing of the antibody response helps, first, to fine tune the specificity of the antibody for its antigen and, second, to direct the humoral immune system to the areas where it is needed. Thus multiple measures of antigen-specific antibodies of different isotypes can inform on the type of immune response taking place. Finally, as described earlier, it is important to acknowledge that immune responses can wane with time, and thus a lack of IgG, for example, does not necessarily mean that memory responses are impaired but may simply represent an immune response that has waned.

One final issue worthy of consideration concerns the measurement of neutralizing antibodies as an alternative to the total and specific antibody assays that have been described. Neutralizing antibody levels give a more specific measure of immunity to a particular virus by assessing sera for their ability to prevent replication of a known amount of virus. A susceptible cell line is inoculated with the target virus *in vitro* in the presence of a particular dilution of the test serum, and the amount of virus replication is assessed by light microscopy or other standard tests for the presence of the virus or virion component. The antibody titre recorded is the reciprocal of the highest dilution that completely inhibits virus replication. In this way, the measurement of neutralizing antibody provides a more accurate measure of the effectiveness of a particular immune response in preventing virus infection or activation than gross measures of antibody levels. However, neutralizing antibody titres have not yet been used extensively in PNI.

Clinical implications It is widely agreed that an increase in antibody titres occurs as a consequence of an increase in viral activity. One of the many hypotheses put forward to explain such increases is that the host has experienced some degree of immune disturbance which has resulted in infection or, in the case of latent viruses, virus react-ivation. In investigations such as these, the increase in antibody titres is construed as a sign of underlying immune dysfunction. However, it could be argued that elevations in antibody titres, far from being a sign of immunosuppression, are in fact characteristic of an effective humoral immune response to the antigen. It should also be recognized that alterations in antibody titres may reflect a virus-specific response and not a general humoral response. Furthermore, compared with other virus-directed methods (e.g. virus isolation), the significance of virus-specific antibody titres is limited by the fact that an increase in antibody titre occurs some time after virus activation and replication commences. Thus, while measurements of antibody levels are informative, clinical implications should be made with caution.

3.3.2. Integrated *in vivo* measures

Thus far, we have provided an overview of many traditional *in vitro* assays. However, we have not explored the relationship between *in vitro* assays and *in vivo* functioning. Unfortunately, this issue is a perennial problem for all investigators of the human immune system as ethical considerations necessarily limit the scope for *in vivo* research in humans. Therefore it is not possible to offer any informed discussion of the relationship between data from *in vitro* assays and *in vivo* functioning. Nonetheless, it is possible to contend that *in vivo* investigations of the immune system offer outcome measures of the greatest clinical relevance because they provide a measure of integrated immune responses. In recognition of this, consideration will be given to the limited number of *in vivo* approaches that have been utilized so far.

3.3.2.1 Delayed hypersensitivity tests

Rationale Hypersensitivity is defined as an exaggerated or inappropriate form of an otherwise adaptive immune response that results in tissue damage. Four types of hypersensitivity have been described: type I (immediate) is clinically observed in conditions such as hay fever, where an IgE response to pollen results in mast cell activation and the release of chemical mediators that can result in asthma or rhinitis; type II is caused by hypersensitivity of antibody-dependent cytotoxic mechanisms; type III is immune complex mediated, where large quantities of antibody–antigen complexes overwhelm the host's ability to clear them, resulting in serum sickness: finally, in type IV (delayed hypersensitivity) the release of lymphokines following a T cell–antigen interaction results in an inflammatory response. Type IV (delayed hypersensitivity) will be the focus of this section as it has been adopted several times as an index of the functional efficacy of cell-mediated immunity to antigenic stimulation.[79–81]

Technical description Delayed hypersensitivity (DTh) is defined as a reaction that takes more than 12 h to develop. There are at least four different types of DTh but we will consider only the tuberculin-type DTh response which has been used most widely in studies of the effects of acute stress on the immune system.[81,82] In human research, the DTh test typically takes the form of the simultaneous intradermal application of one or several DTh antigens. These antigens elicit an immunological reaction involving the release of lymphokines by antigen-sensitized T cells. These lymphokines, in turn, activate macrophages which release inflammatory mediators. The reaction time for tests of this response is approximately 48 h.

Advantages and limitations The advantage of DTh tests of this kind is that they are symptomatic measurements of an *in vivo* process. Indeed, the tuberculin-type hypersensitivity reaction is a recognized measure of previous exposure to a specific antigen and is also considered a suitable assay for determining the presence of particular immunodeficiencies. However, complex mechanisms control the responses involved in DTh reactions, and tests such as these do not allow us to determine where immune system impairment has taken place; nor is it possible to quantify easily the nature of the immune response generated. Finally, responses to the DTh antigens are also likely to be influenced by the recency of previous antigen exposure. Thus this *in vivo* technique is not without its limitations.

3.3.2.2 Responses to live or attenuated virus preparations

Rationale and technical description In these investigations healthy individuals are inoculated with a virus and a range of *in vivo* immunological responses to the virus or viral antigens contained in a vaccine (antibody responses, lymphocyte proliferation, etc.) are examined. Two main approaches have been adopted: inoculation with a live virus[83] and inoculation with a vaccine which contains inactivated or weakened virus preparations.[84–87]

Advantages The most significant advantage conferred by both live virus and vaccine challenge studies is that they enable the researcher to examine the relationship between stress and *in vivo* immunity in the face of a naturalistic pathogen. Thus it is possible to conclude from investigations like that of Kiecolt-Glaser et al.[54] that their elderly caregivers who produced a poor response to an influenza vaccine challenge may in fact be more susceptible to influenza infection. Such a conclusion could not have been reached if the immunological outcome measures had been any of the non-specific in vitro assays described previously.

A further advantage associated with live virus challenge studies (and, to a lesser extent, live vaccine challenge studies) is that they enable the investigator to explore the relationship between stress and clinically verifiable disease. This is demonstrated in the investigation by Cohen et al.[83] who found that, after challenging subjects with one of five respiratory viruses, both respiratory infections and clinical colds increased in a dose–response manner with increases in psychological stress.

Limitations It is evident from these data that live virus challenge studies are among the most pre-eminent investigations that have been conducted in the field. However, there is one caveat worthy of comment. This concerns the fact that immune responses to vaccination can be affected by a range of variables other than psychological stress. In a recent review, Loveren et al.[88] reported on a range of endogenous factors (e.g. age, gender, and genetic status) and exogenous factors (e.g. smoking and diet) that can modulate responses to vaccination. They also noted that the immunological history of the host can also be of importance (e.g. concurrent/past infections and vaccinations). Such considerations demonstrate that an individual's immunological responses to an in vivo challenge do not occur in isolation, but are in fact modulated by other factors. This should be taken into consideration when interpreting data from in vivo investigations.

3.4 Directions for future research

In this chapter we have sought to alert the reader to some of the limitations and strengths of existing in vitro and in vivo assessments of the immune system. Our discussion has focused exclusively on the rationale behind the various assays and the methodological issues which limit the interpretability of the data obtained. Several key considerations for future research are apparent from this discussion. The first concerns the selection of immunological outcome measures. Many investigations into the effects of stress on the immune system adopt a single-outcome measure and then attempt to draw conclusions on the basis of the enumerative or functional status of this single parameter. However, the machinery of the immune system is complex and intimately interconnected, and therefore warrants the assessment of multiple parameters. In the same way that a single trait does not provide an adequate description of an individual's personality, a single immunological index should not be regarded as an adequate marker of the immune system.

A second related issue concerns the choice of immunological parameters. It is evident that various assays are able to inform us about various features of the immune system. Therefore the selection of assays should be closely aligned with the research question being asked and, if relevant, the disease process under investigation. For example, the selection of immune measures relevant for investigations into stress-associated immune changes in inflammatory disorders would differ substantially from those required to evaluate the role of immune mechanisms in viral disease. Indeed, even with viral disease, consideration of what immune measures would be important in primary versus secondary infection would be required. Such issues necessarily introduce another layer of complexity into this debate which is beyond the scope of this review. Suffice to say that we hope that the isolated use of non-specific immunological outcome measures (e.g. non-specific lymphocyte proliferation) will become obsolete.

Thirdly, caution should be exerted when interpreting immunological data. The complex interactions between the various facets of the immune system mean that immunological impairment at one level does not translate into impairment at all other levels. This issue is clearly illustrated by fluctuations in T-cell numbers. An increase in T-cell numbers may indicate the presence of infection and thus at one level indicate a lapse in the functional efficacy of the immune system. However, it also indicates that a cellular response has been mounted.

In addition to the methodological issues that have been identified in this chapter, there are several other factors, the majority of which are external to the assay but intrinsic to the host, which may also confound the results from PNI investigations (e.g. nutritional status, exercise, timing of samples, etc.) These factors are highly relevant to the discussion of how immunological data in such studies should be interpreted. However, they have been explored in previous reviews[88,89] and therefore will not be examined here.

It is evident that the measurement of stress-related immune impairment is an extremely complex issue. However, if adequate consideration is given to the strengths and weaknesses of the assays available, it is possible to delineate the consequences of stress for the immune system and further our understanding of stress–immune interactions.

References

1 Ader R, Cohen N (1975). Behaviourally conditioned immunosuppression. *Psychosom Med* 37: 333–40.
2 Brickman CM (1994). The molecular basis of the human immune system. *J Clin Immunoassay* 17: 85–91.
3 Chigara M (1994). Self and nonself: duality of immune system. *Med. Hypotheses* 43: 6–10.
4 Roitt IM, Brostoff J, Male DK (1989). *Immunology* (2nd edn). London: Churchill Livingstone.
5 Zunich KM, Lane HC (1990). The immunology of HIV infection. *J Am Acad Dermatol* 22: 1202–5.
6 Fitzgerald PA, Mendelsohn M, Lopez C (1985). Human natural killer cells limit replication of herpes simplex virus type 1 *in vitro. J Immunol* 134: 1665–72.
7 Fillion L, Lemyre L, Mandeville R, Piche R (1996). Cognitive appraisal, stress state, and cellular immunity responses before and after diagnosis of breast tumor. *Int J Rehabil Health* 2: 169–87.

8   Kang D-H, Fox C (2000). Neuroendocrine and leukocyte responses and pulmonary function to acute stressors. *Ann Behav Med* **22**: 276–85.

9   Van Rood YR, Bogaards M, Goulmy E, Van Houwelingen HC (1993). The effects of stress and relaxation on the *in vitro* immune response in man: a meta-analytic study. *J Behav Med* **16**: 163–81.

10 Marsland AL, Herbert TB, Muldoon MF, *et al.* (1997). Lymphocyte subset redistribution during acute laboratory stress in young adults: mediating effects of hemoconcentration. *Health Psychol* **16**: 341–8.

11 Boyce WT, Adams S, Tschann JM, Cohen F, Wara D, Gunnar MR (1995). Adrenocortical and behavioral predictors of immune responses to starting school. *Pediatr Res* **38**: 1009–17.

12 Boscarino JA, Chang J (1999). Higher abnormal leukocyte and lymphocyte counts 20 years after exposure to severe stress: research and clinical implications. *Psychosom Med* **61**: 378–86.

13 Mills PJ, Dimsdale JE, Nelesen RA, Dillon E (1996). Psychologic characteristics associated with acute stressor-induced leukocyte subset redistribution. *J Psychosom Res* **40**: 417–23.

14 De Gucht V, Fischler B, Demanet C (1999). Immune dysfunction associated with chronic professional stress in nurses. *Psychiatry Res* **85**: 105–11.

15 Castle S, Wilkins S, Heck E, Tanzy K, Fahey J (1995). Depression in caregivers of demented patients is associated with altered immunity: impaired proliferative capacity, increased CD8+, and a decline in lymphocytes with surface signal transduction molecules (CD38+) and a cytotoxicity marker (CD56+ CD8+). *Clin Exp Immunol* **101**: 487–93.

16 La Via MF, Munno I, Lydiard RB, *et al.* (1996). The influence of stress intrusion on immunodepression in generalized anxiety disorder patients and controls. *Psychosom Med* **58**: 138–42.

17 Dhabhar FS, Miller AH, McEwen BS, Spencer RL (1995). Effects of stress on immune cell distribution: dynamics and hormonal mechanisms. *J Immunol* **154**: 5511–27.

18 Joseph BZ, Beam R, Martin RJ, Borish L (1995). Prednisone inhibits leukocyte granule secretion into the asthmatic airway. *Int J Immunopathol Pharmacol* **8**: 23–30.

19 Kang D-H, Coe CL, McCarthy DO (1996). Academic examinations significantly impact immune responses but not lung function in healthy well-managed asthmatic adolescents. *Brain Behav Immun* **10**: 164–81.

20 Anesi A, Franciotta D, Di Paolo E, *et al.* (1994). PHA-stimulated cellular immune function and T-lymphocyte subsets in major depressive disorders. *Funct Neurol* **9**: 17–22.

21 Pettingale KW (1990). Is stress immunosuppressive? In Whalley LJ, Page ML (eds). *Current Approaches: Stress, Immunity and Disease*. Southampton: Duphar, 10–19.

22 Molbak K, Lisse IM, Aaby PT (1996). Lymphocyte subsets and prolonged diarrhea in young children from Guinea-Bissau. *Am J Epidemiol* **143**: 79–84.

23 Sallusto F, Lenig D, Forster R, Lipp M, Lanzavecchia A (1999). Two subsets of memory T lymphocytes with distinct homing potentials and effector functions. *Nature* **401**: 708–12.

24 Mackay CR (1991). T-cell memory: the connection between function, phenotype and migration pathways. *Immunol Today* **12**: 189–92.

25 Oshimi Y, Oshimi K, Miyazaki S (1996). Necrosis and apoptosis associated with distinct Ca2+ response patterns in target cells attacked by human natural killer cells. *J Physiol* **495**: 319–29.

26 Berke G (1995). The CTL's kiss of death. *Cell* **81**: 9–12.

27 Phillips JH, Lanier LL (1986). Lectin-dependent and anti-CD3 induced cytotoxicity are preferentially mediated by peripheral blood cytotoxic T lymphocytes expressing Leu-7 antigen. *J Immunol* **136**: 1579–85.

28 Benschop RJ, Jabaaij L, Oostveen FG, Vingerhoets AJJM, Ballieux RE (1998). The influence of psychological stress on immunoregulation of latent epstein-barr virus. *Stress Med* **14**: 21–9.

29 Dolbier CL, Cocke RR, Leiferman JA, *et al.* (2001). Differences in functional immune responses of high vs. low hardy, healthy individuals. *J Behav Med* **24**: 219–29.

30 Kiecolt-Glaser JK, Malarkey WB, Chee M, *et al.* (1993). Negative behaviour during marital conflict is associated with immunological down regulation. *Psychosom Med* **55**: 395–409.

31 Morimoto K, Takeshita T, Inoue-Sakuir C, Maruyama S (2001). Lifestyles and mental health status are associated with natural killer cell and lymphokine-activated killer cell activities. *Sci Total Environ* **270**: 3–11.

32 Jung W, Irwin M (1999). Reduction of natural killer cytotoxic activity in major depression: interaction between depression and cigarette smoking. *Psychosom Med* **61**: 263–70.

33 Goodkin K, Blaney N, Feaster D, *et al.* (1992). Active coping style is associated with natural killer cell cytotoxicity in asymptomatic HIV-1 seropositive homosexual men. *J Psychosom Res* **36**: 635–50.

34 Sette A, Alexander J, Ruppert J, *et al.* (1994). Antigen analogs/MHC complexes as specific T cell receptor antagonists. *Annu Rev Immunol* **12**: 413–31.

35 D'Angeac AD, Hale AH (1980). Pretreatment of P815 mastocytoma cells with inhibitors of protein synthesis reduces their susceptibility to lysis by cytotoxic thymus-derived lymphocytes. *Cell Immunol* **55**: 342–54.

36 Walsh CM, Matloubian M, Liu CC, *et al.* (1994). Immune function in mice lacking the perforin gene. *Proc Natl Acad Sci USA* **91**: 10854–8.

37 Franco MA, Tin C, Rott LS, VanCott JL, McGhee JR, Greenberg HB (1997). Evidence for CD8+ T-cell immunity to murine rotavirus in the absence of perforin, fas, and gamma interferon. *J Virol* **71**: 479–86.

38 Ogg GS, Jin X, Bonhoeffer S, *et al.* (1998). Quantitation of HIV-1-specific cytotoxic T lymphocytes and plasma load of viral RNA. *Science* **279**: 2103–6.

39 Tindle RW (1997). Immunomanipulative strategies for the control of human papillomavirus associated cervical disease. *Immunol Res* **16**: 387–400.

40 Herbert TB, Cohen S (1993). Stress and immunity in humans—a meta-analytic review. *Psychosom Med* **55**: 364–79.

41 Fillion L, Belles-Isles M, Lemyre L, Roy R (1994). Reliability of lymphocyte proliferation assays. *Stress Med* **10**: 43–8.

42 Raychaudhuri S, Morrow WJW (1993). Can soluble antigens induce CD8+ cytotoxic T-cell responses? A paradox revisited. *Immunol. Today* **14**: 344–8.

43 Lane HC, Fauci AS (1985). Immunologic abnormalities in the acquired immunodeficiency syndrome. *Annu Rev Immunol* **3**: 477–500.

44 Berger R, Florent G, Just M (1981). Decrease of the lymphoproliferative response to varicella-zoster virus antigen in the aged. *Infect Immun* **32**: 24–7.

45 Feldmann M, Maini RN (2001). Anti-TNF alpha therapy of rheumatoid arthritis: what have we learned? *Annu Rev Immunol* **19**: 163–96.

46 Carteron NL (2000) Cytokines in rheumatoid arthritis: trials and tribulations. *Mol Med Today* **6**: 315–23.

47 Cohen MC, Cohen S (1996). Cytokine function: a study in biologic diversity. *Am J Clin Pathol* **105**: 589–98.

48 Wardle EN (1993). Cytokines: an overview. *Eur J Med* **2**: 417–23.

49 Elenkov IJ, Chrousos GP (1999). Stress hormones, Th1/Th2 patterns, pro/anti-inflammatory cytokines and susceptibility to disease. *Trends Endocrinol Metab* **10**: 359–68.

50 Paik I-H, Toh K-Y, Lee C, Kim J-J, Lee S-J (2000). Psychological stress may induce increased humoral and decreased cellular immunity. *Behav Med* **26**: 139–42.

51 Glaser R, MacCullum RC, Laskowski BF, Malarkey WB, Sheridan JF, Kiecolt-Glaser JK (2001). Evidence for a shift in the Th1 to Th2 cytokine response associated with chronic stress and aging. *J Gerontol* **56A**: M477–82.

52 Gillis AJH, Bird CR (1978). T cell growth factor: parameters of production and a quantitative microassay for activity. *J Immunol* **120**: 2027–32.

53 Gilliland G, Perrin S, Blanchard K, Bunn HF (1990). Analysis of cytokine mRNA and DNA: detection and quantitation by competitive PCR. *Proc Natl Acad Sci USA* **87**: 2725–9.

54 Kiecolt-Glaser JK, Glaser R, Gravenstein S, Malarkey WB, Sheridan J (1996). Chronic stress alters the immune response to influenza virus vaccine in older adults. *Proc Natl Acad Sci USA* **93**: 3043–7.

55 Hu-Liu J, Ohara J, Watson, C, Tsang W, Paul WE (1989). Derivation of a T cell line that is highly responsive to IL-4 and IL-2 (CT.4R) and of an IL-2 hyporesponsive mutant of that line (CT.4S). *J Immunol* **142**: 800–907.

56 von Freeden-Jeffry U, Vieira P, Lucian LA, McNeil T, Burdach SE, Murray R (1995). Lymphopenia in interleukin (IL)-7 gene-deleted mice identifies IL-7 as a nonredundant cytokine. *J Exp Med* **181**: 1519–26.

57 Horak I, Lohler J, Ma A, Smith KA (1995). Interleukin-2 deficient mice: a new model to study autoimmunity and self-tolerance. *Immunol Rev* **148**: 35–44.

58 Decker D, Schondorf M, Bidlingmaier F, Hirner A, von Ruecker AA (1996). Surgical stress induces a shift in the type1-type2 T helper cell balance, suggesting down regulation of cell-mediated and up-regulation of antibody-mediated immunity commensurate to the trauma. *Surgery* **119**: 316–25.

59 Modlin RL (1994). Th1–Th2 paradigm: insights from leprosy. *J Invest Dermatol* **102**: 828–32.

60 Kubiet MA, Gonzales-Rothi RJ, Cottey R, Bender BS (1996). Serum antibody response to influenza vaccine in pulmonary patients receiving corticosteroids. *Chest* **110**: 367–70.

61 Maes M, Hendriks D, Gastel AV, *et al.* (1997). Effects of psychological stress on serum immunoglobulin, complement and acute phase protein concentrations in normal volunteers. *Psychoneuroendocrinology* **22**: 397–409.

62 Bosch JA, De Geus EJC, Kelder A, Veerman ECI, Hoogstraten J, Amerongen AVN (2001). Differential effects of active versus passive coping on secretory immunity. *Psychophysiology* **38**: 836–46.

63 Evans P, Der G, Ford G, Hucklebridge F, Hunt K, Lambert S (2000). Social class, sex and age differences in mucosal immunity in a large community sample. *Brain Behav Immun* **14**: 41–8.

64 Edelman GM, Cunningham BA, Gall WE, Gottlieb PD, Ruithauser U, Waxdal MJ (1969). *Proc Natl Acad Sci USA* **63**: 78–85.

65 Davies DR, Metzger H (1983). Structural basis of antibody function. *Annu Rev Immunol* **1**: 87–117.

66 Stowe RP, Pierson DL, Feeback DL, Barrett ADT (1999). Stress-induced reactivation of Epstein–Barr virus in astronauts. *Neuroimmunomodulation* **8**: 51–8.

67 Glaser R, Friedman SB, Smyth J, *et al.* (1999). The differential impact of training stress and final examination stress on herpes virus latency at the United States Military Academy at West Point. *Brain Behav Immun* **13**: 240–51.

68 Glaser R, Pearson GR, Jones JF, *et al.* (1991). Stress-related activation of Epstein–Barr virus. *Brain Behav Immun* **5**: 219–32.

69 Mouton C, Fillion L, Tawadros E, Tessier R (1989). Salivary IgA is a weak stress marker. *Behav Med* **15**: 179–85.

70 Jabaaij L, Benschop RJ, Vingerhoets AJJM, *et al.* (1993). Daily hassles and symptoms: their relationship to enumarative immunologic measures. *Stress Med* **9**: 259–69.

71 Bosch JA, Ring C, de Geus EJC, Veerman ECI, Amerongen AVN (2002). Stress and secretory immunity. *Int Rev Neurobiol* **52**: 213–53.

72 Yang Y, Koh D, Ng V, *et al.* (2002). Self perceived work related stress and the relation with salivary IgA and lysozyme among emergency department nurses. *Occup Environ Med* **59**: 836–41.

73 Bosch JA, Brand HS, Ligtenberg AJM, Bermond B, Hoogstraten J, Amerongen AVN (1998). The response of salivary protein levels and S-IgA to an academic examination are associated with daily stress. *J Psychophysiol* **12**: 384–91.

74 Sarid O, Anson O, Yaari A, Margalith M (2001). Epstein–Barr virus specific salivary antibodies as related to stress by examinations. *J Med Virol* **64**: 149–56.

75 McDade TW, Stalings JF, Angold A, *et al.* (2000). Epstein–Barr virus antibodies in whole blood spots: a minimally invasive method for assessing an aspect of cell-mediated immunity. *Psychosom Med* **62**: 560–7.

76 Kataoka T, Kawamaki T, Takahashi N, Honjo T (1980). Rearrangement of immunoglobulin γ1-chain gene and mechanism for heavy chain class switch. *Proc Natl Acad Sci USA* **77**: 919–23.

77 Gauchat J-F, Lebman DA, Coffman RL, Gascan H, De Vries JE (1990). Structure and expression of germline ε transcripts in human B cells induced by interleukin 4 to switch to IgE production. *J Exp Med* **172**: 463–73.

78 Jacob J, Kelsoe G, Rajewsky K, Weiss U (1991). Intraclonal generation of antibody mutants in germinal centres. *Nature* **354**: 389–92.

79 Dhabhar FS (2002). A hassle a day may keep the doctor away: stress and the augmentation of immune function. *Integr Comp Biol* **42**: 556–64.

80 Smith GR, Conger C, O'Rourke DF, Steele RW, Charlton RK, Smith SS (1992). Psychological modulation of the delayed hypersensitivity skin test. *Psychosomatics* **33**: 444–51.

81 Vedhara K, Nott KH (1996). The assessment of the emotional and immunological consequences of examination stress. *J Behav Med* **19**: 467–78.

82 Pariante CM, Carpiniello B, Rudas N, Piludu G, del Giacco GS (1994). Anxious symptoms influence delayed-type hypersensitivity skin test in subjects devoid of any psychiatric morbidity. *Int J Neurosci* **79**: 275–83.

83 Cohen S, Tyrrell DAJ, Smith AP (1991). Psychological stress and susceptibility to the common cold. *N Engl J Med* **325**: 606–12.

84 Vedhara K, Cox NK, Wilcock GK, *et al.* (1999). Chronic stress in elderly carers of dementia patients and antibody response to influenza vaccination. *Lancet* **353**: 627–31.

85 Jabaaij L, van Hattum J, Vingerhoets AJJM, Oostveen FG, Duivenvoorden HJ, Ballieux RE (1996). Modulation of immune response to rDNA hepatitis B vaccination by psychological stress. *J Psychosom Res* **41**: 129–37.

86 Vedhara K, McDermott MP, Evans TG, *et al.* (2002). Chronic stress in non-elderly caregivers: psychological, endocrine and immune implications. *J Psychosom Res* **53**: 1153–61.

87 Burns VE, Drayson M, Ring C, Carroll D (2002). Perceived stress and psychological well-being are associated with antibody status after meningitis C conjugate vaccination. *Psychosom Med* **64**: 963–70.

88 Loveren HV, Van Amsterdam JGC, Vandebriel RJ, *et al.* (2001). Vacine induced antibody responses as parameters of the influence of endogenous and environmental factors. *Environ Health Perspect* **109**: 757–64.

89 Kiecolt-Glaser JK, Glaser R (1988). Methodological issues in behavioural immunology research with humans. *Brain Behav Immun* **2**: 67–78.

Chapter 4

Psychoneuroimmunology and ageing

Frank J. Penedo and Jason R. Dahn

4.1 Introduction

4.1.1 Demographics of ageing

The world is experiencing a growing population of older adults which has no historical precedent, and in developing countries this increase is occurring at an exponential rate. By 2030, it is estimated that over 70 million persons in the United States will be 65 or older and roughly 9 million of these individuals will be over 80.[1] The expansion of the ageing population in the United States has primarily reflected the increasing life expectancies of men and women, which are projected to be 74 years and 82 years, respectively, by 2020. However, the dramatic rise in the older adult population over the next 30 years will also be due to the ageing 'baby boomer' generation.[1] The rapid growth in this segment of the population will challenge and strain society's ability to provide for their financial and medical needs.

4.1.2 Myths and realities of ageing

Older adults are often stereotyped as being severely limited in social, physical, and cognitive resources. While this reflects our common fear of the ageing process, it grossly misrepresents the reality of older adulthood. Ageing does impact many facets of life; however, these changes are typically gradual and do not interfere with living a productive and satisfying life. Most older adults live with partners, family, or independently (only 5% reside in nursing homes), and remain employed (30%) or active as volunteers (30%) (less than 10% have a significant limiting physical disability). While there is a range of normative cognitive changes that occur with ageing (e.g. declining processing speed), older adults tend to compensate easily with minor adjustments such that there are few perceptible decrements in overall functioning. While the ageing process does necessitate adjustment to change, these changes are often subtle and occur over many decades.

The impact of ageing on physical health status is highly variable, and understanding individual differences in ageing is quite challenging, given the multiple and complex factors that are involved in the ageing process (e.g. genetics, health behaviours, environmental exposure to toxins, psychosocial factors). Although ageing is not synonymous with disease, most chronic conditions typically manifest in later adulthood (e.g. cardiovascular disease, cancer), revealing the body's underlying frailty and compromising quality of life. Older adults report lower levels of health control, self-efficacy, and self-esteem,[2] and a substantial proportion (18–27%) rate their health status as 'fair' or 'poor'.[3] A similar percentage (26%) between the ages of 65 and 74 report being limited in activities by a chronic health condition, and this increases to 45% for those over age 75.[1] Nonetheless, older adults' self-ratings of well-being indicate that the majority of this group perceive themselves to be in 'good health'.

Because older adults are living longer with chronic disease, it is imperative that we understand the mechanisms for enhancing or maintaining quality of life, and this is particularly true when psychosocial factors may influence disease- and treatment-related processes. In the remainder of this chapter, we will briefly review the health and disease factors which are common to older adults and discuss these issues in the context of age-related declines in immune functioning. Specifically, we will review work which indicates that older adults experience a number of immunological changes such as thymic involution and alterations in the production and function of T lymphocytes, B lymphocytes, cytokines and natural killer (NK) cells, which appear to diminish the capacity of the immune system to fight disease (e.g. infections, HIV, cancer). Similarly, we will address alterations that occur in neuroendocrine functioning, altering the bidirectional communication between the immune and endocrine systems. Both of these systems may be influenced by psychosocial stress (e.g. bereavement) and an individual's internal (e.g. coping) and external (e.g. social support) resources. Finally, we review recent studies employing psychosocial interventions designed to enhance psychosocial factors and disease processes, and discuss the challenges and future directions for psychoneuroimmunology (PNI) research with older adults.

4.2 The clinical context

4.2.1 Health, disease, and disability in older adults

A comprehensive review of health and disease factors is beyond the scope of this chapter. As a result, the following is a cursory glance at a range of factors that affect morbidity and mortality in older adults. Cognitive deterioration, in particular Alzheimer's disease, is a consistent concern raised by older adults.[4] Yet the incidence of all-type dementia is quite low compared with that of depression, a primary predictor of disability and mortality. Older adults are quite vulnerable to symptoms of depression and anxiety with up to 20% having significant depressive symptoms,[5] often with co-occurring symptoms of anxiety.[6] Rates tend to be higher in ethnic minorities, and this is especially true for new immigrants and less acculturated groups in the United States.[7] For instance, elevated levels of depressive symptoms have been found in older Mexican Americans (31.9% and 17.3% for women and men, respectively[8]). A higher burden of depressive symptoms is predictive of lower self-rated health,[9] and depressive symptoms appear to decrease well-being, increase disability, and interfere with appropriate service utilization.[10] Many studies indicate that older adults with depressed mood have more impaired or disrupted sleep.[11,12] Anxiety symptoms have also been related to poor sleep as well as poorer psychosocial functioning, lower personal mastery, and increased need for social support.[6] Cumulatively, these studies indicate that physical and mental health are intricately related and impact on quality of life through their influence on mood, cognition, and behaviour, and that this seems to occur in a sociocultural context.

Heart disease is the leading cause of death for older adults in the United States, followed by cancer, cerebrovascular disease, lung disease, pneumonia and influenza, and finally diabetes-related complications.[13] In older adults, disability is caused primarily by arthritis, accounting for one-third of cases, followed by heart disease, hypertension, and diabetes-related complications.[14] Depression and disability are consistent independent predictors of mortality[15] even after controlling for medical and socioeconomic factors.

Management of chronic disease can diminish quality of life, reduce opportunities for social interaction, and alter illness-related perceptions. The impact of chronic disease is both physical and psychological, affecting an individual's actual functioning as well as their perceptions of health and functioning. Perceived overall health has been shown to predict mortality[15] and declines with increasing comorbid conditions.[16] Among older adults with HIV, 25% report moderate to severe levels of depression, and they also report less social support and reduced access to medical care and social services.[17] In a community sample of older adults, pain was found to be persistent over time and to have a strong longitudinal association with depression,[18] suggesting a reciprocal relationship and being indicative of a poor prognosis. The treatments for many of the diseases of older adulthood serve to manage the disease process rather than cure it, and as a consequence individuals must cope as best they can with the resources available to them.

4.3 Theoretical basis of a role for psychoneuroimmunology

4.3.1 Immunosenescence: ageing of the immune system

The ageing process involves a gradual decline in the integrity of all organ systems, including those involved in the immune response and particularly functional markers of this system.[19] Immunosenescence is characterized by age-related decrements in immune function that involve impairment of several lymphocyte activities and leads to a state of immune dysregulation.[20] This dysregulation tends to be marked by thymic involution, decreased thymic production of lymphoid precursor T and B cells, reduced proliferative capacity of T lymphocytes, increased T-cell apoptosis, reduced responsivity of CD19+ cells and antibody production, and alterations in the production of various cytokines, including decreases in IL-2 and INF-γ, increases in IL-6 and IL-4, and a greater ratio of memory to naive T lymphocytes.[21,22] This cytokine shift has been associated with a naive to memory T-cell predomination. In a recent review by Straub *et al.*,[23] NK cell function, neutrophil phagocytic capacity and respiratory burst, macrophage/dendritic cell traffic, MHC class II expression, and immune complex processing were also shown to decline with age. Although there has been some controversy and disagreement in the literature reporting the specific effects of ageing on the immune system,[22,24] most studies consistently suggest that age-related changes in immunity occur, and that these alterations leave older adults immunocompromised and at a considerable disadvantage in combating neoplasms, infections, and autoimmune pathologies (see Chapters 6, 7, and 8, respectively). Key age-related changes in immune function and their implications are listed in Table 4.1.

4.3.1.1 Age-related alterations in immune functioning

T and B lymphocytes Ageing involves a severe reduction of the thymus, the primary lymphoid organ where T-lymphocyte precursors mature and differentiate into functional T cells (see Chapter 1). In general, age-related involution of the thymus gland compromises T-cell maturation and differentiation, leading to lower production of naive T cells and higher circulating levels of memory T-cell subsets.[25] Perhaps the most widely documented and empirically supported age-related decline in immune function involves marked changes in T-lymphocyte subpopulation counts and functional capacity. Studies indicate that T-cell function is the most sensitive immunological parameter to ageing, although total T-cell counts remain stable throughout the lifespan.

Understanding age-related changes in B-lymphocyte function presents a challenge as it is difficult to establish whether such decrements in B-cell function are merely a reflection of suppressed T-cell activity (e.g. T-cell stimulated B-cell proliferation and antibody secretion).[26] Some studies suggest that the number of B lymphocytes decreases with age, while others argue that these levels remain fairly stable. What is clear is that the quantity of B cells that are responsive to antigen presentation declines with age. However, these same studies show that the amount of antibody produced by activated B lymphocytes does not decrease with age, suggesting that observed reductions in antibody production are a consequence of non-functional B cells. While studies are equivocal, the age-related alterations in cell functioning appear to indicate a diminished capacity to respond to antigens, leaving older adults more vulnerable to infections, neoplasms, and autoimmune disorders.

Cytokines Primarily released by activated immune cells, cytokines serve as communicatory signals in cell–cell interactions. Cytokines act at extremely low concentrations to mediate the steps involved in the immune response, including antigen presentation, T and B lymphocyte activation, differentiation and proliferation, and the recruitment of monocytes. Cytokines can be classified based on two criteria: whether the cytokine promotes cell-mediated or humoral immunity (i.e. Th1 or Th2, respectively), and

Table 4.1 Age-related changes in immune function and key implications

	Age-related change	Key implication
T lymphocytes	↓ Cytolitic capacity	↓ Capacity to fight neoplasms,
	↓ Proliferative response	infections and autoimmune pathology
	↓ CD28 and CD2 surface molecule expression	↓ T-cell activation
	↓ CD69 surface molecule expression	↓ Signal transduction and T-cell activation
	↑ CD95 surface molecule expression	↑ Apoptosis
	↓ Naive T-cell counts	↑ Susceptibility to new infections
	↑ Memory T-cell counts	
B lymphocytes	↓ Reduced B-cell function	↓ Responsiveness to antigen presentation
	↑ IgA and IgG antibody secretion	↑ Autoimmunity
	↓ IgM antibody	↑ Inability to fight infection
Cytokines	↓ IL-2 production	↓ Activation of T cells and macrophages
	↓ IL-2 receptors	↓ Growth and differentiation of LGLs and B cells
	↓ INF-γ production	↓ APC regulation
		↓ B-cell differentiation
		↑ Production of IL-4
	↑ IL-4 production	↑ Apoptosis
		↓ INF-γ production
	↑ IL-6	↓ B-cell differentiation
		↓ IgA antibody production
	↑ IL-10	↓ INF-γ production
		↓ Macrophage and monocyte cell counts
Natural killer cells	Several conflicting studies but most suggest preserved function	Preserved function may compensate for age-related losses in B and T lymphocytes

APC, antigen-presenting cell; LGL, large granular lymphocyte.

whether the cytokine promotes or retards inflammation. The Th1 family includes cytokines such as interferon gamma (INF-γ) and IL-2, while Th2 cytokines include IL-1, IL-6, and IL-10. Th1 cytokines are known to promote cell-mediated immunity and enhance effector-cell functions, including cytotoxic T-lymphocyte and NK cell activity. Th2 cytokines facilitate humoral immunity by stimulating B-cell proliferation and activation, and by triggering production of antibodies.[27] The decrease in calcium observed in the elderly is partly responsible for suppressed production of certain cytokines. This development is exacerbated by a decreased capacity of ageing T cells to produce and respond to key cytokines such as IL-2, thus compromising T-cell proliferation. In contrast, ageing is also characterized by increases in several cytokines associated in promoting a pro-inflammatory response and suppressing cell-mediated immunity. Some have shown that ageing involves a shift from a Th1 cell-mediated to a Th2 humoral immune response.[28] This shift may suppress the Th1 response which is primarily driven by IL-2 and INF-γ. These two cytokines are involved in generating and activating cytotoxic T lymphocytes and NK cells, which in turn are the primary effector cells in cell-mediated responses and play a critical role is host defences including immunity against tumours.[29,30] In contrast, the Th2 response involves production of IL-4 and IL-6, two cytokines that have a downregulatory effect on INF-γ and thus inhibit the Th1 cell-mediated response. Cell-mediated immunity, or Th1-regulated immunity, is associated with the activation of macrophages, NK cells, and cytotoxic T-cell differentiation[31] (see Table 4.1). Although not conclusive, most studies seem to suggest that ageing is associated with a shift from a Th1-dominated cell-mediated immune response to a Th2 non-specific humoral response. This shift may render the older individual more susceptible to infections, neoplasms, and autoimmune disorders.

Natural killer cells The function of NK cells is described in Chapter 1. Although some early findings suggested that NK cell function decreases with age, recent evidence suggests that NK cell counts and functional capacity are preserved, and in some cases enhanced, in older age (see Table 4.1).

4.3.1.2 Clinical presentation and vulnerability to disease

Immunosenescence has been implicated in disease susceptibility and progression in several chronic conditions; however, many chronic illnesses common in older age and their treatment negatively impact immune function in older adults. Consequently, studies establishing causal links between decrements in immune function and disease susceptibility are difficult to establish.

Infectious disease Age-related decreases in antibody production have been linked to reactivation of several latent viruses such as the Epstein–Barr virus (EBV) and herpes zoster. Moreover, elevated incidence and mortality rates in the elderly from influenza, pneumonia, parasitic infections, and tetanus can also be attributed to reduced antibody production in this population. Some studies have documented that up to 40% of healthy elderly individuals do not develop sufficient antibodies following immunization with the influenza vaccine. Moreover, elderly persons with no prior exposure to pathogens such as the hepatitis B virus or pneumococcal infection show a significantly lower antibody production relative to younger individuals.[32,33] Half of the almost 3000 cases of West Nile fever reported in 2002 occurred in persons over age 59, suggesting that the immune system of older adults has a reduced capacity to respond to this new viral pathogen.[34]

HIV/AIDS Older adults living with HIV/AIDS are already coping with primary, and possibly secondary, ageing processes including immunosenescence, reduced ability to fight infections, cognitive decrements, and general decreased functioning of body systems.[35] These processes can be compounded by HIV/AIDS and may be related to shorter survival rates observed in this subgroup.[36] The course of HIV/AIDS involves compromises of many bodily systems including the respiratory and central nervous systems (see Chapter 7). This creates difficulty in distinguishing between age-related and HIV-related disease in older populations. Furthermore, differential diagnosis is complex, given that many age-associated symptoms and diseases (e.g. Alzheimer's disease, respiratory illnesses, impaired memory) resemble the symptoms associated with HIV infection.[37] In addition to these challenges, lipid disorders associated with HIV treatment may place older individuals at a greater risk of suffering strokes or myocardial infarctions.[38] Studies examining disease progression among HIV-positive older adults consistently show that these individuals progress faster, have less desirable health indices at diagnosis (e.g. lower CD4+ cells, higher viral load), have shorter AIDS-free intervals, have a higher number of opportunistic infections, and have shorter survival rates.[39–42] Several age-related factors have been proposed as possible physiological mechanisms underlying faster progression in older adults (e.g. greater production of HIV, preferential infectivity of memory CD4+ cells, impaired replacement of CD4+ cells, more rapid destruction of infected CD4+ cells, and less effective anti-HIV cytotoxicicy).[41,43–50]

Cancer One of the most feared health-related aspects of growing old is the possibility of developing cancer. There is good reason for concern as over 50% of breast cancer cases and 80% of prostate cancer cases are diagnosed among women and men over the age of 65. Age-related impaired recognition and destruction of tumour cells by the immune system may be implicated in cancer development and progression among older adults. Numerous studies have provided evidence suggesting an important role for the immune system in cancer progression. Adequate tumour surveillance and destruction is dependent on optimal specific and non-specific immune responses. Adaptive responses involving CD8+ T-cytolytic activity require antigen presentation by MHC-I proteins on tumour cells and CD4+ T-helper cell presentation, which in turn induces cytokine production.[51] CD8+ T-cytolytic cells inhibit tumour progression and metastasis through their cytolytic activity.[52] Moreover, innate responses involve NK cells which are responsible for tumour surveillance and lysing. Peripheral blood lymphocytes activated with IL-2 in culture, together with NK cells, acquire MHC non-restricted killing which is conventionally designated as lymphokine-activated killer (LAK) activity; these cells have been shown to mediate tumour progression in animal models and cancer patients.[53–55] Additionally, cytokines influence the growth of various tumours through effects on tumour cell differentiation, proliferation, mobility and adherence, and modulation of angiogenesis.[56] Several studies have identified a predominance of Th2 cytokine patterns at tumour sites,[57] and numerous studies have shown suppressed production of IL-2 and INF-γ across various cancer populations.[57–59] Lastly, studies have also described a suppressed Th1 immune response among primarily older cancer patients relative to healthy controls.[28]

Evidence supporting the notion that the immunosuppressive effects of psychosocial factors may interact with immunosenescence to make a possible contribution to disease processes in older adults is quite scarce. A conceptual framework for PNI mechanisms in disease development and progression in older adults is presented in Figure 4.1.

4.3.2 Endocrinosenescence: ageing of the endocrine system

Production of certain hormones is altered as the human body goes through the ageing process. Recently, age-related endocrine changes have received attention, especially given their pathogenesis in disorders of older adulthood (e.g. benign prostatic hyperplasia, osteoporosis, diabetes, etc.). Older adults experience menopause, andropause, and adrenopause, and decreases in circulating levels of oestrogen, testosterone, and dehydroepiandrosterone (DHEA) and its sulphate (DHEAS). There are also observed decreases in substance P, growth hormone (GH), melatonin, and insulin-like growth factor 1 (IGF-1). These hormones have significant specific functions which, under a state of dysregulation, may compromise health status. Senescence also leads to reduced production of calcitonin and vitamin D, and increased release of parathyroid hormone (PTH).[23] Furthermore, decline in pancreatic and thyroid function is also common in elderly men and women. Because thyroid hormones regulate metabolism, age-related reductions in circulating thyroid hormones are implicated in poor metabolic response to cold or caloric needs.[60] However, ageing does not have clinically significant effects on the secretion of the peptide hormone corticotrophin (ACTH) or the glucocorticoid hormone cortisol in humans[61–63] and non-human primates.[64] Salivary cortisol is a sensitive measure of stress in older adults. In response to a laboratory psychosocial stress task, the cortisol response of older men (over 60) is significantly greater than the response of younger men and women.[65] Findings indicate that flat diurnal profiles in older adults may be associated with endocrine dysregulation and related to a range of health impairment indicators

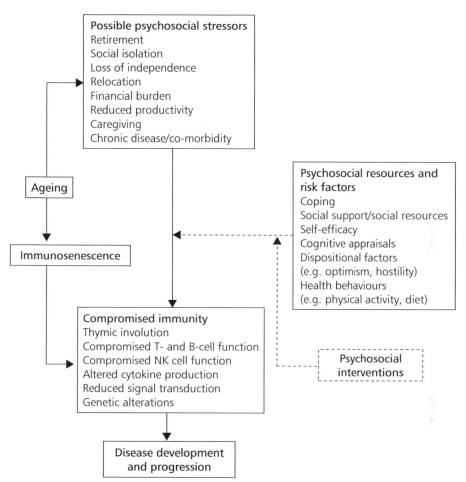

Fig. 4.1 Conceptual framework for PNI mechanisms and immunosenescence in disease development and progression in older adults. The ageing process can be characterized by the possible experience of several psychosocial stressors such as caregiving stress, social isolation, relocation, etc. These commonly experienced stressors have been shown to compromise immunity in older populations and thus could exacerbate already existing decrements in immunity that are a consequence of the normal ageing process. Furthermore, this exacerbation of immunosenescent changes may compromise the immune system's capacity to protect the host against neoplasms, infections, and autoimmune pathologies. Therefore psychosocial factors may indirectly promote disease development and progression. Adequate psychosocial resources such as adaptive coping styles and efficacious social resources, as well as positive health behaviours, may buffer the negative effects of psychosocial stressors on immune function. Psychosocial interventions may modify these resources and risk factors, prevent further decrements in immunity, and ameliorate disease development and progression in older adults.

including elevated body mass index (BMI), blood pressure, and heart rate, lower testosterone, and insulin resistance.[66] Similarly, flat cortisol profiles, associated with stress-induced cortisol dysregulation, have been related to earlier mortality and suppressed NK cell counts among advanced breast cancer patients.[67]

4.3.2.1 Menopause

Generally, around the age of 50 most women go through the menopause, the natural cessation of menstruation. Postmenopausally, secretion of oestradiol (E_2), lutenizing hormone (LH), follicle-stimulating hormone (FSH), and free alpha-subunit (FAS) show marked declines. Gonadotropin-releasing hormone (GnRH) release, while decreasing in pulse frequency, increases in overall amount with ageing. Hall and Gill[68] provide a comprehensive review of the effects of ageing on female neuroendocrine function.

4.3.2.2 Andropause

Age-related changes in male gonadal function are similar to those in females in that oestrogen and testosterone secretion both decrease with age. However, the abrupt halt in gonadal function that occurs in women is not seen in men. In contrast, the diminution of male gonadal function is gradual and shows much higher individual variability. Total plasma testosterone levels and bioactive free testosterone levels decrease by approximately 35% and 55%, respectively, between the ages of 25 and 75.[69] However, concentrations of the active androgen dihydrotestosterone decrease only slightly or are unchanged in male senescence.[70] Although mean testosterone levels decrease with age, there is a high level of inter-individual variability, which may have specific implications for studies addressing testosterone levels in male senescence.[71] Testosterone decline with age in men is well documented,[72,73] and age-related changes in the hypothalamic–pituitary–gonadal (HPG) axis have been proposed to account for this decrease.[74] The degree of testosterone decline appears to depend on health status, as testosterone has negative associations with weight, BMI, serum triglycerides, cholesterol, and glucose.[75] Some have suggested that testosterone stimulates proliferation and growth of androgen-dependent prostate cancer.[76]

4.3.2.3 Adrenopause

DHEA, the most abundant circulating androgen in humans, acts as a buffer hormone and plays numerous roles in physiological processes. Primarily secreted by the adrenal glands, but also by the brain, epidermis, and gonads, DHEA is synthesized from pregnenalone, a derivative of cholesterol, and is quickly sulphated to yield DHEAS, the predominant form of DHEA found in plasma. As the human body ages, DHEA/DHEAS levels are altered.[77] Blood DHEAS levels decline by 1–2% per year after age 30, and by age 70–80 plasma concentrations are approximately 20–30% those of younger persons. Notably, the size of the zona reticularis, the source of DHEAS production, diminishes with age.[62] However, glucocorticoid levels remain comparatively constant across the lifespan in humans[78] and other primates.[64] Thus the ratio of cortisol to DHEA decreases may provide evidence of both physiological and pathological brain ageing. This ratio is much larger in the elderly and is positively correlated with age.

4.3.2.4 Somatopause

Somatopause, or decrease in the GH–IGF-I axis is also part of the natural ageing process.[61] Plasma levels of both GH and IGF-I decrease with ageing in humans aand mice.[79] This decrease may be linked to thymic involution. Moreover, decreases in GH are associated with metabolic dysregulation and suppressed development of lean muscle and bone mass,[79] and lower circulating melatonin is associated with disrupted diurnal cycles.[80]

4.3.2.5 Associated disease processes

These age-related changes in endocrine function may be associated with several disease processes including hyper- and hypothyroidism, non-insulin dependent diabetes mellitus (NIDDM), and arthritis. Hormone replacement therapy (HRT) as an intervention to compensate for age-related changes in circulating hormones has received much attention in the past few years and is currently quite controversial given its documented risks.[81]

4.3.3 Links between endocrinosenescence and immunosenescence

Neuroendocrine and immune interactions involve a complex bidirectional communicatory process (see Chapter 1). The ageing process is characterized by a dysregulation of circulating hormones (e.g. decreased DHEA, altered circadian cortisol rhythm), a condition that is further exacerbated by stress.[28] Stress hormones such as catecholamines (e.g. epinephrine and norepinephrine) and cortisol have been shown to have immunosuppressive effects.[82] One pathway through which stress hormones may modulate the immune response involves the shift from Th1 to Th2 cytokine production observed following elevated cortisol and catecholamine levels. This shift promotes a reduction in cell-mediated immune responses and increases in humoral responses, thus increasing susceptibility to infectious agents and reduced antitumour immunity.[83]

Activation of the hypothalamic–pituitary–adrenal (HPA) axis is generally characterized by the release of hormones with immunosuppressive effects.[84] Lymphocytes express receptors for glucocorticoids, ACTH, and corticotrophin-releasing hormone (CRH), and the immunosuppressive effects of these hormones are well established.[85–87] Exposure to chronic stress leads to chronically elevated glucocorticoid release, promoting a shift from a T-helper Th1 to a Th2 response.[88,89]

4.4 Empirical evidence

4.4.1 Psychosocial stressors and immunity

The association between psychosocial stress and a decline in immune function across several immunological parameters has been well established. Acute stress may enhance immune response, preventing infection and facilitating injury recovery (see Chapter 11). Various studies suggest that immune changes may mediate the relationship between stress and illness[90–93](see Chapters 5–8). Most stress-induced decrements in immunity mimic age-related immunosuppression. One can argue that older adults facing a chronic stressor may be at a psychosocial and physiological disadvantage. Furthermore, the progressive decrease in size of the thymus that occurs during ageing is correlated with increased glucocorticoid levels.[32] There is also evidence that CRH can act centrally to suppress immune responses independent of circulating glucocorticoids[94] in addition to direct action on immune cells with proper receptors.[95]

Although highly variable in their incidence and impact on psychological well-being, several age-related factors or lifestyle changes (e.g. retirement, social isolation, loss of independence, relocation, financial burden, less productivity, caregiving, chronic disease) may have a negative impact on the overall quality of life of an older adult. Several of these psychosocial stressors have been specifically shown to influence immunity in older populations. Bereavement among older adults has been associated with compromised lymphocyte proliferative responses to mitogen stimulation and suppressed NK cell cytotoxicity.[96] Depression has been associated with suppressed lymphocyte response to mitogens[97] and suppressed NK cytotoxicity.[98] The immuno-suppressive effects of caregiving have been widely studied in older individuals, and studies consistently suggest that providing care for a chronically ill spouse may lead to marked immune dysfunction including suppressed lymphocyte proliferation and NK cell cytotoxicity, increased antibody titres to latent herpes viruses, lowered T-cell subset counts, and lower expression of surface signal transduction molecules.[99,100] Some studies have also supported the notion that older adults show marked impairments relative to younger individuals when faced with stressors and depressive illness.[101]

4.4.2 Impact of psychosocial factors on immune and endocrine function

An abundance of information suggests that psychosocial factors have a role in disease progression via their effects on immune and endocrine functioning; however, a thorough review of this literature is beyond the scope of this chapter. Instead, we focus on the few studies that have studied these processes specifically in older adults, even though findings are sometimes difficult to interpret given the plethora of variables which affect the immune and endocrine functioning of older adults (e.g. ageing-related changes, disease processes and comorbid conditions, access to health care, changes in social support, etc.).

4.4.2.1 Mood and quality of life

Depression rates among older adults have been reported to be in the range 10–21%.[102] Studies comparing older depressed populations with younger counterparts have shown that older depressed individuals show significantly lower proliferative response to PHA and lower IL-2 stimulated NK cell cytotoxicity.[51] McGuire et al.[103] reported that, compared with non-depressed peers, community-dwelling older adults with chronic mild depressive symptoms had poorer lymphocyte proliferation to multiple mitogens over an 18-month period, and the response was poorest among the oldest of the depressed participants. Assessing the impact of a moderate life stressor on older adults, Lutgendorf et al.[104] found that individuals in the process of a voluntary housing relocation had reduced vigour and more intrusive thoughts than non-moving peers. In addition, movers demonstrated diminished NK cell counts relative to controls. However, at 3-month follow-up differences between the groups were no longer significant. In regression analyses controlling for relevant covariates, greater vigour was significantly associated with higher NK cell counts across all study time points.

4.4.2.2 Bereavement

Several studies have shown that depression resulting from mourning the loss of a spouse or a close relative is associated with suppressed lymphocyte proliferative response to several mitogens including PHA, ConA, and PWM.[105] Lower NK cell cytotoxicity in older adults has been documented following the death of a spouse, while pre-bereavement acceptance among spouses of terminally ill patients was associated with greater proliferative response to PHA.

4.4.2.3 Cognitions

Lutgendorf et al.[106] reported that older adults with more intrusive thoughts had higher levels of cortisol irrespective of their housing relocation status (i.e. movers versus non-movers), and housing relocation status and intrusive thoughts both independently predicted occurrence of illness episodes. The findings support the general notion that stress as indicated by ruminative intrusive thoughts results in higher levels of circulating neuroendocrine hormones in older adults, as it does in other populations.

4.4.2.4 Coping

Stowell et al.[107] related the coping styles of older adults to the number and percentage of CD3+, CD4+, and CD8+ T lymphocytes and to the proliferative response of blood leucocytes to mitogens. They found that the association between coping and mitogen-induced proliferation depended on stress level and that the relationship was strongest for participants endorsing high stress. Proliferation to the mitogens was differentially affected by the interaction of stress level and coping style. At high stress levels, greater proliferation to mitogens was predicted by active coping. In general, avoidance coping was less consistently related to proliferation but, surprisingly, at low stress levels it was related to increased proliferation, suggesting that avoidance may be adaptive under certain circumstances. Results suggest that active strategies may be more beneficial when stress is elevated, while avoidant strategies, which are usually discouraged, may be useful during periods of low stress.

4.4.2.5 Social resources

In a review[108] of over 20 marital interaction studies that included physiological measures, only one focused primarily on older adults (age 55–75). Findings from this review indicated that older men and women who showed more negative behaviour during a conflict task had poorer immune responses during the task. These individuals also tended to characterize their disagreements as more negative relative to persons with better immune responses.[99]

4.4.2.6 Personality

In a prospective study, a pessimistic explanatory style was predictive of coronary heart disease[109] while a more optimistic outlook appeared to be protective. The authors suggest that explanatory style may alter the perception of stressful situations and/or lead to more adaptive coping responses (e.g. seeking social support) which may reduce inflammatory responses that cause or worsen endothelial damage. In a study of caregivers, perceiving change as a challenge and having control over one's life appeared to protect individuals from symptoms of depression and fatigue.[110] Lower perceived control has been associated with lower proliferative response to the PHA mitogen and lower NK cell cytotoxicity among older populations.[111] Similarly, greater optimism or a positive outlook and less emotional suppression has been related to higher NK cell cytotoxicity and cell number among older men treated for cancer.[112]

4.4.2.7 Summary

While often studied separately, these findings, when considered cumulatively, suggest a decisive link between psychological processes (i.e. mood, cognitions, personality disposition) and immune functioning. They are consistent with the reports on younger adults and support a growing literature indicating that older adults may be differentially affected by the experience of stress.

4.4.3 Health behaviours and immune and endocrine function in older adults

4.4.3.1 Sleep

Older adults often report poor sleep and incidence of insomnia varies from 15% to 20%.[12] Severe sleep problems are endemic in caregivers who also evidence high rates of clinical depression.[113] Following a mild stress task, healthy older adults have higher cortisol as well as impaired sleep (e.g. lower sleep efficiency).[114] More recent results compared the impact of cortisol on the sleep profiles of younger and older adults. Relative to their younger counterparts, older adults slept poorly with more wake time and early-stage sleep.[115] They also evidenced higher 24-h secretions of IL-6 and cortisol, suggestive of HPA axis activation, which were both positively related to poor sleep. These findings suggest that older adults may be more vulnerable to sleep disturbances, given the increasing amounts of circulating neuroendocrine hormones.

Sleep appears to be related to the immune system via bidirectional pathways, with sleep loss resulting in decreased NK cell counts and sleep functioning regulated by both stimulatory and inhibitory cytokines.[116]

4.4.3.2 Physical activity

While the role of physical activity in the development of disease processes has been studied extensively, findings are often disease specific and even within a disease are sometimes equivocal.[117] Some of the strongest results indicate that physical activity protects an individual from cardiovascular disease, especially coronary heart disease, secondary to improvements in known risk factors (e.g. blood pressure). In a review of the effects of physical activity on immune functioning in older adults, the authors conclude that, while physically active older adults appear to have higher *in vitro* measures of immune functioning, most studies have been flawed by small sample sizes, short follow-up periods, limited number of immune parameters, and uncontrolled potential confounders.[118] More recently, older adults who exercised vigorously were found to have greater peripheral blood mononuclear cell proliferation to influenza vaccination than their moderately active or sedentary peers.[119]

4.4.3.3 Nutrition

Proper immune functioning is related to adequate nutrition from birth to older adulthood.[120] Approximately 35% of the healthy elderly have nutrient deficiencies which may impact on immune and cognitive functioning. Specifically, antioxidant nutrients may alter cell-mediated immunity and buffer the decrements in immune functioning normally associated with ageing.[121,122]

4.4.3.4 Substance use/abuse

Estimated prevalence rates of drug use among adults aged between 55 and 59 indicate that about 2% had used illicit drugs in the past month and approximately 16% engaged in binge alcohol use.[123] Rates for individuals aged over 65 drop substantially to 0.3% and 6.1% for illicit drug use and binge alcohol use, respectively. It is anticipated that these rates will increase dramatically with the ageing of the 'baby boom' generation who have demonstrated higher rates of drug and alcohol use at all ages. Alcohol use is known to suppress immune functioning and may act directly or indirectly through its effect on gonadal steroid hormones.[124] Similarly, cocaine appears to suppress immune responsiveness by altering the function of NK cells, T cells, neutrophils, and macrophages, and by dysregulating the production of cytokines.[125]

4.4.4 Psychosocial interventions and psychoneuroimmunology in older adults

Intervention studies focusing on enhancing psychosocial factors, such as coping, social support, and cognitive restructuring, and promoting relaxation in older adults are very limited. In part, this reflects the difficulty and challenge of engaging and delivering interventions to older individuals who may be physically ill, burdened by caregiving and financial responsibilities, or socially isolated.[126] While limited evidence exists documenting the effects of psychosocial interventions on immune and endocrine function specifically with older populations, recent studies have attempted to address the criticisms related to previous work (e.g. use of specific immune measures and utilization of standardized interventions).[127] For example, adults aged over 60 years participating in an alternative medicine intervention, Tai Chi Chih, reported improved quality of life on measures of role limitations and physical functioning compared with a wait-list control group.[128] Additionally, participants in the programme demonstrated a 50% increase from baseline to 1 week post-intervention in varicella zoster virus-specific cell-mediated immunity, an essential component of memory immunity protecting against reinfection in the event of subsequent exposure to the virus. Values for the control group were unchanged.

4.4.4.1 Cancer

Older stage I/II melanoma patients who participated in a psychosocial intervention demonstrated reduced distress, improved coping, and altered NK lymphoid cell system relative to controls at 6-month follow-up,[129,130] and intervention participants had improved survival relative to controls. Fawzy et al.[131] recently conducted a 10-year follow-up of this earlier work, reporting that the intervention remained a significant predictor of survival. Results suggest that altering the affective and coping response of cancer survivors may have consequences for immune functioning and that this may reduce morbidity and mortality. Unfortunately, while many other studies have attempted to replicate these findings in other patient populations (e.g. breast cancer), the results have been equivocal (see Chapter 6).

4.4.4.2 Caregiving

Caregiving research represents a unique model for assessing the confluence of both ageing-related changes in physiological processes and the increasing limitations in physical well-being and functioning, social support, and financial resources that characterize older adulthood. Relative to age-matched controls, female caregivers of dementia patients demonstrate poorer proliferative responses to ConA and PHA and a lower percentage of NK cell cytotoxicity,[132] which is consistent with prior research.[133] Subsequent research has found that elderly caregivers exhibit increased levels of distress, greater salivary cortisol, blunted lymphocyte proliferation to PHA mitogen, and reduced lymphocyte sensitivity to glucocorticoids compared with control participants.[134] Moreover, cortisol levels were negatively related to indices of proliferation, indicating that HPA activation has a suppressive effect on immune functioning. The findings confirm that caregiving results in significant distress, and extends prior work by suggesting that such distress may result in immune dysregulation causing a physiological vulnerability that may hasten morbidity and mortality.

Garand *et al.*[135] provided an intervention to older dementia caregivers (mean age 65.5 ± 10.8 years) to strengthen psychological resources and facilitate management of behavioural problems and compared them with a group receiving similar support but less specific information. No group by time interactions were detected for mood measures, NK cell cytotoxicity, or T-cell proliferative responses to PHA or ConA; however, the intervention group did show stronger proliferative responses to both mitogens from baseline to post-intervention and then again at 6-month follow-up. In this study, immune responsiveness may have been mediated by factors independent of mood such as increased self-efficacy (i.e. while the mood of caregivers remained the same, they may have felt more capable of performing the tasks of daily caregiving) and this may translate into improved immunity. In a recent intervention study with relatively younger caregivers (mean age 54.7 ± 4.4 years), participants in a five-session structured stress management programme reported less depression, anxiety, fatigue, and confusion.[136] In addition, they demonstrated significantly increased NK cell activity after the intervention.

Using an antibody response model, Vedhara *et al.*[137] recently reported that distressed elderly caregivers who participated in an 8-week cognitive–behavioural stress management intervention demonstrated enhanced antibody responses to influenza vaccination relative to a control group of caregivers and a non-caregiving control group. Half of the intervention participants evidenced a fourfold increase in antibody titres compared with only 7% of caregiving control group members and 29% of those control members without caregiving responsibilities.

The evidence is quite abundant that caregiving results in distress and altered immune functioning, and caregiver strain appears to result in increased risk of mortality.[138] Risk may be conferred through the direct effects on health behaviours or indirectly via alterations in the immune system. In a recent epidemiological study, women who fulfilled caregiving duties for a disabled or ill spouse had increased risk of coronary heart disease,[139] even after controlling for numerous risk factors including smoking history, alcohol intake, BMI, medical history, and menopausal status. The authors suggest that the increased risk of coronary heart disease may be the result of immune and endocrine alterations that are caused by caregiving distress. They note that similar findings were not found for caregiving related to disabled or ill parents or others, and suggest that caring for a spouse or partner may be unavoidable, provide fewer opportunities for respite, and be more financially draining.

4.5 Directions for future research

4.5.1 Challenges for psychoneuroimmunology research in older adults

Many of the challenges encountered in conducting PNI research in older populations parallel those found in younger and middle-aged adults (e.g. selection bias, health behaviours, clinical significance of findings, etc.). However, the older population faces some unique age-related challenges that can cause difficulties in studying relationships between psychosocial factors and immune and endocrine function. For instance, the average elderly individual manages about three concurrent chronic conditions (e.g. hypertension, arthritis, diabetes) for which he or she must take medication. Some reports suggest that individuals over the age of 65 can fill up to 13.5 medication prescriptions per year. This elevated number of prescriptions, as well a possible physical limitations imposed by chronic conditions such as arthritis, can negatively impact immunological and endocrine parameters in older adults. Therefore PNI studies must carefully assess and control for such factors when attempting to establish relationships between psychological factors and immune and endocrine measures.

In an effort to provide guidelines for conducting PNI research among older adults, the SENIEUR Protocol was developed by Ligthart *et al.*[140] This protocol provides a strict set of inclusion criteria for studies evaluating immune function in the elderly (e.g. no current infection, inflammation, or malignancy; normal glucose and haemoglobin levels) and ideally provides the 'optimally aged' healthy control group. However, the guidelines may also be used to study disease populations. For instance, SENIEUR guidelines aim to exclude individuals facing diseases or under medication regimens that are known to impact on immune function, but when studying ageing and disease, the protocol also provides recommendations for inclusion of disease populations and rigorous methodology. Since its development, over 200 studies have followed these guidelines for inclusion into their protocols. In a relatively recent report,[141] use of the SENIEUR protocol has resulted in several studies challenging previously reported age-related changes in the immune systems; attributing these earlier findings to be a consequence of underlying disease rather than normal ageing processes. However, much work is still needed to provide conclusive and comprehensive evidence countering accepted age-related decrements in immunity. Moreover, adhering to the SENIEUR protocol poses challenges as only 15–20% of the elderly population may meet the criteria.

4.6 Conclusions

The ageing process is characterized by changes in several components of the immune system that occur at all levels, from chemical intracellular changes (e.g. impaired signal transduction) to alterations in entire organs (e.g. thymic involution). Most of these changes appear to promote a state of immune and neuroendocrine dysregulation, and the majority of research in this area suggests that immunocompetence declines with age. Although studies reporting such age-related decrements are fairly consistent, significant limitations and possible confounders in the existing literature remain. Many of the reported age-related decrements have been identified in animal models or in human studies with relatively small sample sizes and lacking adequate control for other factors that may affect immune and endocrine function (e.g. health behaviours, nutritional status). Furthermore, the distinction between changes that occur as a result of the ageing process and those that occur as a consequence of disease and its related treatment also remains difficult to establish. It is worth noting that not all components of the immune or endocrine system are compromised as a consequence of ageing. For instance, although the functional capacity of T cells is impaired in older adults, other immune system components that play a critical role in host defences, such as NK cell function, are well preserved and possibly even enhanced. Use of strict inclusion guidelines for studies in healthy older adults has also challenged some of the previously accepted age-related changes in immunity such a decreased production of certain cytokines; however, many of these studies are biased as they have been conducted among centenarians and thus are not representative of the general older population. Carefully designed studies that adequately control for possible confound measures known to impact the immune system, such as those proposed by the SENIEUR Protocol, including a healthy aged-matched control group if studying disease populations and adequate sample sizes studied prospectively, will provide more conclusive relationships between ageing and decrements in immune and endocrine function.

A wealth of burgeoning research is delineating pathways through which psychosocial factors can impact on immune and neuroendocrine function in healthy and diseased populations, and some limited but promising work is linking these relationships to clinical outcomes. One of many questions remaining to be answered is whether psychosocial factors, such as stressful events, coping, social support, and personality resources, exacerbate age-related decrements in immunocompetence. A number of studies have documented the immunosuppressive effects of stress and other psychosocial factors in primarily younger populations. The ageing population may be faced with a myriad of potential psychosocial stressors including, but not limited to, retirement, social isolation, loss of independence, relocation, low income, sense of lack of productivity, caregiving burdens, and comorbidities. These potential stressors, in combination with age-related decrements in immunity, may place older adults not only at a psychosocial disadvantage, but possibly at risk of further decline in immune defences. This compromised position may be of particular importance among chronically ill older adults. Some limited research has established associations between psychosocial factors, such as negative affect, bereavement, caregiving stress, and negative health behaviours, and impaired B-cell, T-cell, and NK-cell function and suppressed cytokine production in older populations. Furthermore, some work has shown that psychosocial interventions aimed at providing relaxation training among stressed healthy older adults can not only reduce perceived stress, but also enhance immune function. Although much work is needed to establish the clinical relevance of such enhancement in older populations, this work is promising. Regardless of immunosenescent changes that are taking place in older adults, psychosocial factors may positively (or negatively) impact immunity in this population. Given ageing trends throughout the world and the emphasis on extending life, the field of psychoneuroimmunology may provide a critical contribution in establishing psychosocial and physiological mechanisms by which older adults may buffer the impact of psychosocial stressors on health and disease.

References

1 **US Department of Health and Human Services, Administration on Aging** (2002). *A Profile of Older Americans* Washington, DC: US Department of Health and Human Services.

2 **Schieman S, Campbell JE** (2001). Age variations in personal agency and self-esteem: the context of physical disability. *J Aging Health* **13**:155–85.

3 **Roberts RE, Kaplan GA, Shema SJ, Strawbridge WJ** (1997). Prevalence and correlates of depression in an aging cohort: the Alameda county study. *J Gerontol B Psychol Sci Soc Sci* **52B**: S252–8.

4 **Kukull WA, Higdon R, Bowen JD, et al.** (2002). Dementia and Alzheimer disease incidence: a prospective cohort study. *Arch Neurol* **59**: 1737–46.

5 **Gallo JJ, Lebowitz BD** (1999). The epidemiology of common late-life mental disorders in the community: themes for the new century. *Psychiatry Serv* **50**: 1158–66.

6. **Mehta KM, Simonsick EM, Penninx BWJH, et al.** (2003). Prevalence and correlates of anxiety symptoms in well-functioning older adults: findings from the health aging and body composition study. *J Am Ger Soc* **51**: 499–504.

7 **Gonzalez HM, Haan MN, Hinton L** (2001). Acculturation and the prevalence of depression in older Mexican Americans: baseline results of the Sacramento area latino study on aging. *J Am Geriatr Soc* **49**: 948–53.

8 **Black SA, Markides KS, Millar TQ** (1998). Correlates of depressive symptomatology among older community-dwelling Mexican Americans: the Hispanic EPESE. *J Gerontol B Psychol Sci Soc Sci* **53B**: S198–208.

9 **Han B** (2002). Depressive symptoms and self-rated health in community-dwelling older adults: a longitudinal study. *J Am Geriatr Soc* **50**: 1549–56.

10 **Beekman ATF, Penninx BWJH, Deeg DJH, de Beurs E, Geerlings SW, van Tilburg W** (2002). The impact of depression on the well-being, disability and use of services in older adults: a longitudinal perspective. *Acta Psychiatr Scand* **105**: 20–7.

11 **Blazer DG, Hays JC, Foley DJ** (1995). Sleep complaints in older adults: a racial comparison. *J Gerontol A Bio Sci Med Sci* **50**: M280–4.

12 **Foley DJ, Monjan AA, Izmirlian G, Hays JC, Blazer DG** (1999). Incidence and remission of insomnia among elderly adults in a biracial cohort. *Sleep* **22**: S373–8.

13 **Anderson RN, Smith BL** (2003). Deaths: leading causes for 2001. *Natl Vital Stat Rep* **52(9)**: 1–86.

14 **Verbrugge LM, Patrick DL** (1995). Seven chronic conditions: their impact on US adults' activity levels and use of medical services. *Am J Public Health* **85**: 173–82.

15 **Ganguli M, Dodge HH, Mulsant BH** (2002). Rates and predictors of mortality in an aging, rural, community-based cohort: the role of depression. *Arch Gen Psychiatryiatry* **59**: 1046–52.

16 **Kempen GIJM, Miedema I, van den Bos GAM, Ormel J** (1998). Relationship of domain-specific measures of health to perceived overall health among older subjects. *J Clin Epidemiol* **51**: 11–18.

17 **Heckman TG, Heckman BD, Kochman A, Sikkema KJ, Suhr J, Goodkin K** (2002). Psychological symptoms among persons 50 years of age and older living with HIV disease. *Aging Mental Health* **6**: 121–8.

18 **Geerlings SW, Twisk JWR, Beekman ATF, Deeg DJH, van Tilberg W** (2002). Longitudinal relationship between pain and depression in older adults: sex, age, and physical disability. *Soc Psychiatry Psychiatr Epidemiol* **37**: 23–30.

19 **Burns EA, Goodwin JS** (1990). Immunology and infectious disease. In: Cassel CK, Risenberg DE, Sorensen LB, Walsh JR (eds) *Geriatric Medicine* New York: Springer-Verlag, 312–29.

20 **Weksler ME** (1994). Immune senescence. *Ann Neurol* **35**: S35–7.

21 **Malaguarnera L, Ferlito L, Imbesi RM, et al.** (2001). Immunosenescence: a review. *Arch Gerontol Geriatr* **32**: 1–14.

22 **Miller RA** (1996). Aging and the immune response. In Schneider EL, Rowe JE (eds) *Handbook of the Biology of Aging* (4th edn). San Diego, CA: Academic Press, 335–92.

23 **Straub RH, Miller LE, Scholmerich J, Zietz B** (2000). Cytokines and hormones as possible links between endocrinosenscence and immunosenescene. *J Neuroimmunol* **109**: 10–15.

24 **Pawelec G, Wagner W, Adibzadeh M, Engle A** (1999). T cell immunosenescence *in vitro* and *in vivo*. *Exp Gerontol* **34**: 419–29.

25 **Nakahama M, Mohri N, Mori S, Shindo G, Yokoi Y, Machinami R** (1990). Immunohistochemical and histometrical studies of the human thymus with special emphasis on age-related changes in the medullary epithelial and dendritic cells. *Virchows Arch* **58**: 245–51.

26 **Callard RE, Basten A** (1978). Immune function in aged mice. IV. Loss of T cell and B cell function in thymus-dependent antibody responses. *Eur J Immunol* **8**: 552–8.

27 **Kang D, Fox C** (2001). Th1 and Th2 cytokine responses to academic stress. *Res Nurs Health* **24**: 245–57.

28 **Solomon GF, Morley JE** (2001). Psychoneuroimmunology and aging. In Ader R, Felten DL, Cohen N (eds) *Psychoneuroimmunology* Vol. 2. San Diego: Academic Press, 701–17.

29 **Seder RA, Paul WE** (1994). Acquisition of lymphokine-producing phenotype by CD4+ T cells. *Annu Rev Immunol* **12**: 635.

30 **Yamashita N, Clement LT** (1989). Phenotypic characterization of the post-thymic differentiation of human allantigen-specific CD8+ cytoxic T lymphocytes. *J Immunol* **143**: 1518.

31 **Webster JI, Tonelli L, Sternberg EM** (2002). Neuroendocrine regulation of immunity. *Annu Rev Immunol* **20**: 125–63.

32 **Ginaldi L, De Martinis M, D'Ostilio A, et al.** (1999). The immune system in the elderly: II. Specific cellular immunity. *Immunol Res* **20**: 109–15.

33 **Ginaldi L, Loreto MF, Corsi MP, Modesti M, De Martinis M** (2001). Immunosenescence and infectious diseases. *Microbes Infect* **3**: 851–7.

34 **US Department of Health and Human Services** (2003). *Epidemic/Epizootic West Nile Virus in the United States: Guidelines for Surveillance, Prevention, and Control* (3rd revision). Fort Collins, CO: US Department of Health and Human Services, Centers for Disease Control and Prevention, National Center for Infectious Diseases.

35 **Schneider E, Rowe JW** (1996). *Handbook of the Biology of Aging* New York: Academic Press.

36 **Wallace J, Paauw D, Spach D** (1993). HIV infection in older patients: when to suspect the unexpected. *Geriatrics* **48**: 61–64, 69–70.

37 **Linsk NL** (2000). HIV among older adults: age-specific issues in prevention and treatment. *AIDS Read* **10**: 430–40.

38 **Carr A, Samaris K, Chisholm DJ, Kuper DA** (1998). Pathogenesis of HIV-1 Protease inhibitor-associated peripheral lipodystrophy, hyperlipidemia, and insulin resistance. *Lancet* **352**: 1881–3.

39 **Skiest DJ, Rubinstein E, Carley N, et al.** (1996). The importance of comorbidity in HIV- infected patients over 55: a retrospective case–control study. *Am J Med* **101**: 605–11.

40 **Brosgart C, Hillman D, Neaton J, et al.** (1997). Old age is a predictor of death and progression of HIV disease. *Program and Abstracts of the 4th Conference on Retroviruses and Opportunistic Infections, Washington, DC.*

41 Phillips A, Lee C, Elford J, *et al.* (1991). More rapid progression to AIDS in older HIV-Infected people: the role of CD4[+] T-cell counts. *J Acqir Immune Defic Syndr Hum Retrovirol* **4**: 970–5.

42 Ferro S, Salit I (1992). HIV infections in patients over 55 years of age. *J Acquir Immune Defic Syndr* **5**: 348–53.

43 Wei X, Ghosh SK, Taylor ME, *et al.* (1995). Viral dynamics in human immunodeficiency virus type 1 infection. *Nature* **373**: 117–22.

44 Ho DD, Neumann AU, Perelson AS, *et al.* (1995). Rapid turnover of plasma virions and CD4 lymphocytes in HIV-1 infection. *Nature* **373**: 123–6.

45 Schnittman SM, Lane HC, Greenhouse J, *et al.* (1990). Preferential infection of CD4+ memory T cells by human immunodeficiency virus type 1: evidence for a role in the selective T-cell functional defects observed in infected individuals. *Proc Natl Acad Sci USA* **87**: 6058–62.

46 Mackall CL, Fleisher TA, Brown MR, *et al.* (1995). Age, thymopoiesis and CD4+ T-lymphocyte regeneration after intensive chemotherapy. *N Engl J Med* **332**: 143–9.

47 Adler WH, Baskar PV, Chrest FJ, Dorsey-Cooper B, Winchurch RA, Nagel JE (1997). HIV-1 infection and aging. Mechanism to explain the accelerated rate of progression in the older patient. *Mech Ageing Dev* **96**: 137–55.

48 Harley CB, Futcher AB, Greider CW (1990). Telomeres shorten during ageing of human fibroblasts. *Nature* **345**: 458–60.

49 Wolthers KC, Otto SA, Meyaard L, *et al.* (1996). Accelerated loss of tomere length in HIV infection. *11th International Conference on AIDS, Vancouver, BC.* Abstract We.A.263.

50 Powers DC (1993). Influenza A virus-specific cytotoxic T lymphocyte activity declines with advancing age. *J Am Geriatr Soc* **41**: 1–5.

51 Vile RG (1996). Gene therapy for cancer: the course ahead. *Cancer Metastasis Rev* **15**: 403–10.

52 Shu S, Plautz GE, Krauss JC, Chang AE (1997). Tumor immunology. *JAMA* **278**: 1972–81.

53 Rosenberg SA, Lotze MT, Yang JC, *et al.* (1993). Prospective randomized trial of high-dose interleukin-2 alone or in conjunctionwith lymphokine-activated killer cells for the treatment of patients with advanced cancer. *J Natl Cancer Inst* **85**: 622–32 [Erratum **85**: 1091].

54 Whiteside TL, Herberman RB (1994). Role of human natural killer cells in health and disease. *Clin Diagn Lab Immunol* **1**: 125–33.

55 Whiteside TL, Herberman RB (1995). The role of natural killer cells in immune surveillance of cancer. *Curr Opin Immunol* **7**: 704–10.

56 Murgo AJ, Faith RE, Plotnikoff NP (1999). Neuropeptides, cytokines, and cancer—interrelationships. In Plotnikoff NP, Faith RE, Murgo AJ, Good RA (eds) *Cytokines: Stress and Immunity.* Boca Raton, FL: CRC Press, 133–47.

57 Elsässer-Beile U, von Kleist S, Martin M (1992). Comparison of mitogen- and virus-induced interferon production in whole blood cell cultures of patients with various solid carcinomas and controls. *Tumor Biol* **13**: 358–63.

58 Elsässer-Beile U, von Kleist S, Stähle W, Shurhammer-Fuhrmann C, Schulte Mönting J, Gallati H (1993). Cytokine levels in whole blood cell cultures as parameters of the cellular immunologic activity in patients with malignant melanoma and basal cell carcinoma. *Cancer* **71**: 231–6.

59 Fischer JR, Schindel M, Bulsebruck H, Lahm H, Krammer PH, Drings P (1997). Decrease of interleukin-2 secretion is a new independent prognostic factor associated with poor survival in patients with small-cell lung cancer. *Ann Oncol* **8**: 457–61.

60 Terry LC, Halter JB (1994). Aging of the endocrine system. In Hazzard WR, Bierman EL, Blass JP, Ettinger WH, Halter JB (eds) *Principles of Geriatric Medicine and Gerontology* New York: McGraw-Hill.

61 Lamberts SWJ, van den Beld A, van der Lely A (1997). The endocrinology of aging. *Science* **278**: 419–24.

62 Parker CR Jr (1999). Dehydroepiandrosterone and dehydroepiandrosterone sulfate production in the human adrenal during development and aging. *Steroids* **64**: 640–7.

63 Nawata H, Yanase T, Goto K, Okabe T, Ashida K (2002). Mechanism of action of anti-aging DHEA-S and the replacement of DHEA-S. *Mech Ageing Dev* **123**: 1101–6.

64 Goncharova ND, Lapin BA (2002). Effects of aging on hypothalamic–pituitary–adrenal system function in non-human primates. *Mech Ageing Dev* **123**: 1191–1201.

65 Kudielka BM, Kirshbaum C (2003). Awakening cortisol responses are influenced by health status and awakening time but not by menstrual cycle phase. *Psychoneuroendocrinology* **28**: 35–47.

66 Bjorntorp P, Holm G, Rosmond R (1999). Hypothalamic arousal, insulin resistance and type 2 diabetes mellitus. *Diabet Med* **16**: 355–7.

67 Sephton SE, Sapolsky RM, Kraemer HC, Spiegel D (2000). Diurnal cortisol rhythm as a predictor of breast cancer survival. *J Natl Cancer Inst* **92**: 994–1000.

68 Hall JE, Gill S (2001). Neuroendocrine aspects of aging in women. *Endocrinol Metab Clin North Am* **30**: 631–46.

69 Vermeulen A, Kaufman JM, Giagulli VA (1996). Influence of some biological indexes on sex hormone-binding globulin and androgen levels in aging or obese males. *J Clin Endocrinol Metab* **81**: 1821–6.

70 Vermeulen A (1991). Clinical review 24: androgens in the aging male. *J Clin Endocrinol Metab* **73**: 221–4.

71 Vermeulen A (2000). Andropause. *Maturitas* **34**: 5–15.

72 Morley JE, Patrick P, Perry HM 3rd (2002). Evaluation of assays available to measure free testosterone. *Metabolism* **51**: 554–9.

73 Hermann M, Berger P (1999). Hormone replacement in the aging male? *Exp Gerontol* **34**: 923–33.

74 Hermann M, Berger P (2001). Hormonal changes in aging men: a therapeutic indication? *Exp Gerontol* **36**: 1075–82.

75 Schatzl G, Madersbacher S, Temml C, *et al.* (2003). Serum androgen levels in men: impact of health status and age. *Urology* **61**: 629–33.

76 Bok RA, Small EJ (2002). Bloodborne biomolecular markers in prostate cancer development and progression. *Nat Rev Cancer* **2**: 918–26.

77 Ferrari E, Casarotti D, Muzzoni B, *et al.* (2001). Age-related changes of the adrenal secretory pattern: possible role in pathological brain aging. *Brain Res Rev* **37**: 294–300.

78 Ferrari E, Cravello L, Muzzoni B, *et al.* (2001). Age-related changes of the hypothalamic–pituitary–adrenal axis: pathophysiological correlates. *Euro J Endocrinol* **144**: 319–29.

79 Burgess W, Liu Q, Zhou J, *et al.* (1999). The immune–endocrine loop during aging: role of growth hormone and insulin-like growth factor-I. *Neuroimmunomodulation* **6**: 56–68.

80 Touitou Y (2001). Human aging and melatonin. Clinical relevance. *Exp Gerontol* **36**: 1083–1100.

81 Manson JE, Hsia J, Johnson KC, *et al.* (2003). Estrogen plus progestin and the risk of coronary heart disease. *N Engl J Med* **349**: 523–34.

82 Rabin BS, Cohen S, Ganguli R, Lysle DT, Cunnick JE (1989). Bidirectional interaction between the central nervous system and the immune system. *Crit Rev Immun* **9**: 279–312.

83 Brunda MJ, Luistro L, Warrier RR, *et al.* (1993). Antitumor and antimetastatic activity of interleukin 12 against murine tumors. *J Exp Med* **178**: 1223–30.

84 Munck A, Guyre PM (1986). Glucocorticoid physiology, pharmacology and stress. *Adv Exp Med Biol* **196**: 81–96.

85 Smith PC, Hobisch A, Lin DL, Culig Z, Keller ET (2001). Interleukin-6 and prostate cancer progression. *Cytokine Growth Factor Rev* **12**: 33–40.

86 Reichlin S (1993). Neuroendocrine–immune interactions. *N Engl J Med* **329**: 1246–53.

87 Savino W, Dardenne M (1995). Immune–neuroendocrine interactions. *Immunol Today* **14**: 318–22.

88 Derijk R, Michelson D, Karp B, *et al.* (1997). Exercise and circadian rhythm-induced variations in plasma cortisol differentially regulate interleukin-1 beta (IL-1 beta), IL-6, and tumor necrosis factor-alpha (TNF alpha) production in humans: high sensitivity of TNF alpha and resistance of IL-6. *J Clin Endocrinol* **82**: 2182–91.

89 Elenkov IJ, Chrousos GP (1999). Stress hormones, Th1/Th2 patterns, pro/anti-inflammatory cytokines and susceptibility to disease. *Trends Endocrinol Metab* **10**: 359–68.

90 Baum A, Posluszny D (1999). Health psychology: mapping biobehavioral contributions to health and illness. *Annu Rev Psychiatr* **50**: 137–63.

91 Glaser R, Rabin B, Chesney M, Cohen D, Natelson B (1999). Stress-induced immunomodulation: Implications for infectious diseases? *JAMA* **281**: 2268–70.

92 Maier S, Watkins L (1998). Cytokines for psychologists: implications of bi-directional immune-to-brain communication for understanding behavior, mood, and cognition. *Psychol Rev* **105**: 83–107.

93 McEwen B (1998). Protective and damaging effects of stress mediators. *N Engl J Med* **338**: 171–9.

94 Tsagarakis S, Grossman A (1994). Corticotropin-releasing hormone: interactions with the immune system. *Neuroimmunomodulation* **1**: 329–34.

95 Radulovic M, Dautzenberg FM, Sydow S, Radulovic J, Spiess J (1999). Corticotropin-releasing factor receptor 1 in mouse spleen: expression after immune stimulation and identification of receptor-bearing cells. *J Immunol* **162**: 3013–21.

96 Bartrop RW, Luckhurst E, Lazarus L, Kiloh LG, Penny R (1977). Depressed lymphocyte function after bereavement. *Lancet* i: 834–6.

97 Schleifer SJ, Keller SE, Bond RN, Cohen J, Stein M (1989). Major depressive disorder and immunity: role of age, sex, severity, and hospitalization. *Arch Gen Psychiatryiatry* **45**: 81–9.

98 Irwin M, Brown M, Patterson T, Hauger R, Mascovich A, Grant I (1992). Neuropeptide Y and natural killer activity. Findings in depression and Alzheimer caregiver stress. *FASEB J* **5**: 3100–7.

99 Kiecolt-Glaser JK, Glaser R, Cacioppo JT, *et al.* (1997). Marital conflict in older adults: endocrinological and immunological correlates. *Psychosom Med* **59**: 339–49.

100 Castle S, Wilkins S, Heck E, Tanzy K, Fahey J (1995). Depression in caregivers of demented patients is associated with impaired proliferative capacity, increased CD8+, and a decline in lymphocytes with surface signal transduction molecules (CD38+) and a cytotoxicity marker (CD56+CD8+). *Clin Exp Immunol* **101**: 487–93.

101 Kiecolt-Glaser JK, Glaser R (1999). Chronic stress and mortality among older adults. *JAMA* **282**: 2259–60.

102 Koenig HG, George LK, Peterson BL, Pieper CF (1997). Depression in medically ill hospitalized older adults: prevalence, characteristics and course of symptoms according to six diagnostic schemes. *Am J Psychiatry* **154**: 1376–83.

103 McGuire L, Kiecolt-Glaser JK, Glaser R (2002). Depressive symptoms and lymphocyte proliferation in older adults. *J Abnorm Psychol* **111**: 192–7.

104 Lutgendorf SK, Reimer TT, Harvey JH, *et al.* (2001). Effects of housing relocation on immunocompetence and psychosocial functioning in older adults. *J Gerontol A Bio Sci Med Sci* **56A**: M97–105.

105 Schleifer SJ, Keller SE, Camerino M, Thornton J, Stein M (1983). Suppression of lymphocyte stimulation following bereavement. *JAMA* **250**: 374–7.

106 Lutgendorf SK, Reimer TT, Schlechte J, Rubenstein LM (2001). Illness episodes and cortisol in healthy older adults during a life transition. *Ann Behav Med* **23**: 166–76.

107 Stowell JR, Kiecolt-Glaser JK, Glaser R (2001). Perceived stress and cellular immunity. *J Behav Med* **24**: 323–39.

108 Kiecolt-Glaser JK, Newton TL (2001). Marriage and health: his and hers. *Psychol Bull* **127**: 472–503.

109 Kubzansky LD, Sparrow D, Vokonas P, Kawachi I (2001). Is the glass half empty or half full? A prospective study of optimism and coronary heart disease in the normative aging study. *Psychosom Med* **63**: 910–16.

110 Clark PC (2002). Effects of individual and family hardiness on caregiver depression and fatigue. *Res Nurs Health* **25**: 37–48.

111 Esterling BA, Kiecolt-Glaser JK, Bodnar JC, Glaser R (1994). Chronic stress, social support, and persistent alterations in the natural killer cell response to cytokines in older adults. *Health Psychol* **13**: 291–8.

112 Penedo FJ, Dahn J, Kinsinger D, *et al.* (2005). Anger suppression mediates the relationship between optimism and natural killer cell cytotoxicity in men treated for localized prostate cancer. Under review. *J Psychom Res.*

113 Carter PA (2003). Family caregivers' sleep loss and depression over time. *Cancer Nurs* **26**: 253–9.

114 Prinz PN, Bailey SL, Woods DL (2000). Sleep impairments in healthy seniors: roles of stress, cortisol, and interleukin-1 beta. *Chronobiol Int* **17**: 391–404.

115 Vgontzas AN, Zoumakis M, Bixler EO, *et al.* (2003). Impaired nighttime sleep in healthy old versus young adults is associated with elevated plasma interleukin-6 and cortisol levels: physiologic and therapeutic indications. *J Clin Endocrinol Metab* **88**: 2087–95.

116 Irwin M (2002). Effects of sleep and sleep loss on immunity and cytokines. *Brain Behav Immun* **16**: 503–12.

117 US Department of Health and Human Services (1996). *Physical Activity and Health: A Report of the Surgeon General.* Atlanta, GA: US Department of Health and Human Services, Centers for Disease Control and Prevention, National Center for Chronic Disease Prevention and Health Promotion.

118 Woods JA, Lowder TW, Keylock KT (2002). Can exercise training improve immune functioning in the aged? *Ann NY Acad Sci* **959**: 117–27.

119 Kohut ML, Cooper MM, Nickolaus MS, Russell DR, Cunnick JE (2002). Exercise and psychosocial factors modulate immunity to influenza vaccine in elderly individuals. *J Gerontol A Bio Sci Med Sci* **57**: M557–62.

120 Chandra RK (2002). Nutrition and the immune system from birth to old age. *Eur J Clin Nutr* **56**: S73–6.

121 Hughes DA (1999). Effects of dietary antioxidants on the immune function of middle-aged adults. *Proc Nutr Soc* **58**: 79–84.

122 High KP (1999). Micronutrient supplementation and immune function in the elderly. *Clin Infect Dis* **28**: 717–22.

123 Substance Abuse and Mental Health Services Administration (2001). *Summary of Findings from the 2000 National Household Survey on Drug Abuse.* NHSDA Series H-13; DHHS Publication No. SMA 01–3549. Rockville, MD: US Department of Health and Human Services.

124 Kovacs EJ, Messingham KA (2002). Influence of alcohol and gender on immune response. *Alcohol Res Health* **26**: 257–63.

125 **Baldwin GC, Roth MD, Tashkin DP** (1998). Acute and chronic effects of cocaine on the immune system and the possible link to AIDS. *J Neuroimmunol* **83**: 133–8.

126 **Nokes KM, Chew L, Altman C** (2003). Using a telephone support group for HIV-positive persons aged 50+ to increase social support and health-related knowledge. *AIDS Patient Care STDS* **17**: 345–51.

127 **Miller GE, Cohen S** (2001). Psychological interventions and the immune system: a meta-analytic review and critique. *Health Psychol* **20**: 47–63.

128 **Irwin MR, Pike JL, Cole JC, Oxman MN** (2003). Effects of a behavioral intervention, Tai Chi Chih, on varicella-zoster virus specific immunity and health functioning in older adults. *Psychosom Med* **65**: 824–30.

129 **Fawzy F, Cousins N, Fawzy N, *et al.*** (1990). A structured psychiatric intervention for cancer patients. I. Changes over time in methods of coping and affective disturbance. *Arch Gen Psychiatry* **47**: 720–8.

130 **Fawzy F, Kemeny M, Fawzy NW, Elashoff R** (1990). A structured psychiatric intervention for cancer patients. II.Changes over time in immunological measures. *Arch Gen Psychiatry* **47**: 729–35.

131 **Fawzy F, Canada AL, Fawzy NW** (2003). Malignant melanoma: effects of a brief structured psychiatric intervention on survival and recurrence at 10-year follow-up. *Arch Gen Psychiatry* **60**: 100–3.

132 **Cacioppo JT, Poehlmann KM, Kiecolt-Glaser JK, *et al.*** (1998). Cellular immune responses to acute stress in female caregivers of dementia patients and matched controls. *Health Psychol* **17**: 182–9.

133 **Glaser R, Kiecolt-Glaser JK** (1994). *Handbook of Human Stress and Immunity*. San Diego, CA: Academic Press.

134 **Bauer ME, Vedhara K, Perks P, Wilcok GK, Lightman SL, Shanks N** (2000). Chronic stress in caregivers of dementia patients is associated with reduced lymphocyte sensitivity to glucocorticoids. *J Neuroimmunol* **103**: 84–92.

135 **Garand L, Buckwalter KC, Lubaroff D, Tripp-Reimer T, Frantz RA, Ansley TN** (2002). A pilot study of immune and mood outcomes of a community-based intervention for dementia caregivers: the PLST intervention. *Arch Psychiatr Nurs* **16**: 156–67.

136 **Hosaka T, Sugiyama Y** (2003). Structured intervention in family caregivers of the demented elderly and changes in their immune function. *Psychol Clin Neurosci* **57**: 147–51.

137 **Vedhara K, Bennett PD, Clark S, *et al.*** (2003). Enhancement of antibody responses to influenza vaccination in the elderly following a cognitive–behavioural stress management intervention. *Psychother Psychosom* **72**: 245–52.

138 **Schultz R, Beach SR** (1999). Caregiving as a risk factor for mortality: the caregiver health effects study. *JAMA* **282**: 2215–19.

139 **Lee S, Colditz GA, Berkman LF, Kawachi I** (2003). Caregiving and risk of coronary heart disease in U.S. women. *Am J Prev Med* **24**: 113–19.

140 **Ligthart GH, Corberand JX, Fournier C, *et al.*** (1984). Admission criteria for immunogerontological studies in man: the SENIEUR Protocol. *Mech Ageing Dev* **28**: 45–55.

141 **Ligthart GH** (2001). The SENIEUR Protocol after 16 years: the next step is to study the interaction of ageing and disease. *Mech Ageing Dev* **22**: 136–40.

Chapter 5

Psychoneuroimmunology and coronary heart disease

Andrew Steptoe and Lena Brydon

5.1 **Introduction**

A decade ago, there would have been no place for a chapter on coronary heart disease (CHD) in a book on psychoneuroimmunology. Research on the pathways through which psychosocial factors affect CHD was focused on cardiovascular stress reactivity, high blood pressure, lipids, and myocardial ischaemia, and the role of immune processes was not yet understood. However, recent years have witnessed a revolution in knowledge about the causes of atherosclerosis (the disease underlying CHD). It is now recognized that vascular inflammation is central to atherosclerosis, and that T lymphocytes, monocytes, and inflammatory cytokines are all involved. Inflammatory processes are also implicated in the acute manifestations of CHD, including myocardial infarction and unstable angina pectoris. Psychoneuroimmunology has progressed in parallel, with evidence that stress and depression are associated not only with white blood cell counts, but also with cytokine release and even gene expression.

The aim of this chapter is to provide an introduction to this complex and intriguing new topic. We begin by giving a brief description of CHD, its incidence in the population, and the risk factors for the illness. We summarize current understanding of the development of atherosclerosis, emphasizing the role of immunological and vascular inflammatory processes. The psychosocial factors that contribute to CHD risk will then be outlined. Subsequent sections discuss evidence for the impact of psychoneuroimmunological factors in CHD by considering epidemiological and experimental data relating stress and other psychosocial factors to vascular inflammation. The last major section focuses on the links between depressive symptoms, immune factors, and prognosis in patients with advanced CHD. Research in this exciting field is still at an early stage, but is likely to become increasingly prominent in the literature on psychoneuroimmunology over the next decade.[1] In order to provide a framework for understanding the pathophysiological processes relating psychosocial factors to CHD risk, a summary of the relevant pathways is provided in Figure 5.1.

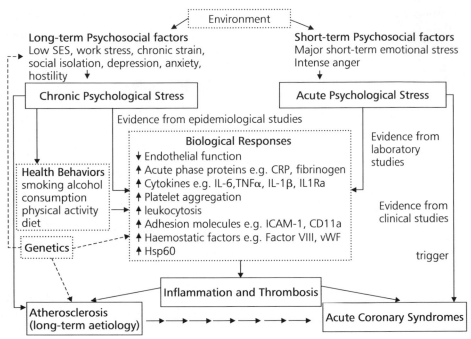

Fig. 5.1 Pathophysiological model of the relationship between chronic and acute psychological stress and coronary artery disease (SES, socioeconomic status). Evidence from epidemiological studies indicates that chronic psychological stress accelerates the long-term progression of atherosclerosis. Results from laboratory studies of acute psychological stress, as well as epidemiological studies, indicate that stress accelerates atherosclerosis by activating biological factors which promote inflammation and thrombosis. Clinical research has also demonstrated that short-term psychological stress can trigger acute coronary syndromes in people with advanced atherosclerosis, most likely through activation of the same biological factors. Genetic vulnerability, adverse health behaviours, and other environmental risk factors are likely to contribute to the extent to which stress influences coronary artery disease risk in a given individual.

5.2 The clinical context: coronary heart disease

Diseases of the heart and circulation are the main cause of death in developed nations, and account for more than 16 million deaths each year throughout the world. At the turn of the millennium, about 40% of deaths in both the United States and the United Kingdom were due to cardiovascular diseases. The main forms of cardiovascular disease are CHD and stroke, and CHD alone is the leading single cause of death in Europe and the United States. Although CHD becomes more common as people grow older, it is also responsible for nearly a quarter of premature deaths.

The disorder underlying CHD is atherosclerosis, a process involving inflammation of the lining of blood vessels leading to progressive accumulation of lipid, macrophages,

T lymphocytes, platelets, and smooth muscle cells in the walls of the coronary arteries. This results in a narrowing of conduit blood vessels such as the coronary arteries, so that blood supply to the working heart muscle can become impaired. In later stages, plaque forms on vessels and contributes to the development of clumps of cells and other material called thrombi. Atherosclerosis starts early in life and continues for decades without any clinical consequences. The disease typically comes to light at an advanced stage when the coronary arteries become partly or completely blocked, and the muscle of the myocardium fails to be supplied with energy and becomes ischaemic. At this point, the person may experience angina pectoris (acute chest pain), a myocardial infarction (heart attack), or death. Sadly, about half of all CHD deaths are sudden cardiac deaths, occurring within a few minutes of onset, often in people who have had no previous diagnosis of heart disease.

The major risk factors for CHD are cigarette smoking, high blood pressure, and high blood levels of cholesterol, particularly low-density lipoprotein cholesterol (LDL-cholesterol). These factors increase risk for CHD, but the disease is not inevitable even in those people with a high risk profile and many people with only one or no risk factors also die of heart disease.[2] Other risk factors include a positive family history, obesity and overweight, and diabetes. There are also important ethnic differences between black, white, and Hispanic Americans, and between white, black, and South Asian people in the United Kingdom. CHD risk is strongly determined by lifestyle, since smoking, food choice, and physical inactivity all contribute to the risk profile. These risk factors operate throughout life, accelerating the development of subclinical atherosclerosis.

An important distinction can be made between the long-term aetiology of CHD and the occurrence of acute coronary syndromes (myocardial infarction and advanced or unstable angina). Psychosocial factors may contribute to the long-term development of atherosclerosis and the progressive narrowing of arteries in the same way as other risk factors, operating in essentially healthy people. Acute cardiac syndromes, in contrast, typically occur in individuals with well-established atherosclerosis, and involve the rupture of plaques in the vessel wall and thrombus formation. Psychological factors may be involved in the triggering of acute coronary syndromes as well as in long-term aetiology.

5.2.1 The role of inflammation in coronary atherosclerosis

An important feature of the development of atherosclerotic lesions is the gradual accumulation of lipid in the artery wall. This used to be regarded as a largely passive process, depending on the concentration of cholesterol in the blood. However, recent evidence has shown the disease to be much more complex and has highlighted the pivotal role of inflammation. Indeed, each atherosclerotic lesion contains a variety of different cells, with highly specific inflammatory responses to lipid storage and vascular injury. For this reason, atherosclerosis has been redefined as a chronic inflammatory response to injury.[3]

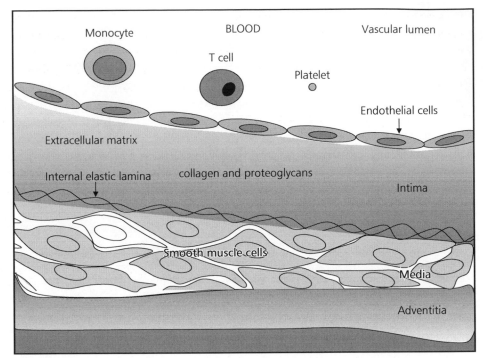

Fig. 5.2 Structure of a normal large artery. (Adapted from A. J. Lusis (2000) *Nature* **407**: 233–41.)

Figure 5.2 outlines the physiological structure of the artery. The innermost lining of the arterial wall is the endothelium, a single layer of cells. Outside this is the intimal layer consisting of extracellular connective tissue matrix, primarily collagen and proteoglycans. This is bounded by a sheet of elastic fibres, the internal elastic lamina, on its peripheral side. The media, the middle layer, consists of smooth muscle cells. The outer layer, or adventitia, consists of connective tissue with interspersed fibroblasts and smooth muscle cells. Blood, containing red blood cells, white blood cells such as monocytes and T lymphocytes, and platelets, circulates through the vascular lumen. As atherosclerosis develops, the different layers of the arterial wall become progressively affected. The processes are very complex, and so only an outline is provided here.[4]

5.2.1.1 Initiating events: damage to the endothelium and LDL modification

The initial stage of atherosclerosis is characterized by functional alterations of the endothelium. The endothelium is an active tissue which normally helps maintain cardiovascular health by producing antiplatelet, anticlotting, and fibrinolytic factors which prevent cells from adhering to its surface, and by regulating vascular tone through the production of molecules such as nitric oxide. Endothelial injury can arise from a variety of sources, including high levels of circulating cholesterol (hypercholes-terolaemia) and modified LDL-cholesterol, elevated levels of homocysteine (an amino acid), free radicals, and vasoactive amines, and the presence of infectious microorganisms. This leads to endothelial dysfunction, in which this protective layer of cells develops pro-inflammatory/pro-thrombotic properties, secreting vasoactive molecules, inflammatory cytokines, and growth factors. It also becomes more perme-able to lipoproteins such as LDL that start to accumulate in the subendothelial matrix. LDL diffuses passively through junctions between endothelial cells and is retained in the vessel wall. Trapped LDL undergoes oxidation as a result of exposure to the oxidat-ive waste of vascular cells, producing minimally oxidized LDL species (mOx-LDL) with proinflammatory activity.

5.2.1.2 Recruitment of monocyte–macrophages, T lymphocytes, and platelets

Endothelial dysfunction also results in recruitment and adhesiveness of leucocytes (specifically monocytes and T lymphocytes) and small circulating cells called platelets to vulnerable sites at the vessel wall (Fig. 5.3). This process is mediated by upregula-tion of molecules known as 'cell adhesion molecules' (CAMs) on endothelial cells, leucocytes, and platelets. CAMs are a family of specific cell surface receptors which mediate adhesive interactions between these cells. mOx-LDL stimulates overlying endothelial cells to increase the expression of CAMs at specific 'atherosclerosis-prone' sites of the arterial wall. A number of proinflammatory cytokines and chemoattrac-tant molecules (chemokines) produced by the endothelium, smooth muscle cells, and leucocytes, including interferon gamma (IFN-γ), interleukin 1 (IL-1), IL-6, IL-8, tumour necrosis factor alpha (TNF-α), and monocyte chemotactic protein-1 (MCP-1), also stimulate upregulation of CAMs and promote leucocyte recruitment and adhesion. Atherosclerosis-prone sites include arterial branches, bifurcations, and curvatures where there are characteristic alterations in the flow of blood, including decreased shear stress and increased turbulence. They are present in many parts of the body, but the particular sites involved in CHD are the coronary arteries. Changes in blood flow stimulate the expression of genes for adhesion molecules, and reduced shear stress also lowers production of endothelium-derived nitric oxide, an anti-inflammatory vasodilator molecule which normally limits expression of these adhesion molecules.

The first step in adhesion, the 'rolling' of leucocytes along the endothelial surface, is mediated by a family of adhesion molecules called selectins, which are expressed on leucocyte and endothelial cell surfaces. Firm adhesion of leucocytes to the vessel wall and their subsequent transmigration into the intima is governed largely by the interac-tion between other complementary adhesion molecules expressed on the endothelium and leucocytes. The immunoglobulin-related adhesion molecules ICAM-1 (intercellu-lar adhesion molecule 1) and VCAM-1 (vascular cell adhesion molecule 1) are

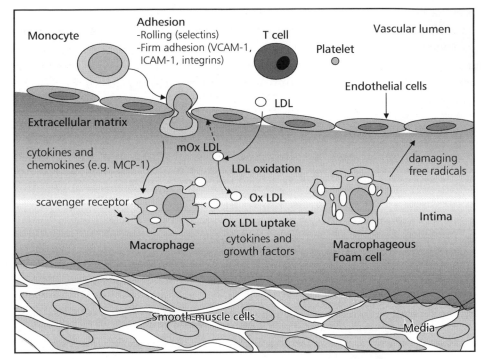

Fig. 5.3 Initial stages of atherosclerotic lesion development. Endothelial dysfunction results in an increased permeability of the endothelium to lipoproteins and recruitment and adhesiveness of monocytes, T lymphocytes, and platelets to the vessel wall. LDL diffuses passively through junctions between endothelial cells and is subject to oxidative modifications in the subendothelial space, progressing from minimally mOx-LDL to Ox-LDL. mOx-LDL, inflammatory cytokines, and chemokines stimulate adhesion molecule expression on endothelial cells, leucocytes, and platelets. Interaction between complementary adhesion molecules expressed on these cells results in firm adhesion of leucocytes and platelets to the vessel wall and their subsequent migration into the intima. On reaching the intima, monocytes are stimulated by cytokines and macrophage chemotactic protein 1 (MCP-1) to differentiate into macrophages. Foam cells are formed when macrophages take up oxidized LDL via their scavenger receptors.

expressed on the endothelium. These molecules bind to other adhesion molecules called integrins (including CD11a and VLA-4) expressed on the cell surface of leucocytes. Specifically, ICAM-1 binds to CD11a on lymphocytes and VCAM-1 binds to VLA-4 on monocytes. The continued attachment and transmigration of monocytes and T cells through gaps between endothelial cells results in a gradual accumulation of leucocytes in the intima. Platelets also adhere and aggregate at the vulnerable arterial sites, binding to leucocytes to form platelet–leucocyte aggregates. Activated platelets release their granules which contain more cytokines and growth factors that reinforce the migration and proliferation of leucocytes in the blood vessel walls.

5.2.1.3 Foam cell formation and smooth muscle migration

Once resident in the arterial wall, monocytes, T lymphocytes, and platelets participate in and perpetuate a local proinflammatory prothrombotic response that develops the lesion (Fig. 5.3). Upon entering the intimal layer of the blood vessel wall, monocytes rapidly proliferate and differentiate into macrophages. Macrophages are scavenging and antigen-presenting cells, which use their scavenger receptors to ingest highly oxidized LDL (ox-LDL), leading to formation of macrophageous foam cells. The activity of macrophages and the regulation of their scavenger receptors is dependent on cytokines (TNF-α and IFN-γ) and other factors including monocyte chemotactic protein 1 (MCP-1). Macrophages promote atherosclerosis by producing cytokines and growth factors, enhancing the transportation and oxidation of LDL-cholesterol, and generating toxic products of lipid oxidation known as free radicals which damage the intima. With time the foam cells die, contributing their lipid-filled contents to the necrotic core of the lesion.

T cells are also important contributors to the progression of atherosclerosis when activated immunologically by macrophages, oxidized lipoproteins, viral infections (herpes types and cytomegalovirus), and proinflammatory cytokines (Fig. 5.4). Activated T cells, in turn, produce other inflammatory cytokines, such as TNF-α, IL-1, IL-6, and IFN γ, which stimulate macrophages as well as vascular endothelial cells, thus amplifying the inflammatory process. Cytokines and growth factors released by activated macrophages, T cells, endothelial cells, and platelets stimulate the migration of smooth muscle cells from the medial layer of the blood vessel wall into the intimal layer. These smooth muscle cells proliferate and become intermixed with the area of inflammation (Fig. 5.4). They may also take up modified lipoproteins, contributing to foam cell formation (as smooth muscle cell derived foam cells), and are stimulated by cytokines and growth factors to secrete fibrous elements, leading to the formation of a dense extracellular matrix of fibrous tissue (fibrous cap).

These processes—the migration of new leucocytes from the blood, foam cell formation, migration and proliferation of smooth muscle cells, extracellular matrix production, and accumulation of extracellular lipid—continue throughout adult life. Plaques (clumps of atheromatous material) form on the surface of the arterial wall, intruding into the lumen. The thickening of the arterial wall does not necessarily lead immediately to narrowing of the lumen of the vessel through which the blood flows because the artery compensates by dilating ('remodelling'). However, eventually the artery can no longer compensate by dilation, and the lesion may then intrude into the lumen and obstruct the flow of blood.

5.2.1.4 Plaque rupture and thrombosis

Acute cardiac events occur when the supply of blood through the coronary arteries to the working muscle of the heart is reduced or stopped altogether. This can happen with progressive narrowing of the lumen of the artery. More commonly,

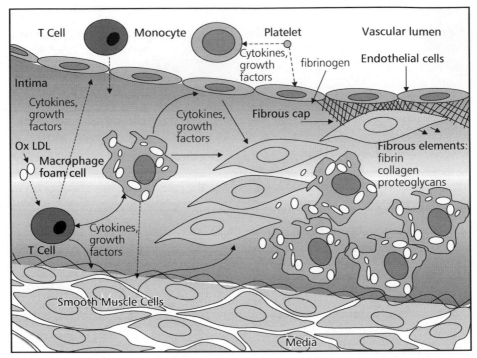

Fig. 5.4 Atherosclerotic lesion progression. Interactions between macrophageous foam cells and T cells lead to a chronic inflammatory process. Cytokines and growth factors released by activated macrophages, T cells, endothelial cells, and platelets stimulate the migration of smooth muscle cells from the medial portion of the arterial wall to the intima where they proliferate and secrete fibrous elements that form a fibrous cap.

however, acute cardiac events involve rupture of vulnerable plaque, exposing the underlying layers to circulating platelets which then aggregate to form a blood clot (thrombus). Inflammatory processes are again involved at this stage, interacting with molecules involved in coagulation and haemostasis, including von Willebrand factor (vWF), tissue factor, factor VIII, fibrin D-dimer, and plasminogen activator inhibitor (PAI).

Vulnerable plaques generally have thin fibrous caps and increased numbers of inflammatory cells. The maintenance of the fibrous cap depends on the balance of matrix production and degradation, and products of inflammatory cells are likely to affect both processes. For example, activated T cells produce IFN-γ which inhibits collagen synthesis by smooth muscle cells, limiting their capacity to renew the collagen that reinforces the plaque. Activated T cells also stimulate macrophages to produce enzymes called metalloproteinases which degrade the extracellular matrix that strengthens the plaque's protective fibrous cap, thereby rendering the cap thin, weak, and susceptible to rupture. Macrophages also promote thrombus formation by

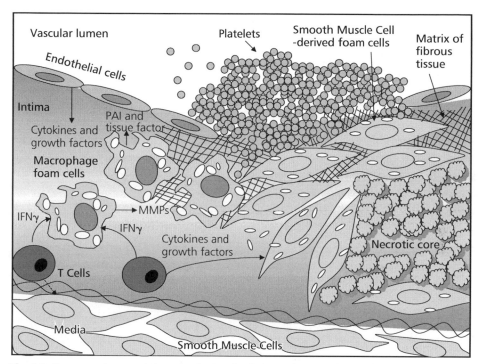

Fig. 5.5 Plaque rupture and thrombosis. Death of macrophage and smooth muscle cell derived foam cells leads to the formation of a necrotic core and accumulation of extracellular lipid. Production of IFN-γ by T cells and subsequent macrophage secretion of matrix metalloproteinases (MMPs) contributes to weakening of the fibrous plaque. Plaque rupture exposes underlying layers to circulating platelets, which then aggregate to form a blood clot (thrombus). Macrophages promote thrombus formation by secreting tissue factor and plasminogen activator inhibitor (PAI) proteins with a key role in the blood clotting process.

secreting PAI as well as tissue factor, a key protein in the initiation of the coagulation cascade–clotting process (Fig. 5.5).

Additionally, molecules called acute phase proteins come into play. Acute phase proteins, including C-reactive protein (CRP) and fibrinogen, have an active role in the inflammatory atherosclerotic process. CRP stimulates the expression of tissue factor on macrophages, smooth muscle cells, and endothelial cells in and around coronary artery plaques. It also stimulates the production of the proinflammatory cytokines IL-1, IL-6, and TNFα from monocytes–macrophages, induces monocyte recruitment into arterial wall, facilitates the uptake of LDL by macrophages, and induces the expression of adhesion molecules. Fibrinogen is thought to promote atherosclerosis by promoting platelet aggregation, enhancing release of endothelial-derived growth factors, stimulating smooth muscle cell proliferation, and increasing plasma and whole blood viscosity. It may also increase the development of thrombi (thrombogenesis) through its role in blood clotting; fibrinogen is cleaved by thrombin to produce fibrin, the most abundant component of clots.

5.2.2 Inflammation and the heart

The pathological process that we have described concerns atherosclerosis and plaque rupture in the coronary arteries. Ultimately, however, these are important because they cause damage to the myocardium by restricting energy supplies to working muscle. It turns out that proinflammatory cytokines are also expressed by the myocardium itself in response to injury. Animal studies have shown rapid increases in inflammatory cytokines such as IL-1, IL-6, and TNF-α when the heart is injured. Why might this be? One possibility is that proinflammatory cytokines are stimulated as part of a protective response, and certainly the complete absence of these cytokines (e.g. in genetic 'knock-out' models) increases cardiac vulnerability.[5] However, intense and prolonged inflammatory cytokine production has damaging effects, as will be seen in the next section.

5.2.3 Population and clinical evidence

The previous section provided a brief summary of the biological processes involved in atherosclerosis and the triggering of acute cardiac events. What is the evidence that these inflammatory and associated haemostatic factors are relevant to the risk of cardiovascular disease in the population? It has to be admitted that intervention trials which demonstrate that modifying these factors has direct effects on the development of CHD have not yet been carried out. Many clinicians also remain unconvinced that knowledge about these factors will necessarily be helpful to the management of individual patients.[6] Nonetheless, data from several prospective studies have shown that elevated levels of circulating inflammatory markers among apparently healthy men and women predict future cardiovascular events. Furthermore, increases in inflammatory markers commonly accompany acute coronary syndromes and correlate with the prognosis of patients who have suffered an acute coronary event. High-sensitivity CRP and fibrinogen have been the most widely studied inflammatory markers. There is robust evidence from epidemiological studies, backed up by meta-analyses, that higher levels of CRP and fibrinogen predict future myocardial infarction, stroke, and cardiovascular death among middle-aged men and women.[7] For example, analysis of deaths or non-fatal myocardial infarctions in a sample of British men followed over 9 years showed an odds ratio of 2.13 for those in the top third of CRP concentration at baseline compared with those in the bottom third.[8] Interestingly, this effect was independent of traditional risk factors such as blood pressure, LDL-cholesterol concentration, and body mass, indicating that understanding the inflammatory components does provide additional information about disease processes. Elevated CRP and fibrinogen levels at the time of hospital admission are also predictors of new coronary events or poor clinical outcome in patients with acute coronary syndromes.[7,9]

Because this is a comparatively new field of investigation, the epidemiological evidence relating other inflammatory processes to future CHD is less strong. Nevertheless, there have been at least three prospective studies showing that elevated plasma IL-6 is associated with an increased risk of CHD in apparently healthy middle-aged and elderly men and women.[9] TNF-α has not yet been studied extensively in this respect, except in older cohorts.[10] Simple markers of immune function such as leucocyte counts are also related to the development of CHD. A meta-analysis of 19 prospective studies reported a risk ratio of 1.4 for healthy people with total leucocyte counts in the top of the population distribution compared with those in the bottom third.[11] Interestingly, levels of circulating soluble adhesion molecules such as ICAM-1 have been found to predict future coronary disease in a small number of studies.[12] The presence of these molecules, probably shed from activated leucocytes, endothelial cells, and/or smooth muscle cells, is thought to be indicative of an ongoing inflammatory process. Furthermore, a number of haemostatic factors linked with inflammation have been found to be predictive of future CHD. Meta-analyses of population-based prospective studies have shown that vWF, factor VIII, plasma viscosity, haematocrit, t-plasminogen activator, and fibrin D-dimer all appear to be independent predictors of CHD.[13–15] It is likely that as science develops in this field, more associations between inflammatory and haemostatic markers in healthy populations and future CHD will be observed.

The evidence for the elevation of inflammatory cytokines elevated in acute coronary syndromes is far stronger. Circulating levels of inflammatory cytokines such as IL-6, IL-1β, IL-1 receptor antagonist (IL-1Ra), and IL-18 are all raised in patients with acute coronary syndromes compared with patients with stable angina or healthy matched controls.[9] Other work shows that high levels of inflammatory cytokines on admission predict a poor outcome. For example, patients with higher IL-6 on admission have more in-hospital cardiac events, a worse 30-day outcome, and greater longer-term mortality.[16,17] Similarly, high TNF-α and increasing levels of IL-1Ra during the first 2 days in hospital are associated with a higher risk of in-hospital coronary events and future infarction.[17,18] One possible explanation is that patients with these characteristics exhibit more intense inflammatory reactions than others, and this increases their chances of further plaque rupture and thrombosis. Importantly, these effects are again independent of standard clinical markers of the severity of cardiac events taken on admission to hospital.

5.2.4 Does infection play a role?

If inflammatory and immune processes are involved in atherosclerosis, the question arises as to what causes the activation of these responses. One possibility that has been seriously entertained over recent years is that chronic low level infection initiates the inflammatory response. It has been proposed that several different microorganisms are associated with atherosclerosis, including *Chlamydia pneumoniae*, *Helicobacter pylori*, and herpes viruses (cytomegalovirus and herpes simplex virus). *Chlamydia pneumoniae* has attracted the greatest scientific interest, since this microorganism is present within atherosclerotic lesions and is known to stimulate innate immune cells like macrophages, leading to the expression of factors that could maintain the inflammatory response. Several early studies in the literature compared CHD patients with healthy controls, and found evidence for a greater prevalence of antibodies against *C. pneumoniae, H. pylori,* and other microorganisms in the serum of patients. However, these studies were often small scale and did not control properly for age, cardiovascular risk factors, and socioeconomic status. More recent case–control studies have not yielded strong results. A meta-analysis of 10 studies of *C. pneumoniae* antibodies showed a very modest association with CHD, and analyses of *H. pylori* have also been negative.[19,20] In addition, well-conducted trials of antibiotic treatment of patients with acute coronary syndromes have not shown benefits in terms of cardiac prognosis,[21] although it is possible that, by this advanced stage, it is too late to alter the course of disease by modifying infection.

An alternative perspective on the role of infection has been proposed by Epstein *et al.*[22] They suggested that instead of a particular infectious organism being important, the crucial factor was 'total pathogen burden', or the number of pathogens to which people had been exposed in their lifetimes. For example, one study tested for antibodies for six microorganisms (including cytomegalovirus, hepatitis A, and herpes simplex virus types 1 and 2) in the serum of 890 patients with coronary artery disease. After controlling for other risk factors, the number of organisms to which the patient had antibodies predicted future myocardial infarction or death.[23] A similar study in Germany found that, over a period of 3 years, cardiovascular mortality was 7.0% in patients with advanced atherosclerosis and seropositivity for no to three pathogens, but 20% in patients who were seropositive for six to eight pathogens.[24] These ideas are very interesting but have yet to be widely tested, and it is unclear how infections (some of which may be inactive) acquired at different stages in a person's life can act in concert to produce vascular inflammation. For the present, the jury is still out on whether infectious agents are important factors in atherosclerosis and acute coronary syndromes.

5.3 Theoretical basis for a role for psychoneuroimmunology

5.3.1 Psychosocial factors in the aetiology of CHD

There is a large scientific literature exploring the role of psychosocial factors in the development of CHD, with research using animal models, experimental and clinical techniques, and large-scale epidemiological surveys. Considerations of space prevent a detailed coverage of this work, but thorough reviews are available.[25–27] Some of the most convincing evidence comes from prospective epidemiological studies in which large healthy populations are evaluated at baseline with measures of both biological and psychosocial risk factors. These populations are then tracked over many years, during which some people develop CHD. The relationship between baseline psychosocial factors and future CHD can then be evaluated, taking account of other influences on the disease process. The results of such studies are not all consistent, but perhaps this is inevitable given the subtle nature of many psychosocial factors, the difficulty in measuring them, and the context in which they operate. However, the strongest evidence obtained so far is for the following factors.

5.3.1.1 Low socioeconomic position

CHD is more common among people of lower socioeconomic status, as measured by income, education, or occupational prestige.[28] There is a gradient rather than a simple difference between rich and poor, so that individuals in the middle of the social spectrum are at higher risk than those at the top, but at lower risk than less affluent groups.

5.3.1.2 Work stress

Work stress can be defined in many different ways, but there is good evidence that people with low control at work are at increased CHD risk, particularly when this is coupled with high levels of work demand.[29] Low control and high demands have also been linked with high blood pressure in many studies.[30] An imbalance between the effort people put into work and the rewards they gain also contributes to risk.

5.3.1.3 Other forms of chronic strain

Other forms of chronic strain have not been evaluated as much as work stress, but there is evidence linking marital strain with CHD, and for increased risk among caregivers of dementing relatives[31] and in people who live in threatening neighbourhoods that lack social cohesion.[32]

5.3.1.4 Social isolation

Individuals who have few intimate relationships or social contacts and are not well integrated into their communities are at increased risk for premature mortality from CHD. This association has been identified in both men and women from several countries.[27] There is less evidence concerning the impact of low social support on CHD, though it does influence survival in individuals who have experienced a myocardial infarction.[33]

5.3.1.5 Depression and anxiety

A positive association between depressive symptoms and future CHD has now been documented in more than 15 prospective studies.[27] For example, in one study depression was measured using a standard questionnaire in nearly 9000 men and women without CHD who were enrolled in the first National Health and Nutrition Examination Survey in the United States.[34] After adjusting for standard risk factors, including age, poverty, smoking, diabetes, and body mass, depressed men and women were more likely to develop CHD over the next 10 years. However, it has to be admitted that some researchers have found no effects, while in other studies the relationship was stronger when CHD was measured in terms of angina rather than other cardiac events. This is important, because both depressive symptoms and the reporting of angina could be influenced by a common bias towards high levels of complaint. Evidence linking anxiety with CHD is sparse, but suggestive of a positive association. The role of depression in acute coronary syndromes is discussed in section 5.4.6.

5.3.1.6 Hostility

The data linking hostility with CHD are more equivocal than for other factors. Hostility is a central element of type A behaviour, the construct developed in the 1950s by cardiologists Friedman and Rosenman. The early results demonstrating associations between type A behaviour and CHD have not been replicated in more recent studies, and the population-based evidence on hostility is not consistent either.[27,35]

It is interesting that the factors most consistently associated with the long-term development of CHD are all chronic experiences or personal characteristics. Occurrences such as acute stressful life events do not have a powerful role. This makes sense in the context of an aetiological process that progresses over years and decades. People's experiences through the years may have small but cumulative effects. One cigarette has a negligible impact on CHD, but one cigarette every 2 h for 20 years has a marked effect. The same may be true of psychosocial factors.

5.3.2 Psychosocial influences on acute cardiac events

The psychosocial factors that contribute to the triggering of acute coronary syndromes in patients with advanced CHD are rather different. There is now substantial experimental evidence that mental stress can provoke acute myocardial ischaemia in susceptible individuals, resulting in a transient degradation of cardiac function.[36] Myocardial ischaemia is the phenomenon that follows reduced blood flow to the working muscle of the heart, which causes disruption of smooth and orderly contractions with each heart beat.

Two psychosocial factors stand out as possible triggers of cardiac events in clinical studies. The first is the experience of major short-term stress. Some of the most convincing evidence has come from studies of people living through earthquakes. For example, an analysis was carried out of sudden cardiac deaths in Los Angeles County in the period surrounding the Northridge earthquake in 1994.[37] There was a marked increase in the number of sudden cardiac deaths on the day of the earthquake. These mostly occurred in people with advanced heart disease and were not the result of physical exertion but emotional stress. Other research has shown associations between cardiac events and emotionally charged situations such as exciting football matches, anniversaries, and other important events in the calendar. The second trigger factor that has been identified in studies of survivors of acute myocardial infarction is the experience of intense anger.[38] It has been shown that high levels of anger are associated with an increased risk of acute myocardial infarction over the following 2 h. Heightened psychophysiological stress reactions may stimulate plaque rupture and the occlusion (blockage) of coronary arteries, and possibly also the disruption of the rhythm of cardiac contractions and the development of damaging cardiac arrhythmias. There is both experimental and clinical evidence that cardiac arrhythmias can be provoked by emotional stress.[39]

5.3.3 Potential mediating pathways

This brief overview outlines the context in which psychoneuroimmunological influences on CHD may operate. Some of the effects of psychosocial factors may be mediated through changes in behaviour: smoking, alcohol consumption, physical activity, and dietary choice. Another possibility is that more direct psychobiological responses are involved, and this notion is supported by the new understanding of the development of atherosclerosis that has emerged over recent years.

5.4 The empirical evidence

5.4.1 Psychoneuroimmunological studies of CHD risk

Psychoneuroimmunological research into CHD is not yet very advanced, but two basic methods have been used to address the possibility that psychosocial influences on the disease are mediated through inflammatory and thrombotic processes. The first is to discover whether inflammatory and thrombotic processes are sensitive to psychological stress by carrying out acute mental stress testing. This involves monitoring biological responses to emotional or behavioural tasks such as simulated public speaking, mental arithmetic, and problem solving. The advantage of this method is that sophisticated biological measures can be obtained under standardized experimental conditions in which the impact of extraneous factors such as physical activity, smoking, or age can be controlled. Mental stress testing has been used in the past to evaluate responses in haemodynamic variables such as blood pressure and heart rate, in neuroendocrine factors like cortisol, and in many other biological measures. Of course, these responses are acute and transient, and are obtained under artificial conditions. Nonetheless, individual differences in blood pressure reactions to standardized stress in the laboratory have been shown to predict the development of high blood pressure, while CHD patients who show stress-induced myocardial ischaemia are at increased risk for future cardiac events.[36,40]

The second research method is to study the inflammatory correlates of the psychosocial factors implicated in the aetiology of CHD in epidemiological or population cohorts. The hypothesis tested in these studies is that apparently healthy people who are exposed to psychosocial adversity will display increased inflammatory activity that might be indicative of the ongoing atherosclerotic process. Sometimes these two methods have been combined, assessing, for example, acute fibrinogen responses in people reporting high and low chronic work stress. Finally, these same methods can be applied to people with diagnosed CHD so as to discover whether stress-induced inflammatory responses are accentuated in people with more advanced atherosclerosis.

The following sections of this chapter will illustrate these methods and the findings that have been obtained so far.

5.4.2 Acute stress and vascular inflammatory responses

Acute psychological stress has been shown to alter several biological factors central to inflammation and atherosclerosis. For example, a stressful speech task induced transient endothelial dysfunction in healthy men for a period of up to 4 h post-stress.[41] Acute mental stress can also activate platelets and stimulate increases in circulating levels of inflammatory cytokines. Our group observed that mental stress induced by two behavioural tasks (colour–word interference and mirror tracing) caused significant increases in the number of circulating leucocyte–platelet aggregates, a sensitive marker of platelet activation, in a group of healthy men.[42] The same tasks also induced significant increases in plasma levels of the inflammatory cytokines IL-6 and IL-1Ra, as well as blood pressure and heart rate, in healthy volunteers.[43] Raised levels of cytokines persisted for 2 h following stress exposure, showing that even short-term stress can have prolonged physiological effects. A similar study found that a stressful interview caused increases in plasma IL-1β, IL-10, TNF-α, cortisol, and norepinephrine in a group of healthy women.[44] Another recent study demonstrated that psychological stress can affect cytokine production at the level of gene expression. Acute psychological stress induced increases in IL-1β gene expression in peripheral blood mononuclear cells of healthy volunteers, and these increases were positively associated with stress-induced elevations in plasma IL-6.[45]

Several studies have shown that acute psychological stressors (e.g. public speaking tasks) lead to a redistribution of leucocytes in the peripheral circulation of healthy individuals, so that there is a marked increase in the number of circulating leucocytes, the most pronounced increases occurring in the cytotoxic T-cell and natural killer (NK) cell subsets.[46] This rapid redistribution is thought to be mediated by altered expression of CAMs and by chemotaxis (selective attraction of leucocytes by chemokines). Notably, acute psychological stressors have been found to induce significant changes in the levels of adhesion molecules expressed on the surface of leucocytes. Specifically, acute psychological stress leads to (i) a preferential increase in the number of lymphocytes not expressing L-selectin (CD62L$^-$) versus CD62L$^+$ cells (especially among cytotoxic CD8+ T cells and NK cells), (ii) a decrease in the lymphocyte cell surface density of L-selectin, and (iii) an increase in the lymphocyte cell surface density of the integrins CD11a and macrophage associated antigen 1 (Mac-1).[47–49] Similarly, a number of studies have reported an increase in the number of circulating leucocytes expressing ICAM-1 following acute stress.[48,50] In addition, a recent study by

Redwine et al.[49] demonstrated that acute psychological stress increases chemotaxis of peripheral blood mononuclear cells in healthy volunteers. This is the first observation of such an effect in humans, although acute stress has previously been shown to increase mononuclear cell chemotaxis in rodents.[51]

It has been suggested that the increase in CD62L$^-$ leucocytes observed following acute stress is predominately due to a preferential release of CD62L$^-$ cells into the circulation.[52,53] However, Redwine et al.[49] also found that acute stress increased plasma levels of soluble L-selectin as well as increasing the number of circulating CD62L$^-$ cells. This indicates that shedding of L-selectin from the leucocyte cell surface may contribute to the increase in circulating CD62L$^-$ cells. Indeed, molecular biology studies suggest that activation of leucocytes leads to rapid shedding of L-selectin.[54] Shedding of L-selectin coincides with increased expression of the integrins CD11a and Mac-1 which are crucial for the process of leucocyte adhesion.[55] Supporting the idea of a shedding mechanism, a variety of acute psychological stressors (oral presentation, driving licence examination, dynamic exercise) have been found to increase soluble ICAM-1 levels in the plasma of healthy volunteers.[56,57]

Finally, acute mental stress activates haemostatic factors linked to inflammation and atherosclerosis. This literature has recently been reviewed, and shows that stress activates both coagulation (i.e. fibrinogen, factor VIII, or vWF) and fibrinolysis (i.e. tissue-type plasminogen activator) in healthy individuals.[58] It is thought that, in patients with atherosclerosis and impaired endothelial function, procoagulant responses to acute stressors outweigh anticoagulant mechanisms, thereby promoting a hypercoagulable state.

5.4.3 Psychosocial risk factors for CHD

5.4.3.1 Low socioeconomic position

The socioeconomic gradient in CHD is only partially accounted for by traditional risk factors and health-related behaviours such as smoking and food choice. Lower socio-economic position is thought to constitute a source of chronic psychological stress, with lower control at work, more negative social interactions, more crowding, and greater community stress.[59] Psychobiological pathways may play a significant role in mediating the association between low socioeconomic position and cardiovascular disease risk.

Several epidemiological studies have found a positive association between low socioeconomic position (as indexed by grade of employment, educational attainment, or income) and biological factors implicated in the inflammatory process. These associations persist after adjustment for traditional risk factors and health-related behaviours. For example, studies of the Whitehall II cohort (a sample of British civil servants who have been monitored since 1985 for cardiovascular disease) have demonstrated that higher plasma levels of the acute phase proteins CRP and fibrinogen are associated with lower socioeconomic status.[60,61] Analyses of other cohorts have found a similar association between fibrinogen and socioeconomic position.[62,63] People in lower socioeconomic positions have significantly higher levels of circulating heat shock protein 60 (Hsp 60) than their higher-status counterparts.[64] Human Hsp60 activates vascular endothelium, smooth muscle cells, and macrophages, thus promoting the pathophysiology of atherosclerosis. Associations are also present between lower socioeconomic position and haemostatic factors, including vWF, factor VIII, and plasma viscosity.[65,66] Furthermore, we have shown that platelet activation under resting conditions is heightened in lower status groups.[42]

Less is known about socioeconomic position and other immune parameters, but at least one study has shown raised total lymphocyte, T-lymphocyte, and NK cell counts in healthy lower-status individuals.[61] Analysis of a subsample of the Whitehall II cohort showed that plasma IL-6 concentration is higher in lower-status individuals,[67] and a random population sample from south London found a positive correlation between serum IL-6 concentrations and paternal socioeconomic background.[68]

Our group has investigated whether inflammatory responses to acute mental stress vary with socioeconomic position. In a recent study, we found that increases in plasma IL-6 following mental stress were prolonged in civil servants in lower occupational grades compared with their higher-grade counterparts.[69] It has also been shown that stress-induced increases in clotting factor VIII and blood viscosity are more prolonged in people from lower socioeconomic positions. One possibility is that repeated or chronic exposure to everyday life stressors primes the immune and cardiovascular systems so that subsequent exposure to challenge results in an exaggerated or more prolonged inflammatory/cardiovascular response. McEwen and Seeman[70] have argued that lower-status individuals experience chronic allostatic load (the damage to biological regulatory systems that occurs following repeated attempts to adapt to life's demands) which increases vulnerability to insulin resistance, obesity, and CHD.

5.4.3.2 Work stress

Several studies have now shown a positive association between work stress and levels of the acute phase protein fibrinogen. For example, a cross-sectional study of middle-aged women in Pittsburgh found that those experiencing high job stress had elevated plasma levels of fibrinogen.[71] Similarly, chronic work stress was associated with elevated levels of fibrinogen in a study of healthy middle-aged male middle managers in Germany, and comparable associations have been described in Sweden and Belgium.[72] A particularly interesting study in The Netherlands assessed the relationship between overcommitment at work (a pattern of high involvement and preoccupation with work) and clotting factors. Middle-aged white-collar workers with high overcommitment scores had impaired fibrinolytic systems, as reflected by decreased tissue-type plasminogen activator activity levels and increased PAI-1 antigen levels throughout the working week.[73] The association between overcommitment and fibrinolytic factors remained significant after controlling for conventional CHD risk factors.

Few studies have assessed the impact of chronic work stress on inflammatory responses to acute mental stress. Nevertheless, one study has examined fibrinogen levels and showed that men reporting low job control had larger stress-induced increases in fibrinogen than those with high control at work.[74]

5.4.3.3 Other forms of chronic strain

Several other forms of chronic or episodic life stress have been associated with raised circulating levels of the proinflammatory cytokine IL-6. A cross-sectional study of healthy older women found that the chronic stress of caring for a relative with Alzheimer's disease was associated with significant elevations in plasma IL-6, over and above the rise associated with normal ageing.[75] More recent work has found that, compared with non-caregivers, carers for dementing spouses had a fourfold higher rate of IL-6 increase over a period of 6 years.[76] This association was independent of relevant chronic health problems, medications, or health behaviours. Similarly, plasma IL-6 levels are elevated in people suffering from post-traumatic stress disorder, university students anticipating academic examinations, and people undergoing driving examinations.[77–79]

5.4.3.4 Social support and social networks

Social support and social networks are distinct though overlapping constructs. Social supports are interactions that provide emotional, confiding, and practical support, and may help to buffer the impact of psychosocial stress. Social networks refer to the size, diversity, and reciprocal nature of social contacts, and socially isolated individuals are those with small social networks.[80] Associations between positive social contact and lower fibrinogen levels have been described. For example, in two studies of employed middle-aged adults, fibrinogen was negatively associated with the extent of participation in pleasurable social activities in men[62] and with perceived support from the boss in women,[71] after controlling for smoking, body mass, physical activity, socioeconomic status, and cholesterol. In contrast, negative or socially undermining relationships involving criticism, intrusiveness, and exploitation have been related to elevated fibrinogen.[81] As might be expected, greater social isolation is positively correlated with fibrinogen.[74] Another cardiovascular risk factor which has been linked with social isolation is Hsp60, since Lewthwaite et al.[64] found higher plasma Hsp60 levels in more socially isolated people.

There is substantial evidence that social support and social isolation relate to cardiovascular and neuroendocrine stress responsivity.[82] However, studies relating these factors to inflammatory responses have been limited. A recent analysis of data from 240 participants in the Whitehall II study found that loneliness, a psychological experience related to social isolation and perceived lack of companionship, was associated with heightened fibrinogen and NK cell responses to an acute laboratory stressor, independently of covariates.[83] Other laboratory studies have attempted to model the impact of social support by comparing the physiological reactions of people tested in isolation with those tested in the presence of supporting others. Responses varied according to the participant's relationship with the supporting individual, with reduced physiological responsivity when support was active and encouraging rather than being conveyed passively by mere presence during testing.[84]

5.4.3.5 Depression and anxiety

The literature relating depression and anxiety to immune and inflammatory processes will not be detailed here, since it is addressed in Chapter 10. The impact of depression on prognosis of patients with established CHD is discussed in section 5.3.6.

5.4.4 Pathways mediating the effect of psychosocial factors on inflammation

There is robust evidence from epidemiological studies and acute stress studies that psychosocial stress activates the inflammatory system. However, the biochemical pathways mediating these effects are not well understood. Psychological stress stimulates the sympathetic nervous system (SNS), which regulates heart rate and release of catecholamines, and the hypothalamic–pituitary–adrenal (HPA) axis, which regulates release of corticosteroids.

The effects of acute stress on leucocyte redistribution and adhesion molecule expression are thought to be driven by the SNS, since they can be mimicked by infusion of the β-adrenergic agonist isoproterenol and diminished by the β-blocker propanolol in healthy individuals.[52,85] A meta-analysis of eight studies of women found that stress-induced increases in NK cell counts were consistently correlated with heart rate responses to stress.[86] Furthermore, a study by Farag et al.[87] showed that decreased leucocyte expression of L-selectin in response to acute stress occurred predominantly in individuals whose blood pressure responses to an acute stressor were caused by an elevation in cardiac output (cardiac reactors) rather than by increased peripheral resistance (vascular reactors). Since cardiac output is mediated by β-adrenergic receptor activation whereas peripheral resistance is mediated by activation of α-adrenergic receptors, these results support the idea that stress-induced reduction in leucocyte L-selectin expression is mediated by β-adrenergic activation. Further evidence for a role of β-adrenergic receptors in stress-induced leucocytosis comes from the recent study by Redwine et al.[49] who found that stress-induced increases in catecholamine levels were positively associated with lymphocyte expression of Mac-1 and negatively associated with L-selectin expression. This suggests that the stress-induced alteration in the expression of these adhesion molecules is mediated by adrenergic receptors.

Similar observations have been made for stress-induced activation of platelets and cytokines. Increases in leucocyte–platelet aggregates following stress are associated with systolic blood pressure stress responsivity.[42] Increases in cytokines such as IL-6, TNF-α, and IL-1Ra in response to acute stress have been found to correlate with cardiovascular stress responses,[43,88] and we recently found that stress-induced increases in leucocyte IL-1β gene expression were positively correlated with heart rate reactivity.[45] Accordingly, infusion with the β-adrenergic agonist isoproterenol induced increases in plasma IL-6 in a group of healthy volunteers.[89]

One mechanism which might be mediating the cytokine response to stress is activation of nuclear factor κB (NF-κB). NF-κB is a transcription factor which upregulates the expression of a number of inflammatory molecules including cytokines. Acute psychological stress has been shown to upregulate NF-κB expression in peripheral blood mononuclear cells of healthy volunteers.[90] Increases in NF-κB expression paralleled stress-induced increases in catecholamines and cortisol, suggesting that both sympathetic and HPA pathways were involved in this response. In contrast, other studies have reported that catecholamines and corticosteroids inhibit the production of cytokines from mononuclear cells. One recent study found that the capacity of a synthetic glucocorticoid hormone to suppress *in vitro* production of IL-6 was significantly reduced in blood samples taken from adults under serious stress (parents of children with cancer) compared with controls.[91] The authors suggested that one mechanism through which chronic stress raises IL-6 levels might be impairment of the immune system's capacity to respond to hormonal signals that terminate inflammation. Other stress-responsive neuroendocrine mediators which could participate in inflammatory responses to stress are substance P and angiotensin II, which stimulate cytokine production from mononuclear cells. This area of research is rapidly evolving, and it is likely that new findings will clarify these mechanisms over the next few years.

5.4.5 Psychoneuroimmunological responses in CHD patients

Psychoneuroimmunological studies of cardiac patients are complicated by two factors. First, patients with CHD already have activated inflammatory systems by virtue of their clinical condition, and so discriminating the influence of psychological factors is difficult. Secondly, CHD patients are typically medicated with drugs such as aspirin and statins, both of which have anti-inflammatory effects. They are frequently prescribed cardioprotective β-blockers as well, and these reduce sympathetic nervous system activation.

There is a large literature concerning cardiovascular and neuroendocrine responses related to stress and other psychosocial factors in CHD patients, but rather little involving psychoneuroimmunological processes. One recent study assessed the white blood cell counts in a group of patients admitted to hospital with acute coronary syndromes. The percentage of monocytes was positively correlated with hostility and negatively correlated with emotional support.[92] This result is intriguing although, given the small and heterogenous sample, it deserves exploration in a larger group of patients.

Another set of relevant findings has related psychosocial factors with platelet activation. As noted in section 5.2, platelets are central to the formation of thrombi and the blockage of diseased arteries in acute coronary syndromes. Unfortunately, comparisons of stress-induced platelet activation in patients with coronary artery disease and healthy controls have produced variable results, with greater or more prolonged responses from patients in some studies but not in others[93,94] This variability may relate to the different procedures used for controlling medication effects in samples of cardiac patients.

5.4.6 Depression in acute coronary syndromes

The topic that has attracted the greatest attention in clinical studies of CHD over recent years is depression. Depression has emerged as a critical issue in patients admitted to hospital with myocardial infarction or unstable angina. It is not surprising that many patients are upset when they experience a life-threatening cardiac episode requiring hospital admission, and transient anxiety and depression are common. However, more than 15 studies have now demonstrated that these emotional responses are not innocent, since patients experiencing depressive symptoms 4–7 days post-admission are at increased risk for poor clinical outcomes.[95,96] For example, Lésperance et al.[97] measured depression using the Beck Depression Inventory in 430 patients admitted to hospital with unstable angina. Patients with elevated depression scores were more than four times more likely to die or sustain a non-fatal myocardial infarction over the following 12 months than non-depressed patients, with differences remaining significant after controlling for clinical disease severity and other cofactors. This association has not been universally observed,[98,99] and some investigators have argued that the apparent influence of depression is due to residual confounding with severity of clinical condition.[100] Nonetheless, the relationship is thought sufficiently robust to warrant attempts to improve cardiac prognosis by reducing depression, and studies of cognitive–behavioural and pharmacological treatments have now been carried out.[101,102]

A number of mechanisms linking depression in cardiac patients to poor prognosis have been proposed, including disturbed autonomic nervous system tone and failure of adherence to medication.[96] However, in view of the associations between depression, immune responses, and inflammation described in Chapter 10, a serious possibility is that depression accentuates vascular inflammation, thereby impairing cardiac health.

Several lines of evidence support this possibility. Physiological measures of the vascular endothelium have shown impairments in endothelial function in depressed people in the community and in those with clinically diagnosed depression.[67,103] Cardiac patients who report vital exhaustion—a syndrome of fatigue and low mood that is closely associated with depression—have been shown to have higher levels of serum IL-1β, TNF-α, and IL-6 than non-exhausted patients.[104] Apparently healthy individuals with vital exhaustion also have elevated IL-6 and IL-1Ra, together with raised fibrinogen and markers of fibrinolysis.[105] Another study of vitally exhausted men showed particularly impaired fibrinolytic capacity in the early morning.[106] Reduced fibrinolysis implies that thrombus formation could be enhanced. It is interesting that the onset of acute cardiac events also peaks in the early morning, as does the plasma IL-6 circadian rhythm. Disturbances in inflammatory processes related to psychosocial factors might contribute to this diurnal pattern.

Associations have been described between depression and inflammatory markers. For example, Miller *et al.*[107] compared 50 depressed with 50 non-depressed men and women, and found that depressed participants had higher C-reactive protein and IL-6 levels, particularly if they were also overweight or obese. Associations between IL-6 and depressive symptoms within the subclinical range have also been described,[108] although the findings across studies have been mixed.[109,110] Recently, a study of cardiac patients with major depression documented elevations in sICAM-1 levels, although not in IL-6, after adjustment for potential confounders.[111]

Platelet activation is also related to depression. Platelet reactivity is known to be heightened in major depression, probably through serotonergic pathways.[112] Depressed post-myocardial infarction patients also have signs of heightened platelet activation.[113] This mechanism is potentially amenable to therapy, since selective serotonin-reuptake inhibitor (SSRI) antidepressants reduce platelet activation in post-infarction depressed patients.[114] Unfortunately, the one study published to date which assessed the use of SSRIs in the management of depression in cardiac patients showed no significant effects on cardiac prognosis.[102] Nevertheless, the sample size in this study was not large, and it is an intriguing possibility that treating depression in cardiac patients may be beneficial not because of antidepressant effects, but because of influences on inflammatory processes.

5.5 **Future directions and conclusions**

CHD is a comparatively new topic for investigation with psychoneuroimmunological methods. However, the ascendancy of the inflammatory model of the underlying disease atherosclerosis has stimulated the field over the last few years. The way in which the pathways described in this chapter might operate is summarized in Figure 5.1. It should be emphasized that evidence is preliminary, and our understanding is likely to evolve substantially over the coming decade. Nevertheless, psychoneuroimmunological methods have already contributed to knowledge about the pathways mediating psychosocial influences on CHD aetiology, and they also have implications for the management of patients with established CHD.

Acknowledgements

The preparation of this chapter was supported by the British Heart Foundation and the Medical Research Council.

References

1 Kop WJ (2003). The integration of cardiovascular behavioral medicine and psychoneuroimmunology: new developments based on converging research fields. *Brain Behav Immun* **17**: 233–7.

2 Greenland P, Knoll MD, Stamler J, *et al.* (2003). Major risk factors as antecedents of fatal and nonfatal coronary heart disease events. *JAMA* **290**: 891–7.

3 Ross R (1999). Atherosclerosis—an inflammatory disease. *N Engl J Med* **340**: 115–26.

4 Glass CK, Witztum JL (2001). Atherosclerosis. the road ahead. *Cell* **104**: 503–16.

5 Mann DL (2003). Stress-activated cytokines and the heart: from adaptation to maladaptation. *Annu Rev Physiol* **65**: 81–101.

6 Hackam DG, Anand SS (2003). Emerging risk factors for atherosclerotic vascular disease: a critical review of the evidence. *JAMA* **290**: 932–40.

7 Libby P, Ridker PM, Maseri A (2002). Inflammation and atherosclerosis. *Circulation* **105**: 1135–43.

8 Danesh J, Whincup P, Walker M, *et al.* (2000). Low grade inflammation and coronary heart disease: prospective study and updated meta-analyses. *BMJ* **321**: 199–204.

9 Lind L (2003). Circulating markers of inflammation and atherosclerosis. *Atherosclerosis* **169**: 203–14.

10 Cesari M, Penninx BW, Newman AB, *et al.* (2003). Inflammatory markers and onset of cardiovascular events: results from the Health ABC study. *Circulation* **108**: 2317–22.

11 Danesh J, Collins R, Appleby P, Peto R (1998). Association of fibrinogen, C-reactive protein, albumin, or leukocyte count with coronary heart disease: meta-analyses of prospective studies. *JAMA* **279**: 1477–82.

12 Ridker PM, Hennekens CH, Buring JE, Rifai N (2000). C-reactive protein and other markers of inflammation in the prediction of cardiovascular disease in women. *N Engl J Med* **342**: 836–43.

13 Danesh J, Collins R, Peto R, Lowe GD (2000). Haematocrit, viscosity, erythrocyte sedimentation rate: meta-analyses of prospective studies of coronary heart disease. *Eur Heart J* **21**: 515–20.

14 Danesh J, Whincup P, Walker M, Lennon L, Thomson A, Appleby P (2001). Fibrin D-dimer and coronary heart disease: prospective study and meta-analysis. *Circulation* **103**: 2323–7.

15 Whincup PH, Danesh J, Walker M, *et al.* (2002). von Willebrand factor and coronary heart disease: prospective study and meta-analysis. *Eur Heart J* **23**: 1764–70.

16 Lindmark E, Diderholm E, Wallentin L, Siegbahn A (2001). Relationship between interleukin 6 and mortality in patients with unstable coronary artery disease: effects of an early invasive or noninvasive strategy. *JAMA* **286**: 2107–13.

17 Biasucci LM, Liuzzo G, Fantuzzi G, *et al.* (1999). Increasing levels of interleukin (IL)-1Ra and IL-6 during the first 2 days of hospitalization in unstable angina are associated with increased risk of in-hospital coronary events. *Circulation* **99**: 2079–84.

18 Ridker PM, Rifai N, Pfeffer M, Sacks F, Lepage S, Braunwald E (2000). Elevation of tumor necrosis factor-alpha and increased risk of recurrent coronary events after myocardial infarction. *Circulation* **101**: 2149–53.

19 Danesh J, Peto R (1998). Risk factors for coronary heart disease and infection with *Helicobacter pylori*: meta-analysis of 18 studies. *BMJ* **316**: 1130–2.

20 Danesh J, Whincup P, Lewington S, *et al.* (2002). Chlamydia pneumoniae IgA titres and coronary heart disease; prospective study and meta-analysis. *Eur Heart J* **23**: 371–5.

21 Cercek B, Shah PK, Noc M, *et al.* (2003). Effect of short-term treatment with azithromycin on recurrent ischaemic events in patients with acute coronary syndrome in the Azithromycin in Acute Coronary Syndrome (AZACS) trial: a randomised controlled trial. *Lancet* **361**: 809–13.

22 Epstein SE, Zhou YF, Zhu J (1999). Infection and atherosclerosis: emerging mechanistic paradigms. *Circulation* **100**: e20–8.

23 Zhu J, Nieto FJ, Horne BD, Anderson JL, Muhlestein JB, Epstein SE (2001). Prospective study of pathogen burden and risk of myocardial infarction or death. *Circulation* **103**: 45–51.

24 Espinola-Klein C, Rupprecht HJ, Blankenberg S, *et al.* (2002). Impact of infectious burden on extent and long-term prognosis of atherosclerosis. *Circulation* **105**: 15–21.

25 Institute of Medicine (2001). *Health and Behavior: The Interplay of Biological, Behavioral, and Societal Influences.* Washington, DC: National Academy of Sciences.

26 Stansfeld SA, Marmot MG (eds) (2002). *Stress and the Heart: Psychosocial Pathways to Coronary Heart Disease.* London: BMJ Books.

27 Hemingway H, Kuper H, Marmot M (2003). Psychosocial factors in the primary and secondary prevention of coronary heart disease: an updated systematic review of prospective cohort studies. In Yusuf S, Cairns JA, Camm AJ, Fallen EL, Gersh BJ (eds) *Evidence-Based Cardiology* (2nd edn). London: BMJ Books, 181–218.

28 Kaplan GA, Keil JE (1993). Socioeconomic factors and cardiovascular disease: a review of the literature. *Circulation* **88**: 1973–98.

29 Kivimaki M, Leino-Arjas P, Luukkonen R, Riihimaki H, Vahtera J, Kirjonen J (2002). Work stress and risk of cardiovascular mortality: prospective cohort study of industrial employees. *BMJ* **325**: 857.

30 Schnall PL, Belkic K, Landsbergis P, Baker D (eds) (2000). *The Workplace and Cardiovascular Disease. Occupational Medicine State of the Art Reviews.* Philadelphia, PA: Hanley & Belfus.

31 Lee S, Colditz GA, Berkman LF, Kawachi I (2003). Caregiving and risk of coronary heart disease in US women: a prospective study. *Am J Prev Med* **24**: 113–19.

32 Diez Roux AV, Merkin SS, Arnett D, *et al.* (2001). Neighborhood of residence and incidence of coronary heart disease. *N Engl J Med* **345**: 99–106.

33 Berkman LF, Leo-Summers L, Horwitz RI (1992). Emotional support and survival after myocardial infarction. *Ann Intern Med* **117**: 1003–9.

34 Ferketich AK, Schwartzbaum JA, Frid DJ, Moeschberger ML (2000). Depression as an antecedent to heart disease among women and men in the NHANES I study. *Ann Intern Med* **160**: 1261–8.

35 Miller TQ, Smith TW, Turner CW, Guijarro ML, Hallet AJ (1996). A meta-analytic review of research on hostility and physical health. *Psychol Bull* **119**: 322–48.

36 Strike PC, Steptoe A (2003). Systematic review of mental stress-induced myocardial ischaemia. *Eur Heart J* **24**: 690–703.

37 Leor J, Poole WK, Kloner RA (1996). Sudden cardiac death triggered by an earthquake. *N Engl J Med* **334**: 413–19.

38 Mittleman MA, Maclure M, Sherwood JB, *et al.* (1995). Triggering of acute myocardial infarction onset by episodes of anger. *Circulation* **92**: 1720–5.

39 Hemingway H, Malik M, Marmot M (2001). Social and psychosocial influences on sudden cardiac death, ventricular arrhythmia and cardiac autonomic function. *Eur Heart J* **22**: 1082–1101.

40 Treiber FA, Kamarck T, Schneiderman N, Sheffield D, Kapuku G, Taylor T (2003). Cardiovascular reactivity and development of preclinical and clinical disease states. *Psychosom Med* **65**: 46–62.

41 Ghiadoni L, Donald AE, Cropley M, *et al.* (2000). Mental stress induces transient endothelial dysfunction in humans. *Circulation* **102**: 2473–8.

42 Steptoe A, Magid K, Edwards S, Brydon L, Hong Y, Erusalimsky J (2003). The influence of psychological stress and socioeconomic status on platelet activation in men. *Atherosclerosis* **168**: 57–63.

43 Steptoe A, Willemsen G, Owen N, Flower L, Mohamed-Ali V (2001). Acute mental stress elicits delayed increases in circulating inflammatory cytokine levels. *Clin Sci* **101**: 185–92.

44 Altemus M, Rao B, Dhabhar FS, Ding W, Granstein RD (2001). Stress-induced changes in skin barrier function in healthy women. *J Invest Dermatol* **117**: 309–17.

45 Brydon L, *et al.* (In press). Psychological stress activates interleukin-1 beta gene expression in human mononuclear cells. *Brain Behav Immun*.

46 Zorrilla EP, Luborsky L, McKay JR, *et al.* (2001). The relationship of depression and stressors to immunological assays: a meta-analytic review. *Brain Behav Immun* **15**: 199–226.

47 Mills PJ, Dimsdale JE (1996). The effects of acute psychologic stress on cellular adhesion molecules. *J Psychosom Res* **41**: 49–53.

48 Goebel MU, Mills PJ (2000). Acute psychological stress and exercise and changes in peripheral leukocyte adhesion molecule expression and density. *Psychosom Med* **62**: 664–70.

49 Redwine L, Snow S, Mills P, Irwin M (2003). Acute psychological stress: effects on chemotaxis and cellular adhesion molecule expression. *Psychosom Med* **65**: 598–603.

50 Mills PJ, Maisel AS, Ziegler MG, *et al.* (2000). Peripheral blood mononuclear cell-endothelial adhesion in human hypertension following exercise. *J Hypertens* **18**: 1801–6.

51 Dhabhar FS, McEwen BS (1999). Enhancing versus suppressive effects of stress hormones on skin immune function. *Proc Natl Acad Sci USA* **96**: 1059–64.

52 Mills PJ, Goebel M, Rehman J, Irwin MR, Maisel AS (2000). Leukocyte adhesion molecule expression and T cell naive/memory status following isoproterenol infusion. *J Neuroimmunol* **102**: 137–44.

53 Dopp JM, Miller GE, Myers HF, Fahey JL (2000). Increased natural killer-cell mobilization and cytotoxicity during marital conflict. *Brain Behav Immun* **14**: 10–26.

54 Marschner S, Freiberg BA, Kupfer A, Hunig T, Finkel TH (1999). Ligation of the CD4 receptor induces activation-independent down-regulation of L-selectin. *Proc Natl Acad Sci USA* **96**: 9763–8.

55 Tohya K, Kimura M (1998). Ultrastructural evidence of distinctive behavior of L-selectin and LFA-1 (alphaLbeta2 integrin) on lymphocytes adhering to the endothelial surface of high endothelial venules in peripheral lymph nodes. *Histochem Cell Biol* **110**: 407–16.

56 Dugue B, Leppanen E, Grasbeck R (1999). Preanalytical factors (biological variation) and the measurement of serum soluble intercellular adhesion molecule-1 in humans: influence of the time of day, food intake, and physical and psychological stress. *Clin Chem* **45**: 1543–7.

57 Heinz A, Hermann D, Smolka MN, *et al.* (2003). Effects of acute psychological stress on adhesion molecules, interleukins and sex hormones: implications for coronary heart disease. *Psychopharmacology* **165**: 111–17.

58 von Kanel R, Mills PJ, Fainman C, Dimsdale JE (2001). Effects of psychological stress and psychiatric disorders on blood coagulation and fibrinolysis: a biobehavioral pathway to coronary artery disease? *Psychosom Med* **63**: 531–44.

59 Evans GW, Kantrowitz E (2002). Socioeconomic status and health: the potential role of environmental risk exposure. *Annu Rev Public Health* **23**: 303–31.

60 Brunner E, Davey Smith G, Marmot M, Canner R, Beksinska M, O'Brien J (1996). Childhood social circumstances and psychosocial and behavioural factors as determinants of plasma fibrinogen. *Lancet* **347**: 1008–13.

61 Owen N, Poulton T, Hay FC, Mohamed-Ali V, Steptoe A (2003). Socioeconomic status, C-reactive protein, immune factors, and responses to acute mental stress. *Brain Behav Immun* **17**: 286–95.

62 Rosengren A, Wilhelmsen L, Welin L, Tsipogianni A, Teger-Nilsson AC, Wedel H (1990). Social influences and cardiovascular risk factors as determinants of plasma fibrinogen concentration in a general population sample of middle aged men. *BMJ* **300**: 634–8.

63 Wilson TW, Kaplan GA, Kauhanen J, *et al.* (1993). Association between plasma fibrinogen concentration and five socioeconomic indices in the Kuopio Ischemic Heart Disease Risk Factor Study. *Am J Epidemiol* **137**: 292–300.

64 Lewthwaite J, Owen N, Coates A, Henderson B, Steptoe A (2002). Circulating human heat shock protein 60 in the plasma of British civil servants: relationship to physiological and psychosocial stress. *Circulation* **106**: 196–201.

65 Kumari M, Marmot M, Brunner E (2000). Social determinants of von Willebrand factor: the Whitehall II study. *Arterioscler Thromb Vasc Biol* **20**: 1842–7.

66 Wamala SP, Murray MA, Horsten M, *et al.* (1999). Socioeconomic status and determinants of hemostatic function in healthy women. *Arterioscler Thromb Vasc Biol* **19**: 485–92.

67 Hemingway H, Shipley M, Mullen MJ, *et al.* (2003). Social and psychosocial influences on inflammatory markers and vascular function in civil servants (the Whitehall II study). *Am J Cardiol* **92**: 984–7.

68 Mendall MA, Patel P, Asante M, *et al.* (1997). Relation of serum cytokine concentrations to cardiovascular risk factors and coronary heart disease. *Heart* **78**: 273–7.

69 Brydon L, Edwards S, Mohamed-Ali V, Steptoe A (2004). Socioeconomic status and stress-induced increases in interleukin-6. *Brain Behav Immun* **18**: 281–90.

70 McEwen BS, Seeman T (1999). Protective and damaging effects of mediators of stress: elaborating and testing the concepts of allostasis and allostatic load. *Ann NY Acad Sci* **896**: 30–47.

71 Davis MC, Matthews KA, Meilahn EN, Kiss JE (1995). Are job characteristics related to fibrinogen levels in middle-aged women? *Health Psychol* **14**: 310–18.

72 Kittel F, Leynen F, Stam M, *et al.* (2002). Job conditions and fibrinogen in 14226 Belgian workers: the Belstress study. *Eur Heart J* **23**: 1841–8.

73 Vrijkotte TG, van Doornen LJ, de Geus EJ (1999). Work stress and metabolic and hemostatic risk factors. *Psychosom Med* **61**: 796–805.

74 Steptoe A, Kunz-Ebrecht S, Owen N, *et al.* (2003). Influence of socioeconomic status and job control on plasma fibrinogen responses to acute mental stress. *Psychosom Med* **65**: 137–44.

75 Lutgendorf SK, Garand L, Buckwalter KC, Reimer TT, Hong S-Y, Lubaroff DM (1999). Life stress, mood disturbance, and elevated interleukin-6 in healthy older women. *J Gerontol: Med Sci* **54A**: M434–9.

76 Kiecolt-Glaser JK, Preacher KJ, MacCallum RC, Atkinson C, Malarkey WB, Glaser R (2003). Chronic stress and age-related increases in the proinflammatory cytokine IL-6. *Proc Natl Acad Sci USA* **100**: 9090–5.

77 Maes M, Song C, Lin A, *et al.* (1998). The effects of psychological stress on humans: increased production of pro-inflammatory cytokines and a Th1-like response in stress-induced anxiety. *Cytokine* **10**: 313–18.

78 Maes M, Lin AH, Delmeire L, *et al.* (1999). Elevated serum interleukin-6 (IL-6) and IL-6 receptor concentrations in posttraumatic stress disorder following accidental man-made traumatic events. *Biol Psychiatry* **45**: 833–9.

79 Dugue B, Leppanen E, Grasbeck R, Benoit D, Esa L, Ralph G (2001). The driving license examination as a stress model: effects on blood picture, serum cortisol and the production of interleukins in man. *Life Sci* **68**: 1641–7.

80 Berkman LF, Glass TA (2000). Social integration, social networks, social support and health. In Berkman LF, Kawachi I (eds) *Social Epidemiology*. New York: Oxford University Press, 137–73.

81 Davis MC, Swan PD (1999). Association of negative and positive social ties with fibrinogen levels in young women. *Health Psychol* **18**: 131–9.

82 Uchino BN, Cacioppo JT, Kiecolt-Glaser JK (1996). The relationship between social support and physiological processes: a review with emphasis on underlying mechanisms and implications for health. *Psychol Bull* **119**: 488–531.

83 Steptoe A, Owen N, Kunz-Ebrecht S, Brydon L (2004). Loneliness and neuroendocrine, cardiovascular, and inflammatory stress responses in middle-aged men and women. *Psychoneuroendocrinology* **29**: 593–611.

84 Lepore SJ (1998). Problems and prospects for the social support—reactivity hypothesis. *Ann Behav Med* **20**: 257–69.

85 Benschop RJ, Rodriguez-Feuerhahn M, Schedlowski M (1996). Catecholamine-induced leukocytosis: early observations, current research, and future directions. *Brain Behav Immun* **10**: 77–91.

86 Benschop RJ, Greenen R, Mills PJ, *et al.* (1998). Cardiovascular and immune responses to acute psychological stress in young and old women: a meta-analysis. *Psychosom Med* **60**: 290–6.

87 Farag NH, Nelesen RA, Dimsdale JE, Loredo JS, Mills PJ (2002). The effects of acute psychological stress on lymphocyte adhesion molecule expression and density in cardiac versus vascular reactors. *Brain Behav Immun* **16**: 411–20.

88 Owen N, Steptoe A (2003). Natural killer cell and proinflammatory cytokine responses to mental stress: associations with heart rate and heart rate variability. *Biol Psychol* **63**: 101–15.

89 Mohamed-Ali V, Flower L, Sethi J, *et al.* (2001). Beta-adrenergic regulation of IL-6 release from adipose tissue: In vivo and in vitro studies. *J Clin Endocrinol Metab* **86**: 5864–9.

90 Bierhaus A, Wolf J, Andrassy M, *et al.* (2003). A mechanism converting psychosocial stress into mononuclear cell activation. *Proc Natl Acad Sci USA* **100**: 1920–5.

91 Miller GE, Cohen S, Ritchey AK (2002). Chronic psychological stress and the regulation of pro-inflammatory cytokines: a glucocorticoid-resistance model. *Health Psychol* **21**: 531–41.

92 Gidron Y, Armon T, Gilutz H, Huleihel M (2003). Psychological factors correlate meaningfully with percent-monocytes among acute coronary syndrome patients. *Brain Behav Immun* **17**: 310–15.

93 Wallen NH, Held C, Rehnqvist N, Hjemdahl P (1997). Effects of mental and physical stress on platelet function in patients with stable angina pectoris and healthy controls. *Eur Heart J* **18**: 807–15.

94 Steptoe A, Strike P, Magid K, *et al.* (2003). Mental stress-induced platelet activation and increases in C-reactive protein concentration in coronary artery disease. In Lewis BS, Halon DA, Flugelman MY, Gensini GF (eds) *Frontiers in Coronary Artery Disease*. Bologna: Monduzzi Editore, Bologna.

95 Ziegelstein RC (2001). Depression in patients recovering from a myocardial infarction. *JAMA* **286**: 1621–7.

96 Carney RM, Freedland KE, Miller GE, Jaffe AS (2002). Depression as a risk factor for cardiac mortality and morbidity: a review of potential mechanisms. *J Psychosom Res* **53**: 897–902.

97 Lésperance F, Frasure-Smith N, Juneau M, Theroux P (2000). Depression and 1-year prognosis in unstable angina. *Ann Intern Med* **160**: 1354–60.

98 Mayou RA, Gill D, Thompson DR, *et al.* (2000). Depression and anxiety as predictors of outcome after myocardial infarction. *Psychosom Med* **62**: 212–19.

99 Lane D, Carroll D, Ring C, Beevers DG, Lip GY (2001). Mortality and quality of life 12 months after myocardial infarction: effects of depression and anxiety. *Psychosom Med* **63**: 221–30.

100 Lane D, Carroll D, Ring C, Beevers DG, Lip GY (2002). In-hospital symptoms of depression do not predict mortality 3 years after myocardial infarction. *Int J Epidemiol* **31**: 1179–82.

101 Berkman LF, Blumenthal J, Burg M, *et al.* (2003). Effects of treating depression and low perceived social support on clinical events after myocardial infarction: the Enhancing Recovery in Coronary Heart Disease Patients (ENRICHD) Randomized Trial. *JAMA* **289**: 3106–16.

102 Glassman AH, O'Connor CM, Califf RM, *et al.* (2002). Sertraline treatment of major depression in patients with acute MI or unstable angina. *JAMA* **288**: 701–9.

103 Broadley AJ, Korszun A, Jones CJ, Frenneaux MP (2002). Arterial endothelial function is impaired in treated depression. *Heart* **88**: 521–3.

104 Appels A, Bar FW, Bar J, Bruggeman C, de Baets M (2000). Inflammation, depressive symptomatology, and coronary artery disease. *Psychosom Med* **62**: 601–5.

105 Van Der Ven A, Van Diest R, Hamulyak K, Maes M, Bruggeman C, Appels A (2003). Herpes viruses, cytokines, and altered hemostasis in vital exhaustion. *Psychosom Med* **65**: 194–200.

106 van Diest R, Hamulyak K, Kop WJ, van Zandvoort C, Appels A (2002). Diurnal variations in coagulation and fibrinolysis in vital exhaustion. *Psychosom Med* **64**: 787–92.

107 Miller GE, Stetler CA, Carney RM, Freedland KE, Banks WA (2002). Clinical depression and inflammatory risk markers for coronary heart disease. *Am J Cardiol* **90**: 1279–83.

108 Dentino AN, Pieper CF, Rao MK, *et al.* (1999). Association of interleukin-6 and other biologic variables with depression in older people living in the community. *J Am Geriatr Soc* **47**: 6–11.

109 Kop WJ, Gottdiener JS, Tangen CM, *et al.* (2002). Inflammation and coagulation factors in persons >65 years of age with symptoms of depression but without evidence of myocardial ischemia. *Am J Cardiol* **89**: 419–24.

110 Steptoe A, Kunz-Ebrecht SR, Owen N (2003). Lack of association between depressive symptoms and markers of immune and vascular inflammation in middle-aged men and women. *Psychol Med* **33**: 667–74.

111 Lésperance F, Frasure-Smith N, Theroux P, Irwin M (2004). The association between major depression, sICAM-1, interleukin-6 and CRP in patients with recent acute coronary syndromes. *Am J Psychiatry* **161**: 271–7.

112 Shimbo D, Child J, Davidson K, *et al.* (2002). Exaggerated serotonin-mediated platelet reactivity as a possible link in depression and acute coronary syndromes. *Am J Cardiol* **89**: 331–3.

113 Kuijpers PM, Hamulyak K, Strik JJ, Wellens HJ, Honig A (2002). Beta-thromboglobulin and platelet factor 4 levels in post-myocardial infarction patients with major depression. *Psychiatry Res* **109**: 207–10.

114 Serebruany VL, Glassman AH, Malinin AI, *et al.* (2003). Platelet/endothelial biomarkers in depressed patients treated with the selective serotonin reuptake inhibitor sertraline after acute coronary events: the Sertraline AntiDepressant Heart Attack Randomized Trial (SADHART) Platelet Substudy. *Circulation* **108**: 939–44.

Chapter 6

Psychoneuroimmunology and chronic malignant disease: cancer

Leslie G. Walker, Victoria L. Green, John Greenman, Andrew A. Walker, and Donald M. Sharp

6.1 Introduction

Cancer is a common disease. It has been estimated that one in every three people in the West will develop cancer, and that one in every four will die from it. Although some cancers can now be cured and treatment can significantly improve the prognosis for many others, the word 'cancer' continues to carry the automatic connotations of pain, loss of dignity, and early death. In addition to the diagnosis itself, treatments are often stressful, and their side effects can have adverse effects on quality of life.

Many patients with cancer now use complementary and alternative medicines (CAMs) to help them to cope with the diagnosis, treatment and prognosis. Estimates of the use of CAMs by cancer patients in the United Kingdom have ranged from 32% in patients undergoing radiotherapy[1] to 16% in unselected oncology patients.[2] In a recent nationally representative telephone random survey of 1204 British adults, 20% had used a complementary treatment in the previous 12 months, and this extrapolates to an annual national expenditure of £1.6 billion.[3] Specifically, many people now pursue these methods specifically to 'boost' their immune system, often encouraged by the media who legitimize these practices in terms of 'the findings of psychoneuroimmunology'.[4]

Therefore the overall aim of this chapter is to provide an objective 'state of the art' resumé of the psychoneuroimmunology of cancer. Having discussed the theoretical basis, and empirical evidence, directions for future psychoneuroimmunological cancer research will then be outlined.

6.2 The biological/clinical context

6.2.1 The nature and prevalence of cancer

The term 'cancer' does not apply to a single disease; rather, it refers to a heterogeneous collection of approximately 200 different diseases, reflecting the multitude of distinct tissues and cell types in humans. Essentially, a cancer forms when cells within the body do not respond appropriately to chemical messages signalling them to stop growing and dividing; the resulting lump is known as a tumour. In addition to uncontrolled proliferation, these cells may gain the ability to spread from their original anatomical site to other organs of the body, where their unchecked growth can form new deposits or metastases. The four most common forms of cancer are lung, breast, colorectal, and prostate.

In 2004, approximately 136 000 people in the USA are expected to develop some form of cancer. In 2001, the latest year for which accurate mortality statistics are available, 553 000 people died from cancer in the USA. This represents 23% of all deaths in the USA, and is second only to deaths from heart disease.[5]

6.2.2 Modern approaches to cancer management

As one would expect for a complex and often disseminated disease, treatments are frequently employed in combination. Conventional treatments include surgery, chemotherapy, radiotherapy, and biological response modifiers. Although every cancer is subtly different, the earlier a growth can be detected, the greater the probability of effective treatment. For example, patients undergoing treatment for early colorectal cancer (Duke's A) have a 5-year survival rate in excess of 95%, whereas patients with advanced disseminated Duke's D tumours have a survival rate of less than 10% at 5 years.[5]

The underlying premise upon which chemotherapy and radiotherapy are based is that the most rapidly dividing cells are also the most vulnerable to the cytotoxic effects of these treatments. Although chemotherapy is effective in the treatment of various haematological and solid cancers (e.g. testicular cancer), and radiotherapy is used successfully for laryngeal and other cancers, these treatments are not universally effective. For example, they have limited effectiveness in advanced lung cancer. Unfortunately, despite recent advances in chemotherapy and radiotherapy, the side effects of these treatments are often considerable and may have a major adverse effect on quality of life. Therefore an important aim of much current research is to minimize adverse effects on quality of life by developing more selective drugs and radiation protocols that spare as much normal tissue as possible.[6]

Since the advent of molecular biology in the mid-1980s, there has been much investigation of the possibility of using biological factors as a means of enhancing the host's anticancer immune response; such factors are broadly termed biological response modifiers (BRMs). A number of such molecules, usually antibody-based, have been licensed for use in various cancers, including breast cancer (trastuzumab) and (in Germany) colorectal cancer (Edrecolomab (17–1A). Bevacizumab is licensed as an anti-angiogenic agent applicable to many solid cancers.[7] Many other such molecules are currently in phase II and III trials and ultimately may offer a range of new therapies for many types of cancer.

A dose-limiting side effect of many types of chemotherapy is myelosuppression (a reduction in red and white blood cells and platelets). In addition to the pharmacological effects of chemotherapy, immunosuppression can also occur as a learned response (classical conditioning).[8,9] Patients may learn to associate various chemotherapy-related cues with immunosuppression, with the result that, over a period of time, exposure to these cues in the absence of chemotherapy can produce conditioned immunosuppression. This is a very clear demonstration of the ability of the brain to modulate host defences in a way that potentially weakens the antitumour immune response.

6.3 Theoretical basis for the role of psychoneuroimmunology in cancer

6.3.1 Rationale

Reviewing the field recently, Turner-Cobb *et al.*[10] point out that for a psychoneuroimmunological perspective of cancer to be valid, it is necessary to demonstrate that tumour development can be regulated by immune defences and that psychosocial factors are capable of altering the immune mechanisms involved in cancer regulation. To this we would wish to add that what holds significance for the onset of the malignant process may not necessarily be relevant to the subsequent progression of the disease. In addition, the mediating role of neurohormonal and endocrine factors needs to be considered fully.

6.3.2 Host defences and cancer onset and progression

The immune system is a complex mixture of cells and soluble factors whose function is to protect the host from infection. In the context of cancer, however, the tumour is derived from host cells and therefore cannot be considered as 'foreign' in the same way as a bacterium or virus. Nevertheless, as a consequence of the changes (mutations) that have occurred during the process of the cell becoming a cancer, these cells possess subtle variations that can be used to distinguish them from their normal counterparts, and it is these variations that enable components of the immune system to identify and target cancerous cells.

The principal components of the immune system which are known to have anticancer properties are natural killer (NK) cells, T lymphocytes, dendritic cells, and, to a lesser extent, antibodies. In addition to these specific components, cytokines (a plethora of soluble factors with diverse roles) present systemically as well as specifically in the local tumour microenvironment, and play a key role in determining the type of immune response that is generated. NK cells are a subset of large granular lymphocytes characterized by expression of cell surface markers, in particular CD56 and CD16. They comprise a group of effectors, and have been the focus of the most attention.[11] NK cells bind to host cells and will only mediate lysis if the former have lost specific major histocompatability complex (MHC) molecules which, when present, provide an inhibitory signal to the NK cell.[12] NK cells, and their more active IL-2-stimulated counterparts lymphokine activated killer (LAK) cells, often identified by expression of the CD57 antigen, have been shown in many studies to mediate tumour cell cytotoxicity. Moreover, *in vivo* their function is generally suppressed in cancer patients, especially in those with advanced disease.

Various T-lymphocyte subsets, in particular CD8+ cytotoxic cells, have also been demonstrated *in vitro* to have potent antitumour cell capabilities as well as exquisite tumour specificity. However, *in vivo*, as with NK cells, their lytic capacity is largely non-functional. This lack of lytic function may be attributed to two factors. First, there may be a lack of co-stimulatory molecules on cells expressing the MHC-cancer specific peptide. Secondly, the cytokine microenvironment may be 'incorrect' due to tumour-derived cytokine secretions, regulatory T cells, or a combination of both factors.[13,14] Using a xenogenic tumour model, in which human colorectal tumours are transplanted into mice, it has been demonstrated clearly that tumour cells constitutively expressing IL-12 cause effective recruitment of T cells into the tumour as well as activation of these cells, thereby causing tumour regression.[15]

Tumour infiltrating lymphocytes (TILs), made up of CD8+ and CD4+ T cells, are found within the tumour mass.[16] Studies have found that TILs are a good prognostic indicator in many types of cancer, including B-cell lymphoma.[17]

Recent interest has focused on the anticancer role of dendritic cells. Dendritic cells are responsible for presenting antigen to T cells, and they are particularly important because they stimulate naive T cells from the host's reservoir.[18] Once activated, dendritic cells significantly upregulate expression of their MHC molecules, as well as the co-stimulatory molecules required for effective T-cell activation. Both *in vivo* and *in vitro*, dendritic cells are capable of recruiting specific anticancer cell-specific cytotoxic T cells. Dendritic cells can be 'immunized' with whole tumour cells or peptide fragments. However, like T cells and NK cells, they are highly dependent on the cytokine environment.[19]

The cytokine environment is largely established through activation of the CD4+ subset of T cells. These can be further subdivided into at least two mature populations (Th1 and Th2) on the basis of the repertoire of cytokines that they produce. The Th1 response is thought to be the predominant response required to mediate an anticancer response. Conversely, Th2 cells secrete a variety of cytokines which are responsible for stimulating a humoral immune response characterized mainly by specific antibody production. Although specific antibodies can be used to target treatment, with the exception of anti-idiotype therapy for B-cell cancers and trastuzumab in a proportion of breast cancers, this approach has not yet proved particularly effective.

A shift in the Th1–Th2 balance has been observed in many cancers. Studies of the IL-12 and IL-10 balance have clearly shown a prevalence of a Th2-type response, especially in advanced tumours.[20,21] However, it is not yet known if this is induced by the cancer or if it is the reason for the progression of some tumours.

The belief that specific BRMs can break T-cell and NK-cell tolerance of the cancer, and promote an antitumour response, is based to a considerable extent on the important multifaceted, functions played by the cytokine network. Currently, it is not clear how individual factors are stimulated, although it is well known that environmental, clinical, and host immune mechanisms all have a part to play. As a clearer understanding emerges of the interactions between the neuroendocrine system (see below), the brain, and the immune system, it is likely that new treatments will be developed, guided by integration of the disciplines of neurology, endocrinology, and immunology.

6.3.3 Psychosocial factors and neuroimmune mechanisms involved in cancer regulation

6.3.3.1 Definitions of stress and coping

In this chapter, stress refers to the circumstances, characteristics, and events (both external and internal to the organism) which constitute, or are perceived to constitute, a threat to survival or well-being. Coping refers to a person's 'response' that is intended to facilitate adaptation to the stressor, thereby incrementing survival chances or minimizing distress, as in the 'fight-or-flight' response. In the case of the fight-or-flight response, the stress response is short term, self-limiting, and usually adaptive, and often leads to a reduction of the threat posed by the stressor and a return of the organism to a resting state. This is the classic process of homeostasis described by the physiologist Claude Bernard.

In an influential book, Lazarus and Folkman[22] defined coping as the 'ongoing cognitive and behavioral efforts to manage specific external and/or internal demands appraised as taxing or exceeding the resources of the person' (p. 141). Therefore coping involves two simultaneous processes of appraisal; an appraisal of the demand (what is the demand and is it a threat?) and an appraisal of the individual's capacity to respond to the demand (can a response be produced that will alleviate or reduce the threat?).

Based on the work of Lazarus and Folkman[22] and Bandura,[23] Anderson and Walker[24] have proposed a model of coping with cancer. The model highlights the following:

♦ the ongoing appraisal of the situation (what is the demand and what are its consequences?)

♦ physiological aspects (the 'stress' response)

♦ affective responses (depression, anxiety, happiness)

♦ coping styles (e.g. fighting spirit, hopelessness, minimization)

♦ perceived self-efficacy (the extent to which the individual believes that he or she can control the disease)

◆ behavioural aspects (compliance with treatment, lifestyle changes such as diet, sleep habits, exercise, and healthy living, relationships with medical staff and the use of complementary therapies).

Anderson and Walker[24] point out that:

> The diagnosis of cancer poses a threat to well-being, and this model of coping explains how psychological interventions may influence the disease process and the behavioural pathways that may be involved. The model also provides a basis for understanding how patients cope with cancer and suggests a framework for timely interventions to enhance mood and quality of life and, potentially, to help patients fight their disease (p. 236)

A diagnosis of cancer and its subsequent treatment can be seen to be an enduring chronic stressor leading to a sustained mobilization of coping resources in the patient. The psychoneuroimmunological implications of this chronic mobilization of the stress response could be of considerable relevance to treatment response, disease progression, and psychological wellbeing.

6.3.3.2 The effect of stress and depression on the immune system

Although NK cell numbers and activity are enhanced immediately after exposure to brief psychological stress, such as cognitive conflict tasks, mental arithmetic, or parachute jumping,[25] stress-induced immunosuppression is now a well-established immunological phenomenon. Situations can arise where stress is prolonged, requiring the organism to produce a more sustained coping response that entails the mobilization of biopsychosocial resources for prolonged periods. Such sustained responses in the face of chronic stress have been shown to be psychologically and biologically taxing and to lead to immunosuppression.[26]

In the past decade, meta-analyses of the effects on immune function of stress[25] and depression[27] have been published. These demonstrated statistically robust alterations in host defences, particularly decreases in functional immune measures such as proliferative responses to mitogens and NK cell activity. Stress was also found to be negatively related to numbers and percentages of circulating white blood cells, immunoglobulin levels, and antibody titres to herpes viruses.[25] Theoretically, these changes could be related to the development and/or progression of cancer.[28–34]

There is a substantial literature demonstrating that social support acts as a buffer against the psychobiological effects of stress in cancer and other diseases.[35] Lutgendorf et al.[36] have studied the effects of social support on vascular endothelial growth factor (VEGF). This cytokine, which plays a pivotal role in regulating tumour angiogenesis, has been associated with poorer survival in patients with ovarian carcinoma. Women with ovarian carcinoma who reported higher levels of social well-being had lower levels of VEGF. Conversely, individuals who reported greater helplessness had higher VEGF levels. Depression was unrelated to VEGF levels. These are interesting observations that may provide an insight into disease progression.

6.3.3.3 The effect of stress and depression on neuroendocrine hormones

The neuroendocrine system is a collection of glands and organs that secrete a diverse array of chemicals affecting all aspects of human physiology. The principal components thought to be involved in the psychosocial regulation of the immune system are the products of the hypothalamus, pituitary, and adrenal glands; commonly termed the HPA axis. Changes in the HPA axis provide probable mechanism(s) by which these psychosocial events will affect the functioning of the immune system in cancer patients (see Chapters 1 and 2).

It has been shown, for example, that some depressed individuals have a hyperactive HPA leading to increased cortisol concentrations, probably due to increased release of corticotrophin-releasing hormone from the hypothalamus and dexamethasone non-suppression.[37] However, the secretion of cortisol can also be erratic due to HPA dysregulation in major depressive disorder[38] and the circadian rhythm of cortisol can become flattened.[39] The secretion of prolactin is lower in women with seasonal affective disorder,[40] and its release can be controlled by serotonin, a monoamine implicated in the pathophysiology of depression.[41] In addition, depressed individuals display an abnormal noradrenergic-mediated growth hormone (GH) release[42] and a delayed nocturnal melatonin peak,[43] although Rabe-Jablonska and Szymanska[44] found that some patients with major depression have elevated melatonin concentration levels during daytime and night-time hours.

In summary, stress and depression alter the circulating levels of neuroendocrine hormones, which in turn have the potential to alter the functioning of the immune system in response to stress.[32,45,46]

6.3.3.4 Effects of neuroendocrine hormones on the immune system

To have a direct effect on cells of the immune system, altered levels of circulating neuroendocrine hormones produced in response to stress need to bind to their appropriate receptors. Receptors for prolactin,[47–51] glucocorticoids,[52–55] catecholamines,[56,57] and melatonin[58–60] are all present on immune cells. In addition, the expression of some of these receptors on lymphocytes is altered during stress and exercise.[61]

The effects of neuroendocrine hormones on the immune system are widespread. They include changes in the proliferative activity of lymphocytes, with prolactin and GH stimulating lymphocyte proliferation,[62–66] whereas glucocorticoids inhibit it.[67] Prolactin, GH, and glucocorticoids can also alter cytokine production in T cells.[68] Catecholamines (epinephrine and norepinephrine) can downregulate proliferation as well as differentiation, modulation of cytokine production and functional activity in immune cells.[69,70] However, in some instances catecholamines have stimulatory effects on B-lymphocyte proliferation.[71,72] In contrast, melatonin increases lymphocyte proliferation, activates T helper cells by increasing IL-2 production, and stimulates monocytes to increase the production of reactive oxygen species and nitric oxide.[73–75] Melatonin also enhances IL-12 production by monocytes, driving T-cell differentiation toward the Th1 phenotype and causing an increase in interferon γ production, with the removal of melatonin causing immunodepression.[76]

There is also evidence that neuroendocrine hormones can modulate immune cells central to the control of cancer cells (e.g. NK and LAK cells).[77] Cortisol directly inhibits NK activity *in vitro* via a calcium-dependent mechanism,[46,78] and the suppressed NK activity observed during acute stress involves catecholamine release from the adrenal glands and subsequent activation of the β-adrenoceptors.[70,79] In contrast, prolactin augments NK and LAK activity *in vitro*,[62,80] and GH reverses the reduced NK activity observed in aged mice[81] as well as increasing low NK activity in GH-deficient patients.[82,83]

Stress is also known to induce lymphocyte apoptosis[84] via the HPA axis in immature T cells and directly by endogenous opioids in mature T cells,[85] and lymphocyte apoptosis is influenced by neuroendocrine hormones. The most widely studied effect is that of induction of lymphocyte apoptosis by glucocorticoids. Glucocorticoids cause immunosuppression partly by induction of lymphocyte apoptosis at concentrations achieved during a stress response,[86–89] and interestingly the apoptosis-inducing effects of glucocorticoids can be inhibited by prolactin.[90] In addition, apoptosis of peripheral blood mononuclear cells can be induced by catecholamines[69,70,91] via induction of a BcP2/Bax and Fas/FasL pathway.[92]

Finally, in addition to their direct effects on lymphocytes, neuroendocrine hormones may also influence the immune system at the genetic level. Prolactin regulates expression of interferon regulatory factor 1, a mediator of diverse immune functions,[93] suppressor of cytokine signalling 2 (SOCS-2) and SOCS-3, and cytokine-inducible *src* homology 2 containing protein, another member of the SOCS family.[94] Glucocorticoids transduce their effects by binding to glucocorticoid response elements that are involved in regulating the expression of numerous genes, including some cytokines.[95,96] In addition, it is thought that hormones of the HPA may promote expression of breast cancer oncogenes.[97]

6.4 Review of empirical evidence in cancer

6.4.1 Cancer-related distress

The emotional and social demands made by the diagnosis and treatment of cancer have been increasingly recognized in the last 25 years. In the United Kingdom, cancer charities and the National Health Service have made a considerable investment in information centres, clinical nurse specialists, and mental health professionals. The illness and treatment can cause wide-ranging problems, including anxiety, depression, sexual problems, body image problems, existential crises, fatigue, nausea, vomiting, pain, and the Damocles' syndrome (i.e. an inability to get on with life here and now because of what *might* happen in the future).[98]

Derogatis *et al.*[99] investigated the prevalence of psychiatric disorders in 215 randomly selected adult cancer patients with varying types and stages of disease in

North America. They found that no less than 47% of these patients were suffering from a diagnosable psychiatric disorder (most commonly adjustment disorders). In a series of studies carried out in the late 1970s and 1980s, Maguire et al.[100] found that between a quarter and a third of women with breast cancer experienced clinically significant anxiety, depression and/or sexual difficulties in the year following surgery. This compares favourably with the findings of a more recent study by Hall et al.[101] in which 50% of 269 women with early breast cancer were clinically anxious and 37% were clinically depressed (as assessed using a structured clinical interview) in the first 3 months after the diagnosis.

Zabora et al.[102] studied 4496 cancer patients with differing types and stages of disease using the Brief Symptom Inventory. Overall, 35% of the sample had clinically significant levels of psychological distress as identified by this measure. Distress for patients with lung cancer was found to be significantly higher than that for other cancers, with the exception of brain, liver, pancreatic, and head and neck cancers. This recent study is important, not only because of its notably large sample size, but also, as Zabora et al.[102] point out, because rates of psychological distress obtained are comparable with those of the earlier studies discussed above.

Although there is evidence that much cancer-related distress can be prevented, these studies make it clear that the diagnosis and treatment continue to cause substantial adverse effects on health-related quality of life, as well as considerable psychosocial and psychiatric morbidity.[98,103]

6.4.2 Immune and neuroendocrine dysregulation in cancer

It has been established that a number of viruses, bacteria, and parasites are carcinogenic. Indeed, Peto[104] has estimated that about 15% of cancers worldwide are caused by known infectious agents. These include *Helicobacter pylori* (stomach cancer), human papilloma viruses (HPV) (cervical and genital cancer, and possibly cancers of the head, neck, oesophagus, and skin), hepatitis B and C (liver cancer), and Epstein–Barr virus (EBV) (various B-cell malignancies and nasopharyngeal cancer). In addition, epidemiological studies have shown that other infections act as significant cofactors for a number of cancers, for example malaria (the major cofactor with EBV for Burkitt's lymphoma in Africa), human T-cell lymphotropic virus type 1 (some T-cell leukaemias and lymphomas), HIV (non-Hodgkin's lymphoma), human herpes virus (Kaposi's sarcoma with HIV), schistosomiasis (bladder and colon cancer), and liver flukes (cholangiosarcoma).[104]

Patients undergoing immunosuppressive therapy have a significantly increased risk of many types of cancer. For example, their risk of non-melanoma skin cancer is almost 25 times that of non-immunosupressed individuals, and the risk is increased significantly for cancers of the thyroid, kidney, bladder, lung, colon, rectum, bladder, and prostate, as well as for melanoma and non-Hodgkin's lymphoma.[104–106] These findings could be a result of the induction of lymphocyte apoptosis by glucocorticoids, leading to a reduction in lymphocyte number and functional ability, thereby weakening the immune system and compromising the surveillance for cancer cells.[85]

Further supporting evidence for the role of host defences comes from social isolation experiments in mice which show that stress enhances tumour metastasis, partly via immunosuppression and reduced immunosurveillance.[107]

Hormones are thought to be important in the onset and progression of a number of cancers, including breast, ovarian, endometrial, and testicular cancer. For example, exogenous oestrogens transiently increase the risk of breast cancer, and the risk is permanently lowered by late menarche, early menopause, early first childbirth, and high parity.[108] Endometrial cancer incidence is also increased by hormone replacement therapy. Ovarian cancer incidence declines with increasing parity, and both endometrial and ovarian cancers are less common in oral contraceptive users.[108]

Endocrine therapy has a well-established place in the treatment of several cancers, including breast and prostate cancers. For example, tamoxifen (a partial oestrogen antagonist) has been shown repeatedly to reduce the risk of recurrence of breast cancer, and there has been considerable recent interest in the role of other compounds such as the third generation of aromatase inhibitors (e.g. anastrazole) in the treatment of women with advanced breast cancer and in post-menopausal women with oestrogen-receptor-positive tumours.[109]

Changes in hormone levels have been associated with different stages and types of cancer. For example, it has been reported that GH serum levels increase with advancing stage of lung cancer,[110] whereas melatonin levels are reduced in patients with primary endocrine-dependent and endocrine-independent tumours.[111]

The main neuroendocrine hormone evaluated in stress-related cancer studies is cortisol. As well as being more distressed, cancer patients with a flattened diurnal cortisol slope exhibit earlier mortality.[112–116] However, the patients involved are often end-stage, and therefore it may be the metastatic cancer which is producing the effects seen in the HPA via the release of factors such as cytokines. In support of a direct effect, female nightshift workers in whom the cortisol rhythm is disturbed are at higher risk of breast cancer.[117,118]

6.4.3 Psychosocial factors and immune mechanisms involved in cancer regulation

A number of studies have attempted to evaluate the prognostic value of depressive symptoms by assessing these at a single time point, usually post-diagnosis. Unsurprisingly, they have yielded conflicting results. Some individuals not depressed at the time of evaluation may have been depressed previously or subsequently. Levy et al.[119] carried out a prospective study of 90 women with early breast cancer and monitored mood and host defences over time (5 days after surgery and 15 months thereafter). Time to recurrence was assessed during a follow-up period of 5–8 years. Prolonged mood disturbance and level of NK cell activity both predicted disease progression. Persistent distress and low NK cell activity after surgery predicted a shorter time to recurrence. However, it should be noted that there was substantial attrition at the 15-month follow up and histological grade was not controlled. It may have been that NK cell activity simply reflected tumour aggressiveness.[24] More recently, however, in a series of 61 patients with early breast cancer, Osborne et al.[120] found that high NK cell activity predicted shorter survival.

Insomnia, a behavioural symptom associated with depression and stress, is more common in newly diagnosed cancer patients compared with normal individuals, and it can persist after cancer treatment has been completed.[121] Moreover, insomnia has been linked to a lower 5-year survival rate in lung cancer patients.[122] There is evidence that insomnia may lead to suppression of the immune system. Higher levels of CD3+, CD4+, and CD8+ cells have been found in good sleepers compared with those suffering from insomnia,[123] and Irwin et al.[124] found that, compared with control subjects, patients with insomnia showed a reduction in NK cell activity. The disruption of the circadian rhythm seen in some patients with cancer may play a role in the alteration of immune system functioning, although further elucidation is required.[125,126]

Therefore there is evidence that stress, depression, and insomnia can induce changes in neuroendocrine hormones which can alter immune system parameters. Alteration of these immune system parameters may be relevant to the onset and/or progression of at least some types of cancer. However, we agree with Turner-Cobb et al.[10] that evidence for stress-induced alterations in immune functions of tumour defence being clinically relevant is 'suggestive rather than conclusive' (p. 57).

6.4.4 Psychosocial interventions and host defences in cancer

A number of randomized controlled trials have demonstrated that a range of psychosocial interventions can modify various aspects of the immune system, although the number of studies in patients with cancer is limited (see reviews by Walker et al.[127] and Turner-Cobb et al.[10]).

In a celebrated study, Fawzy et al.[128] found that a psychosocial intervention altered host defences in 68 patients with good-prognosis malignant melanoma who were randomized to a group psychoeducational intervention or to a control group. Patients randomized to the intervention attended six sessions of weekly group psychotherapy including education about the illness, risk factors, lifestyle, and side effects, stress management including relaxation training, facilitation of adaptive coping strategies, and peer group and professional psychological support. The psychoeducational intervention reduced psychological distress and increased the use of active coping methods. In addition, at the 6-month assessment point, patients in the intervention group had significant increases in the percentage of large granular lymphocytes (defined as CD57+). There were also indications of increased NK cytotoxic activity and a small decrease in the percentage of CD4+ T cells. The authors concluded that the results indicated that a short-term psychiatric group intervention in patients with malignant melanoma with a good prognosis was associated with longer-term changes in affective state, coping, and the NK and lymphoid cell systems.

More recently, a pragmatic randomized controlled trial was carried out to evaluate the immunomodulatory effects of relaxation training and guided imagery in women undergoing multimodality treatment for locally advanced breast cancer.[129] Eighty women with large (>4 cm) or locally advanced (T_3, T_4, T_x, N_2) breast carcinoma participated. Patients underwent primary chemotherapy followed by surgery, hormone therapy, and radiotherapy. Those in the intervention group were taught relaxation and guided imagery. Patients kept daily diaries of the frequency of relaxation practice and imagery vividness. On 10 occasions during the 37 weeks following the diagnosis, blood was taken for immunological assays (enumeration of leucocyte subsets by flow cytometry; T-cell subsets, NK cells, B lymphocytes, and monocytes; cytotoxicity, NK and LAK cell activity; cytokines, IL-1, IL-2, IL-4, and IL-6, and tumour necrosis factor α).

Statistically significant between-group differences were found in the percentage of CD3+, CD25+, and CD56+ T-cell subsets, and patients who rated their imagery vividness highly had elevated levels of NK cell activity at the end of chemotherapy and at follow-up. The authors concluded that relaxation training and guided imagery altered putative anticancer host defences during and after prolonged multimodality therapy in women with breast cancer.[129]

The largest randomized controlled trial published to date evaluated the effects of a group intervention (which included relaxation therapy and various educational components) in 227 women with regional breast cancer.[130] T-cell proliferation in response to polyclonal mitogens remained stable or increased in patients randomized to the intervention, whereas responses decreased in the control group. The intervention did not affect CD3+, CD4+, or CD8+ counts, and CD25+ and CD56+ were not measured. Blood samples were taken only at baseline and 4 months later, thereby precluding detailed sequential analyses. The authors concluded that the intervention had significant, psychological, behavioural, and biological effects.

6.4.5 Psychosocial factors and neuroendocrine hormones in cancer

Several studies suggest that psychotherapy alters the levels of neuroendocrine hormones, especially cortisol. In healthy subjects, stress management training, guided imagery, and music therapy during acute psychosocial stress reduces salivary[131] and plasma[132] cortisol levels, and cognitive–behavioural treatment decreases plasma cortisol levels in couples trying *in vitro* fertilization.[133] In patients with cancer, psychotherapeutic treatment and greater social support can normalize[134–136] or reduce[137] cortisol levels, as well as reducing prolactin levels.[135]

Schedlowski *et al.*[138] studied the effects of an intervention which included relaxation, imagery, information, and coping skills training in 24 women with breast cancer. The intervention took place weekly for 10 weeks. For women receiving the intervention, blood samples were taken before and immediately after the second and tenth sessions. Women in the control group gave blood samples 2 days after the second and tenth sessions of the intervention group. The intervention produced an immediate and persistent reduction in plasma cortisol compared with levels in a control group, and the reduction in cortisol levels was accompanied by an increase in the absolute numbers of white blood cells both immediately following intervention and over the 10-week intervention period. Importantly, however, no significant correlation between cortisol levels and white blood cell numbers was observed.

6.4.6 Psychological factors and cancer incidence

The literature is divided with regard to the putative effects of stressful life events on cancer incidence, not least because of methodological shortcomings in much of the research.[10,139,140] In a meta-analysis of earlier research, Petticrew *et al.*[141] concluded that there was no support for the suggestion of a direct causal relationship between the occurrence of stressful life events and cancer onset. This conclusion, based on a small and unrepresentative sample of studies of poor quality, has been the subject of strong criticism.[10]

In a more recent, and methodologically rigorous, meta-analysis of studies conducted between 1966 and 2002, Duijts *et al.*[142] concluded that there was modest support for an association between stressful life events and breast cancer risk, with death of a spouse showing a particular association. Furthermore, these authors suggested that this association might be explained by the disturbance of immune function precipitated by chronic stress predisposing to malignant growth.

Further support has been given by the findings of a recent large-scale prospective study of 10 808 women in Finland. Lillberg *et al.*[143] found an association between death of a husband or of a close relative or friend and increased risk of breast cancer. They suggested that these stressful life events may influence breast cancer onset through endocrinological and immunological mechanisms.

Although this recent work has suggested a more robust association between cancer onset and stressful life events, there are methodological problems with such prospective cohort studies. Retrospective recall of life events may be inaccurate, and it is usually difficult to determine with any precision the actual date of cancer onset. Particularly in the case of slower-growing tumours, the assessment of life events in cohort studies may be taking place in the presence of as yet undetected cancer which may exert an influence on central nervous system (CNS) or psychological state and thus bias the assessment. Furthermore, it has been suggested[10,24] that it is not the occurrence of the stressful life events *per se* which is important, but the psychological reaction of an individual to these events, particularly with respect to longer-term or chronic stressors.

A number of studies have investigated the role of depression as a risk factor for the development of cancer, again with mixed results. In a large epidemiological study of 2020 male employees of Western Electric in the United States, Shekelle *et al.*[144] showed that depression reported on the Minnesota Multiphasic Personality Inventory was associated with a doubling of risk of death from cancer 17 years later, with a higher than normal incidence of cancer for the first 10 years. This finding was reported as persisting at 20-year follow-up.[145] However, negative findings have also been reported.[146,147]

6.4.7 Psychological factors and cancer progression

It has been suggested that examining the influence of psychological factors on the progression of an identified cancer may be a more fruitful avenue of research. This again would encompass not only the assessment of the occurrence of stressful life events but also the potential influence of psychological response to these events. However, research on life events and cancer progression has also produced inconsistent findings. In an early case–control series, Ramirez *et al.*[148] found that women with breast cancer who had relapsed reported a higher prevalence of major life stressors, such as bereavement and loss of a job, than the control group comprising women with breast cancer who had not relapsed.

In a robust critique of experimental methodologies in this area, Fox[139] pointed out that the retrospective recall of negative life events in case–control series designs could be strongly influenced by the current psychological distress of the subjects who have received a diagnosis of cancer or had been informed of recurrence or relapse, thus biasing results. Fox[139] expressed a strong preference for cohort studies, but noted that few recent cohort studies had been conducted. One cohort study by Barraclough *et al.*[149] found no relationship between the occurrence of stressful life events and breast cancer survival. In discussing these inconsistent findings, Anderson and Walker[24] note that it may not be the occurrence of stressful life events that is important in cancer progression, but the individual's psychological response to them.

A number of studies have found a positive relationship between depression and disease progression in patients with Hodgkin's disease,[150] locally advanced breast cancer,[151] and early breast cancer.[152] However, negative studies have also been reported.[153–155] This work also suffers from methodological limitations in that depression was usually measured at only a single time point. Therefore it is possible that some patients who were not depressed at the time of assessment may have become depressed subsequently, or indeed were depressed prior to the study assessment point. Prospective methods would be more suitable in this situation.

One such prospective study of 90 women with early breast cancer found that prolonged mood disturbance and level of NK cell activity, assessed 5 days after surgery and at 15-month follow-up, predicted disease progression.[119] However, there were high levels of attrition at 15-month follow-up and histological grade was not controlled in this study.

Another method of investigating psychological responses to stressful events is to assess styles of psychological coping. In an important series of studies, Greer and colleagues[156–160] investigated the psychological coping styles of cancer patients. They found that coping styles characterized as a 'fighting spirit' and 'avoidance/denial' were associated with a better prognosis. In contrast, more 'repressive' coping styles have been found to be associated with more rapid cancer progression.[161,162]

It is clear from research on coping styles that the manner of responding to stressful events has implications psychologically and physiologically.[163] The challenge for future psychoneuroimmunology research is to investigate and delineate the psychological, physiological, and immunological links mediating this association.

6.4.8 Psychosocial interventions and survival

To date, 11 randomized controlled trials have attempted to evaluate the impact of psychosocial interventions on survival: six found a statistically significant effect[150,164–168] (Table 6.1) and six found no survival advantage[169–174] (Table 6.2)

Table 6.1 Randomized controlled trials which demonstrate prolonged survival

Study	Cancer	Stage	n	Follow-up	Findings
Spiegel et al.[167]	Breast	Metastatic	86	10 years	Women randomized to weekly supportive–expressive group psychotherapy survived a mean of 36.6 months compared with a mean of 18.9 months in the control group
Richardson et al.[166]	Mixed haematological	Mixed (newly diagnosed)	94	2–5 years	Patients randomized to any of three psychoeducational interventions designed to enhance compliance with treatment survived longer
Fawzy et al.[164,176]	Malignant melanoma	I and II	68	5–6 years	Patients randomized to a brief (six session) psychoeducational group intervention survived longer
Kuchler et al.[165]	Gastrointestinal	All	271	2 years	Patients randomized to psychotherapy survived longer, especially females and patients with stomach, pancreatic, primary liver or colorectal cancer
Ratcliffe et al.[150], Walker et al.[168]	Hodgkin's disease and non-Hodgkin's lymphoma	II, III, and IV	63	5 and 13 years	Patients randomized to relaxation and individual hypnotherapy for chemotherapy side effects survived longer (at 5 year and 13 year follow-ups)

Updated from tables previously published in J. Anderson and L. G. Walker (2002). In C. E. Lewis, R. O'Brien, and J. Barraclough (eds) *The Psychoimmunology of Cancer* (2nd edn). Oxford: Oxford University Press.

Table 6.2 Randomized controlled trials which do not demonstrate prolonged survival

Study	Cancer	Stage	n	Follow-up	Findings
Linn et al.[173]	Mainly lung	End-stage (IV)	120	1 year	Patients randomized to receiving twice-weekly death counselling plus standard medical treatment or medical treatment alone. No difference in survival between the groups
Ilnyckj et al.[172]	Various	Various, but mainly stage I	127	11 years	Patients randomized to one of three intervention groups or to a control group. Interventions were (1) professionally led; (2) professionally led for 3 months, then peer led; (3) peer led. No difference in survival found compared with control group
Cunningham et al.[169]	Breast	Metastatic	66	5 years	Patients randomized to weekly group supportive therapy plus cognitive–behavioural therapy or a home study cognitive–behavioural package. No difference was found in survival between the two groups. The study lacked a non-intervention control group
Edelman et al.[170]	Breast	Metastatic	121	5 years	Cognitive–behaviour therapy versus control. No significant differences between the two groups
Goodwin et al.[171]	Breast	Metastatic	235	Variable	Randomized to weekly supportive-expressive therapy or control. Women in both groups received educational materials and whatever psychosocial support considered necessary. No significant difference in survival
Walker et al.[174]	Breast	Locally advanced	96	3 years	Patients randomized to relaxation plus guided imagery or high level of support. Overall survival in both groups high and non-significantly different

(Strictly speaking, the study by Richardson et al.[166] used pseudo-randomization assignment.) Nine of these studies have been reviewed by Anderson and Walker[24] who concluded that most of the studies reporting no survival benefit had a number of methodological shortcomings (e.g. diagnostically heterogeneous patients, patients with different stages of disease, lack of a defined protocol, control and experimental interventions that may have been equally efficacious).

The studies used a variety of interventions and combinations (cognitive, behavioural, expressive, and educational) as well as patients with different types and stages of disease. Moreover, as Cunningham[175] has pointed out, premorbid psychological characteristics and response to psychotherapy differ substantially between patients. One study suggested that it was only a subgroup of patients, namely those who scored low on assertiveness, who benefited from the intervention.[168] Therefore it is not surprising that inconsistent findings have been reported.

Crucially, from the point of view of this chapter, only two of these psychosocial intervention studies included an evaluation of host defences. Fawzy et al.[176] found that although their intervention enhanced NK activity (see above), this did not emerge as an independent prognostic factor for survival. However, although Walker et al.[174] did not find a survival effect for their intervention (relaxation therapy and guided imagery), they did find that the intervention increased the number of CD56+ cells. Subsequent multivariate analyses revealed that survival was independently predicted by tumour size and change in the number of CD56+ cells during chemotherapy.

We conclude that there is very little current evidence linking intervention-induced enhancement of host defences with prolonged survival.

6.4.9 Effects of host defences on the central nervous system in cancer

It is important to remember that psychoneuroimmunology is concerned not only with the effects of the CNS on host defences, but also with the effects of host defences on the CNS.

With particular reference to cancer, Maier and Watkins[177] suggest that the activation of the brain to immune communication outlined above can lead to behavioural, affective, and cognitive changes which are a direct result of immune system function. This is consistent with a study by Bower et al.[178] who found that fatigued breast cancer survivors had elevated serum markers relevant to pro-inflammatory cytokine activity, as well as lower serum cortisol and NK cell numbers. Further, Maier and Watkins[177] suggest that some of the quality-of-life issues related to cancer and cancer treatment may be at least partly due to the function of the immune system. They propose that some of the side effects of cancer treatments such as chemotherapy may be driven by immune system effects on the CNS.

A number of studies have examined the effects of biological response modifiers on various psychological variables, including mood, cognition, and quality of life.[179] For example, dramatic effects of IL-2 were demonstrated in a randomized controlled trial of patients with advanced colorectal cancer.[180,181] These individuals received chemotherapy [5-fluorouracil plus leukovorin (5FU+L)], or immunochemotherapy (5FU+L plus continuous recombinant IL-2 for 5 days per month). Immunochemotherapy was rated as significantly more distressing than chemotherapy alone, and patients reported a greater incidence of appetite impairment, weight loss, poor concentration, and fever. One patient developed repeated transient psychotic episodes associated with recombinant IL-2 infusions and another regularly became confused. Computerized cognitive assessments revealed that immunochemotherapy produced significant impairment in various tasks, especially reaction time, picture recognition, and vigilance.[180] These effects were not due to sleep deprivation or pyrexia.

6.5 Conclusions and directions for future research

It is clear that the psychoneuroimmunological aspects of cancer have attracted considerable attention recently, and undoubtedly progress has been made. However, there remain a number of important issues that need to be addressed in future research.

Further studies are needed in *Homo sapiens* to clarify the extent to which psychosocial factors can affect the onset and progression of cancer. It is important to appreciate that what holds true for one type of cancer may not hold true for other types of cancer, or indeed stages of disease. It is well known that tumour doubling times can vary greatly even in the same type of cancer.[109] Therefore, as far as onset of disease is concerned, until it becomes possible to date with some precision the onset of the malignant process, further studies attempting to relate life events and mood states to onset are unlikely to be profitable. More promising in the interim will be studies exploring psychoneuroim-munological effects of relatively stable factors (e.g. personality) on disease onset.

The position regarding disease progression is more encouraging because it is feasible to carry out prospective studies to investigate the putative psychoneuroimmunological effects of psychosocial factors on disease progression. One approach to this would be to construct biopsychosocial databases that would enable one to model the independent prognostic value of clinical, genetic, endocrine, immunological, psycho-logical, sociodemographic, and other variables within a single dataset. In Kingston upon Hull, United Kingdom, we have established two such databases, one in colorectal cancer and the other in brain cancer.

However, the most robust approach will be to carry out further randomized controlled trials to investigate the psychoneuroimmunological effects of various psychosocial and other interventions in different types and stages of cancer. It will be important to relate immunological and endocrinological changes induced by interventions to outcome (recurrence, survival), as well as to study the role of individual and other differences (personality, coping, level of immunosuppression, social support, etc.) in mediating these effects. We are currently evaluating the psychoneuroimmunological effects of relaxation and guided imagery in men and women with colorectal cancer, and the effects of reflexology in women with early breast cancer.

Although the psychoneuroimmunology of cancer is an exciting area of research, journalists and others often make claims that cannot be substantiated from existing findings. Not only could this unfairly discredit this field of research, but false promises can undoubtedly have adverse effects on patients and their families. As responsible clinicians, it is important that we promise only that which we can deliver.

References

1 Maher EJ, Young T, Feigel I (1994). Complementary therapies used by patients with cancer. *BMJ* **309**: 671–2.

2 Downer SM, Cody MM, McCluskey P, *et al.* (1994). Pursuit and practice of complementary therapies by cancer patients receiving conventional treatment. *BMJ* **309**: 86–9.

3 Ernst E, White A (2000). The BBC survey of complementary medicine use in the UK. *Complement Ther Med* **8**: 32–6.

4 Simonton OC, Matthews-Simonton S, Sparks TF (1980). Psychological intervention in the treatment of cancer. *Psychosomatics* **21**: 226–7, 231–3.

5 American Cancer Society (2004). *Cancer Statistics* Atlanta, GA: American Cancer Society.

6 DeVita V, Hellman S, Rosenberg S (eds) (2001). *Cancer Principles and Practice of Oncology* (6th edn) Philadelphia, PA: Lippincott–Williams and Wilkins.

7 Harris M (2004). Monoclonal antibodies as therapeutic agents for cancer. *Lancet Oncol* **5**: 292–302.

8 Bovbjerg DH, Redd WH, Maier LA, *et al.* (1990). Anticipatory immune suppression and nausea in women receiving cyclic chemotherapy for ovarian cancer. *J Consult Clin Psychol* **58**: 153–7.

9 Fredrikson M, Furst CJ, Lekander M, Rotstein S, Blomgren H (1993). Trait anxiety and anticipatory immune reactions in women receiving adjuvant chemotherapy for breast cancer. *Brain Behav Immun* **7**: 79–90.

10 Turner-Cobb J, Sephton SE, Spiegel D (2001). Psychosocial effects on immune function and disease progression in cancer: human studies. In Ader C, Felton D, Cohen C (eds) *Psychoneuroimmunology*. New York: Academic Press.

11 Albertsson P, Basse PH, Hokland M *et al.* (2003). NK cells and the tumour microenvironment: implications for NK-cell function and anti-tumour activity. *Trends Immunol* **24**: 603–9.

12 Moretta L, Moretta A (2004). Unravelling natural killer cell function: triggering and inhibitory human NK receptors. *EMBO J* **23**: 255–9.

13 Antonia S, Mule JJ, Weber JS (2004). Current developments of immunotherapy in the clinic. *Curr Opin Immunol* **16**: 130–6.

14 Vicari A, Caux, C, Trinchieri, G (2002). Tumour escape from immune surveillance through dendritic cell inactivation. *Semin Cancer Biol* **12**: 33–42.

15 Nastala CL, Edington HD, McKinney TG, *et al.* (1994). Recombinant IL-12 administration induces tumor regression in association with IFN-gamma production. *J Immunol* **153**: 1697–1706.

16 Malone CC, Schiltz PM, Mackintosh AD, Beutel LD, Heinemann FS, Dillman RO (2001). Characterization of human tumor-infiltrating lymphocytes expanded in hollow-fiber bioreactors for immunotherapy of cancer. *Cancer Biother Radiopharm* **16**: 381–90.

17 Xu Y, Kroft SH, McKenna RW, Aquino DB (2001). Prognostic significance of tumour-infiltrating T lymphocytes and T-cell subsets in *de novo* diffuse large B-cell lymphoma: a multiparameter flow cytometry study. *Br J Haematol* **112**: 945–9.

18 Banchereau J, Steinman RM (1998). Dendritic cells and the control of immunity. *Nature* **392**: 245–52.

19 Cranmer LD, Trevor KT, Hersh EM (2004). Clinical applications of dendritic cell vaccination in the treatment of cancer. *Cancer Immunol Immunother* **53**: 275–306.

20 Neuner A, Schindel M, Wildenberg U, Muley T, Lahm H, Fischer JR (2002). Prognostic significance of cytokine modulation in non-small cell lung cancer. *Int J Cancer* **101**: 287–92.

21 O'Hara RJ, Greenman J, MacDonald AW, *et al.* (1998). Advanced colorectal cancer is associated with impaired interleukin 12 and enhanced interleukin 10 production. *Clin Cancer Res* **4**: 1943–8.

22 Lazarus RS, Folkman S (1984). *Stress, Appraisal and Coping.* New York: Springer.

23 Bandura A (1997). *Self-Efficacy: The Exercise of Control.* New York: Freeman.

24 Anderson J, Walker LG (2002). Psychosocial factors and cancer progression: involvement of behavioural pathways. In Lewis C, O'Brien RM, Barraclough J (eds) *The Psychonueroimmunology of Cancer* (2nd edn) Oxford: Oxford University Press, 235–257.

25 Herbert TB, Cohen S (1993). Stress and immunity in humans: a meta-analytic review. *Psychosom Med* **55**: 364–79.

26 Buckingham J, Gillies GE, Cowell A (1997). *Stress, Stress Hormones and the Immune System* New York: John Wiley.

27 Herbert TB, Cohen S (1993). Depression and immunity: a meta-analytic review. *Psychol Bull* **113**: 472–86.

28 Spiegel D (1996). Cancer and depression. *Br J Psychiatry Suppl* 109–16.

29 Spiegel D (1997). Psychosocial aspects of breast cancer treatment. *Semin Oncol* **24**: S1-36–47.

30 Spiegel D, Sephton SE, Terr AI, Stites DP (1998). Effects of psychosocial treatment in prolonging cancer survival may be mediated by neuroimmune pathways. *Ann NY Acad Sci* **840**: 674–83.

31 Penninx BW, Guralnik JM, Pahor M, *et al.* (1998). Chronically depressed mood and cancer risk in older persons. *J Natl Cancer Inst* **90**: 1888–93.

32 Spiegel D, Giese-Davis J (2003). Depression and cancer: mechanisms and disease progression. *Biol Psychiatry* **54**: 269–82.

33 Yang EV, Glaser R (2003). Stress-induced immunomodulation: implications for tumorigenesis. *Brain Behav Immun* **17** (Suppl 1): S37–40.

34 Sapolsky RM, Donnelly TM (1985). Vulnerability to stress-induced tumor growth increases with age in rats: role of glucocorticoids. *Endocrinology* **117**: 662–6.

35 Kiecolt-Glaser JK, Glaser R (1999). Psychoneuroimmunology and cancer: fact or fiction? *Eur J Cancer* **35**: 1603–7.

36 Lutgendorf SK, Johnsen EL, Cooper B, *et al.* (2002). Vascular endothelial growth factor and social support in patients with ovarian carcinoma. *Cancer* **95**: 808–15.

37 Nemeroff CB, Bissette G, Akil H, Fink M (1991). Neuropeptide concentrations in the cerebro-spinal fluid of depressed patients treated with electroconvulsive therapy. Corticotrophin-releasing factor, beta-endorphin and somatostatin. *Br J Psychiatry* **158**: 59–63.

38 Peeters F, Nicolson NA, Berkhof J (2004). Levels and variability of daily life cortisol secretion in major depression. *Psychiatry Res* **126**: 1–13.

39 Deuschle M, Schweiger U, Weber B, *et al.* (1997). Diurnal activity and pulsatility of the hypothalamus-pituitary-adrenal system in male depressed patients and healthy controls. *J Clin Endocrinol Metab* **82**: 234–8.

40 Partonen T (1994). Prolactin in winter depression. *Med Hypotheses* **43**, 163–4.

41 Nicholas L, Dawkins K, Golden RN (1998). Psychoneuroendocrinology of depression: prolactin. *Psychiatr Clin North Am* **21**: 341–58.

42 Dinan TG (1998). Psychoneuroendocrinology of depression: growth hormone. *Psychiatr Clin North Am* **21**: 325–39.

43 Crasson M, Kjiri S, Colin A, *et al.* (2004). Serum melatonin and urinary 6-sulfatoxymelatonin in major depression. *Psychoneuroendocrinology* **29**: 1–12.

44 Rabe-Jablonska J, Szymanska A (2001). Diurnal profile of melatonin secretion in the acute phase of major depression and in remission. *Med Sci Monit* **7**, 946–52.

45 McEwan B (1998). Protective and damaging effects of stress mediators. *N Engl J Med* **338**: 171–9.

46 Callewaert DM, Moudgil VK, Radcliff G, Waite R (1991). Hormone specific regulation of natural killer cells by cortisol. Direct inactivation of the cytotoxic function of cloned human NK cells without an effect on cellular proliferation. *FEBS Lett* **285**: 108–10.

47 Dohi K, Kraemer WJ, Mastro AM (2003). Exercise increases prolactin-receptor expression on human lymphocytes. *J Appl Physiol* **94**: 518–24.

48 Goffin V, Bouchard B, Ormandy CJ, *et al.* (1998). Prolactin: a hormone at the crossroads of neuroimmunoendocrinology. *Ann NY Acad Sci* **840**: 498–509.

49 Gouilleux F, Moritz D, Humar M, Moriggl R, Berchtold S, Groner B (1995). Prolactin and interleukin-2 receptors in T lymphocytes signal through a MGF-STAT5-like transcription factor. *Endocrinology* **136**: 5700–8.

50 Badolato R, Bond HM, Valerio G, *et al.* (1994). Differential expression of surface membrane growth hormone receptor on human peripheral blood lymphocytes detected by dual fluorochrome flow cytometry. *J Clin Endocrinol Metab* **79**: 984–90.

51 Rapaport R, Sills IN, Green L, *et al.* (1995). Detection of human growth hormone receptors on IM-9 cells and peripheral blood mononuclear cell subsets by flow cytometry: correlation with growth hormone-binding protein levels. *J Clin Endocrinol Metab* **80**: 2612–9.

52 Gotovac K, Sabioncello A, Rabatic S, Berki T, Dekaris D (2003). Flow cytometric determination of glucocorticoid receptor (GCR) expression in lymphocyte subpopulations: lower quantity of GCR in patients with post-traumatic stress disorder (PTSD). *Clin Exp Immunol* **131**: 335–9.

53 Pruett SB, Fan R, Zheng Q (2003). Characterization of glucocorticoid receptor translocation, cytoplasmic IkappaB, nuclear NFkappaB, and activation of NFkappaB in T lymphocytes exposed to stress-inducible concentrations of corticosterone *in vivo. Int Immunopharmacol* **3**: 1–16.

54. Crabtree GM, Smith KA (1981). Glucocorticoid receptor activation and inactivation in cultured human lymphocytes. *J Biol Chem* **256**: 434–41.

55 Steiner AE, Wittliff JL (1986). Concentration of glucocorticoid receptor sites in normal human lymphocytes. *Clin Chem* **32**: 80–3.

56 Landmann R (1992). Beta-adrenergic receptors in human leukocyte subpopulations. *Eur J Clin Invest* **22**(Suppl 1): 30–6.

57 Wahle M, Stachetzki U, Krause A, Pierer M, Hantzschel H, Baerwald CG (2001). Regulation of beta2-adrenergic receptors on CD4 and CD8 positive lymphocytes by cytokines *in vitro. Cytokine* **16**: 205–9.

58 Gonzalez-Haba MG, Garcia-Maurino S, Calvo JR, Goberna R, Guerrero JM (1995). High-affinity binding of melatonin by human circulating T lymphocytes (CD4+). *FASEB J* **9**: 1331–5.

59 Garcia-Perganeda A, Pozo D, Guerrero JM, Calvo JR (1997). Signal transduction for melatonin in human lymphocytes: involvement of a pertussis toxin-sensitive G protein. *J Immunol* **159**: 3774–81.

60 Garcia-Maurino S, Pozo D, Calvo JR, Guerrero JM (2000). Correlation between nuclear melatonin receptor expression and enhanced cytokine production in human lymphocytic and monocytic cell lines. *J Pineal Res* **29**: 129–37.

61 Fujii N, Miyazaki H, Homma S, Ikegami H (1993). Dynamic exercise induces translocation of beta-adrenergic receptors in human lymphocytes. *Acta Physiol Scand* **148**: 463–4.

62 Matera L, Cesano A, Bellone G, Oberholtzer E (1992). Modulatory effect of prolactin on the resting and mitogen-induced activity of T, B, and NK lymphocytes. *Brain Behav Immun* **6**: 409–17.

63 Yamashita N, Hashimoto Y, Honjo M (2000). The effect of growth hormone on the proliferation of human Th cell clones. *Life Sci* **66**: 1929–35.

64 Clark R (1997). The somatogenic hormones and insulin-like growth factor-1: stimulators of lymphopoiesis and immune function. *Endocr Rev* **18**: 157–79.

65 Clevenger CV, Russell DH, Appasamy PM, Prystowsky MB (1990). Regulation of interleukin 2-driven T-lymphocyte proliferation by prolactin. *Proc Natl Acad Sci USA* **87**: 6460–4.

66 Jeay S, Sonenshein GE, Postel-Vinay MC, Kelly PA, Baixeras E (2002). Growth hormone can act as a cytokine controlling survival and proliferation of immune cells: new insights into signaling pathways. *Mol Cell Endocrinol* **188**: 1–7.

67 Rupprecht R, Wodarz N, Kornhuber J, *et al.* (1990). *In vivo* and *in vitro* effects of glucocorticoids on lymphocyte proliferation in man: relationship to glucocorticoid receptors. *Neuropsychobiology* **24**: 61–6.

68 Dimitrov S, Lange T, Fehm HL, Born J (2004). A regulatory role of prolactin, growth hormone, and corticosteroids for human T-cell production of cytokines. *Brain Behav Immun* **18**: 368–74.

69 Bergquist J, Ohlsson B, Tarkowski A (2000). Nuclear factor-kappa B is involved in the catecholaminergic suppression of immunocompetent cells. *Ann NY Acad Sci* **917**: 281–9.

70 Elenkov IJ, Wilder RL, Chrousos GP, Vizi ES (2000). The sympathetic nerve—an integrative interface between two supersystems: the brain and the immune system. *Pharmacol Rev* **52**: 595–638.

71 Edgar VA, Silberman DM, Cremaschi GA, Zieher LM, Genaro AM (2003). Altered lymphocyte catecholamine reactivity in mice subjected to chronic mild stress. *Biochem Pharmacol* **65**: 15–23.

72 Madden KS (2003). Catecholamines, sympathetic innervation, and immunity. *Brain Behav Immun* **17** (Suppl 1): S5–10.

73 Huang YS, Jiang JW, Cao XD, Wu GC (2003). Melatonin enhances lymphocyte proliferation and decreases the release of pituitary pro-opiomelanocortin-derived peptides in surgically traumatized rats. *Neurosci Lett* **343**: 109–12.

74 Carrillo-Vico A, Garcia-Maurino S, Calvo JR, Guerrero JM (2003). Melatonin counteracts the inhibitory effect of PGE2 on IL-2 production in human lymphocytes via its mt1 membrane receptor. *FASEB J* **17**: 755–7.

75 Kuhlwein E, Irwin M (2001). Melatonin modulation of lymphocyte proliferation and Th1/Th2 cytokine expression. *J Neuroimmunol* **117**: 51–7.

76 Maestroni GJ (1993). The immunoneuroendocrine role of melatonin. *J Pineal Res* **14**: 1–10.

77 Shakhar G, Ben-Eliyahu S (1998). In vivo beta-adrenergic stimulation suppresses natural killer activity and compromises resistance to tumor metastasis in rats. *J Immunol* **160**: 3251–8.

78 Matera L, Cardoso E, Veglia F, *et al.* (1988). Effect of cortisol on the native and *in vitro* induced non-MHC restricted cytotoxicity of large granular lymphocytes. *J Clin Lab Immunol* **27**: 77–81.

79 Ben-Eliyahu S, Shakhar G, Page GG, Stefanski V, Shakhar K (2000). Suppression of NK cell activity and of resistance to metastasis by stress: a role for adrenal catecholamines and beta-adrenoceptors. *Neuroimmunomodulation* **8**: 154–64.

80 Cesano A, Oberholtzer E, Contarini M, Geuna M, Bellone G, Matera L (1994). Independent and synergistic effect of interleukin-2 and prolactin on development of T- and NK-derived LAK effectors. *Immunopharmacology* **28**: 67–75.

81 Davila DR, Brief S, Simon J, Hammer RE, Brinster RL, Kelley KW (1987). Role of growth hormone in regulating T-dependent immune events in aged, nude, and transgenic rodents. *J Neurosci Res* **18**: 108–16.

82 Kiess W, Malozowski S, Gelato M, *et al.* (1988). Lymphocyte subset distribution and natural killer activity in growth hormone deficiency before and during short-term treatment with growth hormone releasing hormone. *Clin Immunol Immunopathol* **48**: 85–94.

83 Crist DM, Peake GT, Mackinnon LT, Sibbitt WL, Jr., Kraner JC (1987). Exogenous growth hormone treatment alters body composition and increases natural killer cell activity in women with impaired endogenous growth hormone secretion. *Metabolism* **36**: 1115–17.

84 Yin D, Mufson RA, Wang R, Shi Y (1999). Fas-mediated cell death promoted by opioids. *Nature* **397**: 218.

85 Shi Y, Devadas S, Greeneltch KM, Yin D, Allan Mufson R, Zhou JN (2003). Stressed to death: implication of lymphocyte apoptosis for psychoneuroimmunology. *Brain Behav Immun* **17** (Suppl 1): S18–26.

86 Ashwell JD, Lu FW, Vacchio MS (2000). Glucocorticoids in T cell development and function. *Annu Rev Immunol* **18**: 309–45.

87 Wyllie AH (1980). Glucocorticoid-induced thymocyte apoptosis is associated with endogenous endonuclease activation. *Nature* **284**: 555–6.

88 Evans-Storms RB, Cidlowski JA (1995). Regulation of apoptosis by steroid hormones. *J Steroid Biochem Mol Biol* **53**: 1–8.

89 Hirano T, Horigome A, Takatani M, Oka K (2001). Cortisone counteracts apoptosis-inducing effect of cortisol in human peripheral-blood mononuclear cells. *Int Immunopharmacol* **1**: 2109–15.

90 Krishnan N, Thellin O, Buckley DJ, Horseman ND, Buckley AR (2003). Prolactin suppresses glucocoticoid-induced thymocyte apoptosis *in vivo*. *Endocrinology* **144**: 2102–10.

91 Cioca DP, Watanabe N, Isobe M (2000). Apoptosis of peripheral blood lymphocytes is induced by catecholamines. *Jpn Heart J* **41**: 385–98.

92 Bergquist J, Josefsson E, Tarkowski A, Ekman R, Ewing A (1997). Measurements of catecholamine-mediated apoptosis of immunocompetent cells by capillary electrophoresis. *Electrophoresis* **18**: 1760–6.

93 Yu-Lee L (2001). Stimulation of interferon regulatory factor-1 by prolactin. *Lupus* **10**: 691–9.

94 Dogusan Z, Martens N, Stinissen P, *et al.* (2003). Effects of prolactin on cloned human T-lymphocytes. *Endocrine* **20**: 171–6.

95 Rook GA (1999). Glucocorticoids and immune function. *Baillière's Best Pract Res Clin Endocrinol Metab* **13**: 567–81.

96 Chen HT, Schuler LA, Schultz RD (1998). Growth hormone receptor and regulation of gene expression in fetal lymphoid cells. *Mol Cell Endocrinol* **137**: 21–9.

97 Licinio J, Gold PW, Wong ML (1995). A molecular mechanism for stress-induced alterations in susceptibility to disease. *Lancet* **346**: 104–6.

98 Walker L, Walker MB, and Sharp DM (2003). Psychosocial oncology services for women with breast cancer. *Update Urol Gynaecol Sexual Health* **8**: 25–32.

99 Derogatis LR, Morrow GR, Fetting J, *et al.* (1983). The prevalence of psychiatric disorders among cancer patients. *JAMA* **249**: 751–7.

100 Maguire GP, Lee EG, Bevington DJ, Kuchemann CS, Crabtree RJ, Cornell CE (1978). Psychiatric problems in the first year after mastectomy. *BMJ* **1**: 963–5.

101 Hall A, A'Hern R, Fallowfield L (1999). Are we using appropriate self-report questionnaires for detecting anxiety and depression in women with early breast cancer? *Eur J Cancer* 1: 79–85.

102 Zabora J, Brintzenhofeszoc K, Curbow B, Hooker C, Piantadosi S (2001). The prevalence of psychological distress by cancer site. *Psycho-oncology* 10: 19–28.

103 Walker LG, Walker MB, Sharp DM (2003). The organisation of psychosocial support within palliative care. In Lloyd-Williams M (ed) *Psychosocial Issues in Palliative Care*. Oxford: Oxford University Press, 49–66.

104 Peto J (2001). Cancer epidemiology in the last century and the next decade. *Nature* 411: 390–5.

105 Cohen S, Rabin BS (1998). Psychologic stress, immunity, and cancer. *J Natl Cancer Inst* 90: 3–4.

106 Peracoli MT, Montelli TC, Soares AM, *et al.* (1999). Immunological alterations in patients with primary tumors in central nervous system. *Arq Neuropsiquiatr* 57: 539–46.

107 Wu W, Yamaura T, Murakami K, *et al.* (2000). Social isolation stress enhanced liver metastasis of murine colon 26-L5 carcinoma cells by suppressing immune responses in mice. *Life Sci* 66: 1827–38.

108 IARC (1999). *Hormonal Contraception and Post-Menopausal Hormonal Therapy*. Lyon: IARC.

109 Baum M, Buzdar A (2003). The current status of aromatase inhibitors in the management of breast cancer. *Surg Clin North Am* 83: 973–94.

110 Mazzoccoli G, Giuliani A, Bianco G, *et al.* (1999). Decreased serum levels of insulin-like growth factor (IGF)-I in patients with lung cancer: temporal relationship with growth hormone (GH) levels. *Anticancer Res* 19: 1397–9.

111 Bartsch C, Bartsch H (1999). Melatonin in cancer patients and in tumor-bearing animals. *Adv Exp Med Biol* 467: 247–64.

112 Sephton SE, Sapolsky RM, Kraemer HC, Spiegel D (2000). Diurnal cortisol rhythm as a predictor of breast cancer survival. *J Natl Cancer Inst* 92: 994–1000.

113 Cohen L, de Moor C, Devine D, Baum A, Amato RJ (2001). Endocrine levels at the start of treatment are associated with subsequent psychological adjustment in cancer patients with metastatic disease. *Psychosom Med* 63: 951–8.

114 Touitou Y, Bogdan A, Levi F, Benavides M, Auzeby A (1996). Disruption of the circadian patterns of serum cortisol in breast and ovarian cancer patients: relationships with tumour marker antigens. *Br J Cancer* 74: 1248–52.

115 Touitou Y, Levi F, Bogdan A, Benavides M, Bailleul F, Misset JL (1995). Rhythm alteration in patients with metastatic breast cancer and poor prognostic factors. *J Cancer Res Clin Oncol* 121: 181–8.

116 van der Pompe G, Antoni MH, Heijnen CJ (1996). Elevated basal cortisol levels and attenuated ACTH and cortisol responses to a behavioral challenge in women with metastatic breast cancer. *Psychoneuroendocrinology* 21: 361–74.

117 Davis S, Mirick DK, Stevens RG (2001). Night shift work, light at night, and risk of breast cancer. *J Natl Cancer Inst* 93: 1557–62.

118 Schernhammer ES, Laden F, Speizer FE, *et al.* (2001). Rotating night shifts and risk of breast cancer in women participating in the nurses' health study. *J Natl Cancer Inst* 93: 1563–8.

119 Levy SM, Herberman RB, Lippman M, D'Angelo T, Lee J (1991). Immunological and psychosocial predictors of disease recurrence in patients with early-stage breast cancer. *Behav Med* 17: 67–75.

120 Osborne RH, Sali A, Aaronson NK, Elsworth GR, Mdzewski B, Sinclair AJ (2004). Immune function and adjustment style: do they predict survival in breast cancer? *Psycho-oncology* 13: 199–210.

121 Savard J, Morin CM (2001). Insomnia in the context of cancer: a review of a neglected problem. *J Clin Oncol* **19**: 895–908.

122 Degner LF, Sloan JA (1995). Symptom distress in newly diagnosed ambulatory cancer patients and as a predictor of survival in lung cancer. *J Pain Symptom Manage* **10**: 423–31.

123 Savard J, Laroche L, Simard S, Ivers H, Morin CM (2003). Chronic insomnia and immune functioning. *Psychosom Med* **65**: 211–21.

124 Irwin M, Clark C, Kennedy B, Christian Gillin J, Ziegler M (2003). Nocturnal catecholamines and immune function in insomniacs, depressed patients, and control subjects. *Brain Behav Immun* **17**: 365–72.

125 Sephton S, Spiegel D (2003). Circadian disruption in cancer: a neuroendocrine-immune pathway from stress to disease? *Brain Behav Immun* **17**: 321–8.

126 Bovbjerg DH (2003). Circadian disruption and cancer: sleep and immune regulation. *Brain Behav Immun* **17** (Suppl 1): S48–50.

127 Walker LG, Johnson VC, Eremin O (1993). Modulation of the immune response to stress by hypnosis and relaxation training in normals: a critical review. Contemp Hypn **10**: 19–27.

128 Fawzy FI, Kemeny ME, Fawzy NW, *et al.* (1990). A structured psychiatric intervention for cancer patients. II. Changes over time in immunological measures. *Arch Gen Psychiatry* **47**: 729–35.

129 Eremin O, Walker MB, Simpson E, *et al.* (in preparation). Immuno-modulatory effects of relaxation training and guided imagery in women with locally advanced breast cancer undergoing multimodality therapy: a randomised controlled trial.

130 Andersen BL, Farrar WB, Golden-Kreutz DM, *et al.* (2004). Psychological, behavioral, and immune changes after a psychological intervention: a clinical trial. *J Clin Oncol* **22**: 3570–80.

131 Gaab J, Blattler N, Menzi T, Pabst B, Stoyer S, Ehlert U (2003). Randomized controlled evaluation of the effects of cognitive-behavioral stress management on cortisol responses to acute stress in healthy subjects. *Psychoneuroendocrinology* **28**: 767–79.

132 McKinney CH, Antoni MH, Kumar M, Tims FC, McCabe PM (1997). Effects of guided imagery and music (GIM) therapy on mood and cortisol in healthy adults. *Health Psychol* **16**: 390–400.

133 Facchinetti F, Tarabusi M, Volpe A (2004). Cognitive-behavioral treatment decreases cardiovascular and neuroendocrine reaction to stress in women waiting for assisted reproduction. *Psychoneuroendocrinology* **29**: 162–73.

134 Cruess DG, Antoni MH, McGregor BA, *et al.* (2000). Cognitive-behavioral stress management reduces serum cortisol by enhancing benefit finding among women being treated for early stage breast cancer. *Psychosom Med* **62**: 304–8.

135 van der Pompe G, Duivenvoorden HJ, Antoni MH, Visser A, Heijnen CJ (1997). Effectiveness of a short-term group psychotherapy program on endocrine and immune function in breast cancer patients: an exploratory study. *J Psychosom Res* **42**: 453–66.

136 Turner-Cobb JM, Sephton SE, Koopman C, Blake-Mortimer J, Spiegel D (2000). Social support and salivary cortisol in women with metastatic breast cancer. *Psychosom Med* **62**: 337–45.

137 Heinrichs M, Baumgartner T, Kirschbaum C, Ehlert U (2003). Social support and oxytocin interact to suppress cortisol and subjective responses to psychosocial stress. *Biol Psychiatry* **54**: 1389–98.

138 Schedlowski M, Jacobs R, Stratmann G, *et al.* (1993). Changes of natural killer cells during acute psychological stress. *J Clin Immunol* **13**: 119–26.

139 Fox BH (1998). Psychosocial factors in cancer incidence and progression. In Holland JC (ed) *Psycho-oncology*. New York: Oxford University Press, 110–24.

140 Heffner KL, Loving TJ, Robles TF, Kiecolt-Glaser JK (2003). Examining psychosocial factors related to cancer incidence and progression: in search of the silver lining. *Brain Behav Immun* **17** (Suppl 1): S109–11.

141 Petticrew M, Fraser JM, Regan MF (1999). Adverse life events and risk of breast cancer: a meta-analysis. *Br J Health Psychol* **4**: 1–17.

142 Duijts SF, Zeegers MP, Borne BV (2003). The association between stressful life events and breast cancer risk: a meta-analysis. *Int J Cancer* **107**: 1023–9.

143 Lillberg K, Verkasalo PK, Kaprio J, Teppo L, Helenius H, Koskenvuo M (2003). Stressful life events and risk of breast cancer in 10 808 women: a cohort study. *Am J Epidemiol* **157**: 415–23.

144 Shekelle RB, Raynor WJ Jr, Ostfeld AM, *et al.* (1981). Psychological depression and 17-year risk of death from cancer. *Psychosom Med* **43**: 117–25.

145 Persky VW, Kempthorne-Rawson J, Shekelle RB (1987). Personality and risk of cancer: 20-year follow-up of the Western Electric Study. *Psychosom Med* **49**: 435–49.

146 Hahn RC, Petitti DB (1988). Minnesota Multiphasic Personality Inventory-rated depression and the incidence of breast cancer. *Cancer* **61**: 845–8.

147 Kaplan GA, Reynolds P (1988). Depression and cancer mortality and morbidity: prospective evidence from the Alameda County study. *J Behav Med* **11**: 1–13.

148 Ramirez AJ, Craig TK, Watson JP, Fentiman IS, North WR, Rubens RD (1989). Stress and relapse of breast cancer. *BMJ* **298**: 291–3.

149 Barraclough J, Pinder P, Cruddas M, Osmond C, Taylor I, Perry M (1992). Life events and breast cancer prognosis. *BMJ* **304**: 1078–81.

150 Ratcliffe MA, Dawson AA, Walker LG (1995). Eysenck personality inventory L-scores in patients with Hodgkin's disease and non-Hodgkin's lymphoma. *Psycho-oncology* **4**: 39–45.

151 Walker LG, Walker MB, Ogston K, *et al.* (1999). Psychological, clinical and pathological effects of relaxation training and guided imagery during primary chemotherapy. *Br J Cancer* **80**: 262–8.

152 Watson M, Haviland JS, Greer S, Davidson J, Bliss JM (1999). Influence of psychological response on survival in breast cancer: a population-based cohort study. *Lancet* **354**: 1331–6.

153 Cassileth BR, Lusk EJ, Miller DS, Brown LL, Miller C (1985). Psychosocial correlates of survival in advanced malignant disease? *N Engl J Med* **312**: 1551–5.

154 Jamison RN, Burish TG, Wallston KA (1987). Psychogenic factors in predicting survival of breast cancer patients. *J Clin Oncol* **5**: 768–72.

155 Silberfarb PM, Anderson KM, Rundle AC, Holland JC, Cooper MR, McIntyre OR (1991). Mood and clinical status in patients with multiple myeloma. *J Clin Oncol* **9**: 2219–24.

156 Greer S, Morris T, Pettingale KW (1979). Psychological response to breast cancer: effect on outcome. *Lancet* **ii**: 785–7.

157 Greer S, Morris T, Pettingale KW (1994). *Psychological Response to Breast Cancer: Effect on Outcome. A Reader*. Cambridge: Cambridge University Press.

158 Greer S, Watson M (1985). Towards a psychobiological model of cancer: psychological considerations. *Soc Sci Med* **20**: 773–7.

159 Morris T, Pettingale KW, Haybittle J (1992). Psychological response to cancer diagnosis and disease outcome in patients with breast cancer and lymphoma. *Psycho-oncology* **1**: 105–114.

160 Pettingale KW, Morris T, Greer S, Haybittle JL (1985). Mental attitudes to cancer: an additional prognostic factor. *Lancet* **i**: 750.

161 Kneier AW, Temoshok L (1984). Repressive coping reactions in patients with malignant melanoma as compared to cardiovascular disease patients. *J Psychosom Res* **28**: 145–55.

162 Temoshok L, Heller BW, Sagebiel RW, *et al.* (1985). The relationship of psychosocial factors to prognostic indicators in cutaneous malignant melanoma. *J Psychosom Res* **29**: 139–53.

163 Speigel D (1999). Healing words. Emotional expression and disease outcome. *JAMA* **281**: 1328–9.

164 Fawzy FI, Canada AL, Fawzy NW (2003). Malignant melanoma: effects of a brief, structured psychiatric intervention on survival and recurrence at 10-year follow-up. *Arch Gen Psychiatry* **60**: 100–3.

165 Kuchler T, Henne-Bruns D, Rappat S, *et al.* (1999). Impact of psychotherapeutic support on gastrointestinal cancer patients undergoing surgery: survival results of a trial. *Hepatogastroenterology* **46**: 322–35.

166 Richardson JL, Shelton DR, Krailo M, Levine AM (1990). The effect of compliance with treatment on survival among patients with hematologic malignancies. *J Clin Oncol* **8**: 356–64.

167 Spiegel D, Bloom JR, Kraemer HC, Gottheil E (1989). Effect of psychosocial treatment on survival of patients with metastatic breast cancer. *Lancet* **ii**: 888–91.

168 Walker L, Ratcliffe MA, Dawson AA (2000). Relaxation and hypnotherapy: long term effects on the survival of patients with lymphoma. *Psycho-oncology* **9**: 355–6.

169 Cunningham AJ, Edmonds CV, Jenkins GP, Pollack H, Lockwood GA, Warr D (1998). A randomized controlled trial of the effects of group psychological therapy on survival in women with metastatic breast cancer. *Psycho-oncology* **7**: 508–17.

170 Edelman S, Lemon J, Bell DR, Kidman AD (1999). Effects of group CBT on the survival time of patients with metastatic breast cancer. *Psycho-oncology* **8**: 474–81.

171 Goodwin PJ, Leszcz M, Ennis M, *et al.* (2001). The effect of group psychosocial support on survival in metastatic breast cancer. *N Engl J Med* **345**: 1719–26.

172 Ilnyckyj A, Farber J, Cheang *et al.* (1994). A randomised controlled trial of psychotherapeutic interventions in cancer patients. *Ann R Coll Physicians Surgeons Canada* **27**: 93–6.

173 Linn MW, Linn BS, Harris R (1982). Effects of counseling for late stage cancer patients. *Cancer* **49**: 1048–55.

174 Walker M, Walker L, Simpson E, *et al.* (2000). Do relaxation and guided imagery improve survival in women with locally advanced breast cancer. Abstract, 1999 British Psychosocial Oncology Society Annual Conference. *Psycho-oncology* **9**: 355–64.

175 Cunningham AJ (2002). Group psychological therapy: an integral part of care for cancer patients. *Integr Cancer Ther* **1**: 67–75.

176 Fawzy FI, Fawzy NW, Hyun CS, *et al.* (1993). Malignant melanoma. Effects of an early structured psychiatric intervention, coping, and affective state on recurrence and survival 6 years later. *Arch Gen Psychiatry* **50**: 681–9.

177 Maier SF, Watkins LR (2003). Immune-to-central nervous system communication and its role in modulating pain and cognition: implications for cancer and cancer treatment. *Brain Behav Immun* **17** (Suppl 1): S125–31.

178 Bower JE, Ganz PA, Aziz N, Fahey JL (2002). Fatigue and proinflammatory cytokine activity in breast cancer survivors. *Psychosom Med* **64**: 604–11.

179 Minisini A, Atalay G, Bottomley A, Puglisi F, Piccart M, Biganzoli L (2004). What is the effect of systemic anticancer treatment on cognitive function? *Lancet Oncol* **5**: 273–82.

180 Walker LG, Wesnes KP, Heys SD, Walker MB, Lolley J, Eremin O (1996). The cognitive effects ofrecombinant interleukin-2 (rIL-2). therapy: a controlled clinical trial using computerised assessments. *Eur J Cancer* **32A**: 2275–83.

181 Walker LG, Walker MB, Heys SD, Lolley J, Wesnes K, Eremin O (1997). The psychological and psychiatric effects of rIL-2 therapy: a controlled clinical trial. *Psycho-oncology* **6**: 290–301.

Chapter 7

Psychoneuroimmunology and chronic viral infection: HIV infection

Deidre B. Pereira and Frank J. Penedo

7.1 Introduction

Despite recent advances in immunotherapy for human immunodeficiency virus (HIV) infection, HIV and acquired immunodeficiency syndrome (AIDS) remain serious global health threats. Following initial HIV infection and viraemia, a period of clinical latency generally occurs, commonly followed by a gradual deterioration in immune status and functioning, abnormalities in neuroendocrinological functioning, and the eventual development of HIV-related symptoms and AIDS-related conditions. As with any virally initiated condition that is under surveillance by the immune system, HIV provides a unique and clinically significant paradigm in which to examine psycho-neuroimmunological (PNI) relations. In this chapter we will review the epidemiology, pathophysiology, and treatment of HIV, and we will present an empirically testable theoretical model showing how specific biopsychosocial factors may affect immunity and health outcomes among individuals living with HIV. We then review of some of the most seminal empirical research to date in the PNI of HIV infection, and suggest several directions for future research.

7.2 The biological/clinical context

7.2.1 Epidemiology of HIV infection

Despite recent advances in immunotherapy for HIV infection, HIV and AIDS remain serious global health threats. In the United States, the cumulative number of AIDS cases reported to the Centers for Disease Control and Prevention (CDC) up to December 2001 was 816, 149. Nearly 60% of these individuals belonged to racial and/or ethnic minority groups. Approximately 468, 000 individuals reported with AIDS in the United States have died since the beginning of the epidemic, including 5257 children.[1] Worldwide, HIV infection and AIDS are endemic. Currently, 42 million people are living with AIDS worldwide. During 2002 alone, 3.1 million people died from AIDS across the globe, including 1.2 million women.[2]

Although HIV prevention efforts have had measured success in reducing HIV risk behaviours in men who have sex with men (MSM), this community continues to comprise the greatest number of AIDS cases reported to the CDC each year. Women of colour, especially Black women, and women aged 25–44 years are also at high risk for HIV. Recently, the proportion of all AIDS cases reported among women more than tripled from 7% in 1985 to 25% in 1999.[1]

7.2.2 The HIV-1 virus

HIV belongs to the lentivirus ('slow') subgroup of the retrovirus family. Retroviruses are RNA viruses, i.e. they contain their genetic information in the form of RNA. In order to replicate, RNA viruses use the enzyme reverse transcriptase to convert RNA into DNA, which is then incorporated inside a host cell's genes.[3] The HIV-1 virus particle ('virion') and the life-cycle of HIV are shown in Figure 7.1.

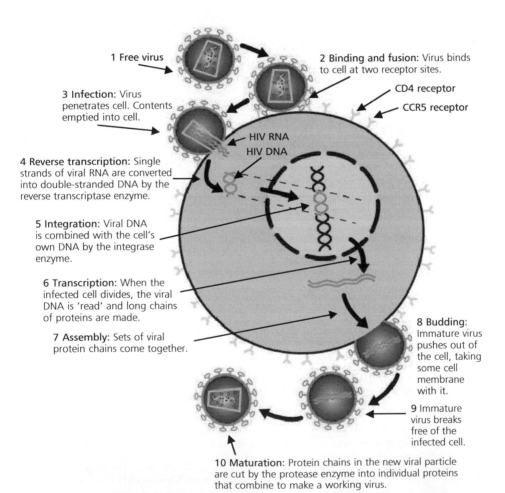

1 Free virus

2 Binding and fusion: Virus binds to cell at two receptor sites.

3 Infection: Virus penetrates cell. Contents emptied into cell.

CD4 receptor

CCR5 receptor

HIV RNA
HIV DNA

4 Reverse transcription: Single strands of viral RNA are converted into double-stranded DNA by the reverse transcriptase enzyme.

5 Integration: Viral DNA is combined with the cell's own DNA by the integrase enzyme.

6 Transcription: When the infected cell divides, the viral DNA is 'read' and long chains of proteins are made.

7 Assembly: Sets of viral protein chains come together.

8 Budding: Immature virus pushes out of the cell, taking some cell membrane with it.

9 Immature virus breaks free of the infected cell.

10 Maturation: Protein chains in the new viral particle are cut by the protease enzyme into individual proteins that combine to make a working virus.

Fig. 7.1 The HIV life-cycle. (Reproduced with permission from New Mexico AIDS InfoNet at http://www.aids.org/factSheets/415-life-cycle.html).

7.2.3 Transmission of HIV from person to person

HIV is transmitted from person to person through sexual contact with an infected individual or contact with HIV-infected blood. Perinatal transmission of HIV (i.e. from mother to child) rarely occurs now, because zidovudine (i.e. AZT), a reverse transcriptase inhibitor, is prescribed for HIV+ pregnant women during the prepartum and intrapartum periods. Breastfeeding is an additional route by which HIV can be transmitted.[3]

7.2.4 Pathogenesis of HIV infection

Once initial exposure to HIV has occurred, the virus quickly infects helper T cells and replicates in the peripheral blood and lymphoid organs. As a result of this explosion in HIV viral load, many infected individuals will experience mild to moderate influenza-like symptoms approximately a month after initial exposure to HIV. Typical symptoms may include low-grade fever, night sweats, headache, and fatigue.[4] The immune system counters this attack by generating cytotoxic T lymphocytes (CTLs) to recognize and kill HIV viral particles. CTL-mediated killing reduces HIV viremia and results in a period of clinical latency that can last for many years.[3] This phase is often referred to as the asymptomatic phase in HIV infection. However, over time, a gradual deterioration of immune status and functioning occurs, resulting in HIV viraemia and the development of HIV-specific symptoms and diseases. AIDS is diagnosed when an individual has a CD4+ CD3+ count <200 cells/ml or at least one AIDS-defining condition is present (Table 7.1).[5]

7.2.5 Mechanisms of deterioration of immune status and functioning in HIV infection

Several mechanisms may explain the deterioration of immunity in HIV infection. First, helper T cells may die when HIV viral particles bud off from the cell surface during the

Table 7.1 Centers for Disease Control and Prevention 1993 revised classification system for HIV infection and expanded surveillance case definition for AIDS among adolescents and adults[5]

CD4+ T-lymphocyte categories		Clinical categories		
		Asymptomatic (A)	Symptomatic[a] (B)	Presence of at least one AIDS-defining illness[b] (C)
≥500 cells/ml	(1)	A1	B1	C1
200–499 cells/ml	(2)	A2	B2	C2
<200 cells/ml	(3)	A3	B3	C3

[a] Examples of conditions in clinical category B include, but are not limited to, the following: candidiasis, oropharyngeal (thrush); candidiasis, vulvovaginal; persistent, frequent, or poorly responsive to therapy; cervical dysplasia (moderate or severe)/cervical carcinoma in situ; constitutional symptoms such as fever (38.5°C) or diarrhoea lasting for more than 1 month.

[b] AIDS-definition conditions included in the 1993 AIDS surveillance case definition are as follows: cervical cancer, invasive; Kaposi's sarcoma; Pneumocystis carinii pneumonia; pneumonia, recurrent; wasting syndrome due to HIV.

HIV replication process. Some infected helper T cells may also undergo programmed cell death, a process known as apoptosis. Surviving infected helper T cells may have inadequate function and fail to proliferate (multiply) adequately in response to stimulation by HIV proteins.[3,4,6] In addition, prolonged HIV infection may lead to the depletion or exhaustion of CTLs. As a result, CTL-mediated killing of viruses and tumours may be impaired.

Secondly, reverse transcriptase may also be implicated in the deterioration of immune status and functioning. Reverse transcriptase is notoriously inaccurate in making DNA copies from HIV RNA, causing the rapid generation of mutations. This leads to impairment in the ability of HIV peptides to bind to class I molecules on antigen-presenting cells, a process that is necessary for an established CTL-mediated killing response to occur.[3,4,6]

Thirdly, immune deterioration may also result from a shift in cytokine production patterns.[7–9] Cytokines are soluble proteins and peptides that modulate immune functioning and relay messages from the immune system to the brain.[10] Research suggests that as HIV progresses, the cytokine production pattern shifts from the production of predominantly type 1 cytokines (Th1) to the production of predominantly type 2 cytokines (Th2) . Th1 cells evoke cellular immunity, while Th2 cells stimulate humoral responses. This is of importance in HIV infection, because Th1 cytokines decrease the vulnerability of lymphocytes to apoptosis, while Th2 cytokines increase susceptibility to apoptosis. Thus this shift in cytokine production may lead to the increased destruction of helper T cells. In addition, research has found that cytokines can have stimulatory effects (e.g. IL-6, a Th2 cytokine), inhibitory effects (e.g. IFN-γ, a Th1 cytokine) or both stimulatory and inhibitory effects (e.g. IL-4) effects on HIV replication.[11]

Fourthly, HIV infection is associated with the impairment of the functioning of CD56+ CD3+ or natural killer (NK) cells over time.[12] NK cells are a subset of lymphocytes that are induced by cytokines to kill tumours and virally infected cells in the absence of induction by a specific antigen.[13] Importantly, NK cells have been found to suppress the replication of HIV as effectively as CTLs.[14] In fact, research suggests that relative preservation of NK cell count and functioning may be associated with maintaining the health of HIV-infected individuals with very low helper T cell counts.[15]

7.2.6 Neuroendocrine abnormalities in HIV infection

In addition to the immune abnormalities mentioned above, HIV infection is also associated with heightened sympathetic nervous system (SNS) activation and functional abnormalities of the hypothalamic–pituitary–adrenal (HPA) and hypothalamic–pituitary–gonadal (HPG) axes.[16–19] Specifically, norepinephrine is associated with an increase in HIV replication up to 11-fold and the suppression of IFN-γ and IL-10, which are immunomodulatory cytokines with antiviral and antitumour functions.[20] In addition, HIV+ individuals, especially those with advanced disease, are known to have hypercortisolaemia and low levels of deoxyhydroepiandrosterone (DHEA), a hormone that counteracts the immunoregulatory functions of cortisol.[8] Importantly, a high cortisol-to-DHEA ratio is associated with a lower number of helper T cells in HIV+ individuals.[21] HIV+ men and women also demonstrate androgen deficiency which is associated with a lower number of helper T cell counts, weight loss, and advanced disease stage.[22,23]

Although few studies have examined the impact of female sex hormones on immune status or functioning in HIV infection, it is known that progesterone and oestrogen control immune cell trafficking, immune functioning, and chemokine receptor expression.[24] CTL functioning is downregulated during the secretory phase of the menstrual cycle, which is characterized by high levels of progesterone and oestrogen.[25] In addition, the periovulatory phase of the menstrual cycle, which is characterized by low progesterone and high oestrogen levels, is associated with decreases in genital HIV viral load.[26]

7.2.7 Overview of the clinical management of HIV-infected individuals

The guidelines for the treatment of HIV-infected individuals are constantly evolving. The Department of Health and Human Services 2002 Guidelines for the Use of Antiretroviral Agents in HIV infected Adults and Adolescents[27] recommends offering antiretroviral therapy to patients with <350 helper T cells/ml or HIV RNA levels >55 000 copies/ml. Treatment success is defined as a $\log_{10}$ decrease in HIV viral load by 8 weeks and >50 copies/ml of HIV RNA by 4–6 months. Reasons for treatment failure include non-adherence, an inadequate or low-potency treatment regimen, and resistance of the virus to the treatment regimen.[27]

To facilitate treatment success, approaching 100% (i.e. >95%) adherence to the anti-retroviral treatment regimen is required. This is difficult for many individuals to achieve. Rates of optimal adherence in published studies vary from 5%[28] to 63%.[29,30] Suboptimal adherence is due to a number of factors. Many of the treatment regimens are complex and costly, and have numerous unpleasant side effects. Some of the regimens have special dietary and refrigeration requirements; many require taking medication several times a day. These are among the factors that make it difficult to keep the regimen and the illness itself concealed from others. Because of the requirement for nearly 100% adherence and the numerous barriers to adherence, much of the recent biopsychosocial research in HIV/AIDS has examined the factors associated with non-adherence to antiretroviral therapy and the efficacy of interventions to improve adherence in HIV-infected individuals.[31] Although not primarily the focus of this chapter, some of the most influential literature on the predictors of antiretroviral adherence is outlined later.

7.3 Theoretical basis for examining psychoneuroimmunological processes in HIV infection

Over the past 20 years, the field of PNI has generated a large body of evidence suggesting a reciprocal relationship between the mind and the body. Some of the earliest and most seminal studies in the field demonstrated relationships between psychosocial factors, including stress, depression, and bereavement, and outcomes such as immunity,[32] neuroendocrine functioning,[33] susceptibility to infectious illnesses,[34] and higher antibody titres to latent viruses, suggesting poorer viral immunosurveillance.[35]

When HIV/AIDS emerged as a serious public health threat in the 1980s, PNI researchers took notice. As knowledge surrounding HIV expanded, it became clear that many of the immune and neuroendocrine outcomes previously studied by PNI researchers were altered or impaired in HIV+ individuals. In addition, clinical research began to document high rates of psychiatric morbidity in HIV+ individuals. HIV-infected individuals experience a high number of severe life stressors such as stigmatization/discrimination based on disease status, sexual orientation, and racial/ethnic group membership, multiple bereavements, homelessness, poverty, unsafe

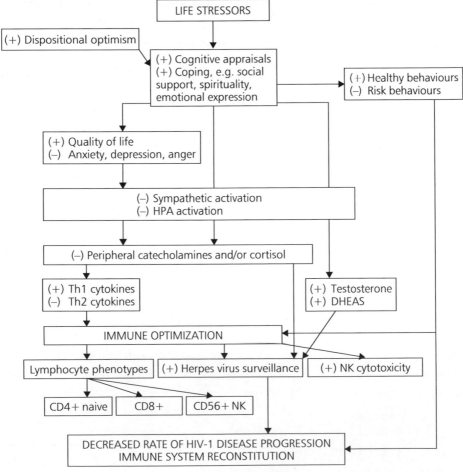

Fig. 7.2 Psychoneuroimmunological processes in HIV infection; a prescription for wellness? (Adapted from M. H. Antoni (2003) *CNS Spectr* **8**: 40–51.)

housing, and immigrant status, to name a few.[36,37] Chronic sorrow and depressive, anxiety, and past/current substance use disorders are also prevalent among HIV+ individuals.[38–40] (However, it is also important to note that in our clinical experience with HIV-infected individuals, we have also noted a great deal of courage, resilience, faith, and positive coping in the face of difficult life circumstances.[36])

Integrating this basic and clinical research, HIV provides a unique and clinically significant paradigm in which to examine PNI relations. Consequently, specific models were developed to provide a framework for testing hypothetical relationships between psychosocial factors, immunity, neuroendocrine, and clinical health outcomes in HIV+ individuals.[41,42] Briefly, these models posit that heightened stress levels cause both SNS and HPA activation in HIV+ individuals. This heightened activation causes a flooding of catecholamines (e.g. norepinephrine) and glucocorticoids (e.g. cortisol). Alterations in hormone production patterns also occur (e.g. decreases in testosterone and DHEA). The flooding of catecholamines and glucocorticoids alters cytokine production patterns (i.e. Th1→Th2 cytokine production pattern), leading to decrements in lymphocyte numbers, CTL functioning, NK cell count, and viral surveillance. HIV viraemia results from this cascade, followed by increased risk of HIV morbidity and mortality (Fig. 7.2).

7.4 Empirical evidence

The relationships between numerous psychosocial constructs and biological and physical outcomes have been examined since the beginning of the HIV epidemic. Generally, these psychosocial variables can be categorized into the following groups: stressful life events, cognitive factors, coping, mood, personality, and health behaviours. Table 7.2 outlines the main psychosocial constructs that have been examined in PNI–HIV research and lists some of the most influential journal articles examining these relations.

7.4.1 The occurrence and impact of negative life events

The occurrence and impact of negative life events have been among the psychosocial factors most consistently associated with biological and physical health markers and survival in HIV+ individuals. In some of the earliest work published in this area, Goodkin et al.[43] reported a significant relationship between greater impact of negative life events and lower total lymphocyte counts, as well as a marginally significant relationship between life events and lower CD4+ CD3+ cell count specifically, among 11 asymptomatic HIV-infected gay men.

Research has also provided compelling evidence for a relationship between stress and immunity prospectively in HIV+ individuals. Evans et al.[44] found that severe life stress was associated with decrements in NK cell and cytotoxic/suppressor T-cell counts among HIV-infected gay men, but not among HIV- uninfected men. Later, Leserman et al.[45] found that asymptomatic HIV-infected gay men with both severe

Table 7.2 PNI and HIV research: empirically researched psychosocial constructs and significant outcomes

Psychosocial construct	Selected references	Significant outcomes		
		Immune	Neuroendocrine	Symptoms, disease progression or survival
The occurrence and impact of negative life events				
Cumulative negative life events	Leserman et al.[53]	☐	☐	☒
	Howland et al.[46]	☒	☐	☐
	Leserman et al.[52]	☐	☐	☒
	Petitto et al.[49]	☒	☒	☐
	Leserman et al.[51]	☐	☐	☒
	Evans et al.[50]	☐	☐	☒
Impact of negative life events	Pereira et al.[55]	☐	☐	☒
	Pereira et al.[56]	☐	☐	☒
	Leserman et al.[45]	☒	☐	☐
	Evans et al.[44]	☒	☐	☐
	Goodkin[74]	☒	☐	☐
Perceived stress	Cruess et al.[79]	☒	☐	☐
	Cruess et al.[113]	☐	☒	☐
	Cruess et al.[112]	☐	☒	☐
Traumatic stress	Kimerling et al.[48]	☒	☐	☐
Stress moderators/mediators				
Cognitive factors				
Coping self-efficacy	Benight et al.[66]	☐	☒	☐
Discovery of meaning	Bower et al.[64]	☐	☐	☒
Intrusion-avoidance of HIV-or trauma-related cognitions	Cruess et al.[70]	☒	☐	☐
	Kimerling et al.[48]	☒	☐	☐
	Lutgendorf et al.[69]	☒	☐	☐
	Antoni et al.[68]	☐	☒	☐
Negative expectancies and causal attributions	Reed et al.[61]	☐	☐	☒
	Segerstrom et al.[63]	☐	☐	☒
	Reed et al.[62]	☐	☐	☒
Coping				
Active, productive coping	Mulder et al.[76]	☐	☐	☒
	Mulder et al.[75]	☐	☐	☒
	Solano et al.[77]	☐	☐	☒
	Goodkin et al.[43]	☒	☐	☐
	Goodkin et al.[74]	☒	☐	☐
Denial[a]	Leserman et al.[52]	☐	☐	☒
	Ironson et al.[78]	☐	☐	☒
	Solano et al.[77]	☐	☐	☒
	Antoni et al.[68]	☒	☐	☐
Social support	Leserman et al.[53]	☐	☐	☒
	Cruess et al.[79]	☒	☐	☐
	Leserman et al.[52]	☐	☐	☒
	Leserman et al.[51]	☐	☐	☒
	Cole et al.[83]	☐	☐	☒

Table 7.2 (*Continued*)

Psychosocial construct	Selected references	Immune	Neuroendocrine	Symptoms, disease progression or survival
	Miller et al.[82]	☐	☐	☒
	Patterson et al.[81]	☐	☐	☒
	Theorell et al.[80]	☐	☐	☒
Spirituality, religiosity Emotional expression, disclosure	Ironson et al.[85]	☐	☒	☒
	Eisenberger et al.[86]	☒	☐	☐
	O'Cleirigh et al.[87]	☒	☐	☒
	Ullrich et al.[90]	☒	☐	☐
	Sherman et al.[91]	☐	☐	☒
	Cole et al.[88]	☐	☐	☒
Mood				
AIDS-related bereavement	Reed et al.[61]	☐	☐	☒
	Goodkin et al.[95]	☒	☐	☐
	Kemeny and Dean[107]	☐	☐	☒
	Kemeny et al.[94]	☒	☐	☐
Anxiety	Evans et al.[92]	☒	☐	☐
	Antoni et al.[109]	☒	☒	☐
Anger	Leserman et al.[53]	☐	☐	☒
Depression, depressive symptoms, dysphoric mood	Leserman et al.[53]	☐	☐	☒
	Evans et al.[92]	☒	☐	☐
	Ickovics et al.[101]	☐	☐	☒
	Antoni et al.[107]	☐	☒	☐
	Leserman et al.[51]	☐	☐	☒
	Leserman et al.[45]	☒	☐	☐
	Lutgendorf et al.[110]	☒	☐	☐
	Mayne et al.[108]	☐	☐	☒
	Patterson et al.[81]	☐	☐	☒
	Kemeny et al.[96]	☒	☐	☐
	Burack et al.[101]	☐	☐	☒
'Distress'/mood disturbance	Cruess et al.[113]	☐	☒	☐
	Cruess et al.[112]	☐	☒	☐
	Vedhara et al.[104]	☐	☐	☒
	Ironson et al.[78]	☐	☐	☒
	Antoni et al. 1990	☐	☒	☐
Personality				
Optimism/pessimism[b]	Tomakowsky et al.[116]	☐	☐	☒
	Cruess et al.[79]	☒	☐	☐
	Byrnes et al.[114]	☒	☐	☐

Studies reporting null findings are not included in the table. Only studies in which a psychosocial factor was associated with an immune, neuroendocrine or clinical health outcome were included. Studies examining the efficacy of a psychosocial intervention on immune, neuroendocrine or clinical health outcomes were included only if intervention-associated changes in psychosocial factors were paralleled by changes in biological or physical health outcomes. References may be listed under more than one category. Studies reporting psychosocial relations to declines in CD4+ CD3+ cell counts over time are categorized under 'Health outcome'.

[a] 'Denial' could also be categorized under 'Cognitions'.

[b] The references in this category could also be listed under 'Negative expectancies and causal attributions'.

stress and depressive symptoms experienced significant decreases in NK cells and CD8+ T lymphocytes from study entry to 2-year follow-up. Although few published studies have examined PNI mechanisms in HIV+ children and adolescents, at least one study suggests that stressful life events are associated with greater declines in helper T cells in this population.[46]

The experience of numerous traumatic stressors is common in the lives of HIV+ individuals. Accordingly, HIV+ individuals have high prevalence rates of post-traumatic stress disorder (PTSD) symptomatology.[47,48] Despite this, very few published research studies have examined the relationship between traumatic stressors, specifically, and immune status in HIV+ individuals. One study by[48] suggests that exposure to traumatic stressors is associated with lower CD4-to-CD8 ratios in HIV+ women. More research in this area is warranted.

Some evidence suggests that the relationship between stress and immunity may be moderated by cortisol production. Specifically, Petitto et al.[49] found that severe life stress was significantly correlated with lower numbers of CD8+ and NK cells and with higher DHEA-sulfate (DHEA-S) concentrations in individuals with high, but not low, cortisol secretion. This suggests that individuals with high cortisol secretion associated with severe life stress may be at increased risk for immunosuppression.

Stressful life events have also been strongly associated with disease progression and survival in HIV+ individuals. Evans et al.[50] examined the relationship between the number of severe life stressors per 6-month study interval and risk for HIV disease progression up to 42-month follow-up among HIV+-asymptomatic gay men. They found that the risk for early HIV disease progression doubled for every severe stressor experienced per 6-month study interval. Among a subset of participants who remained in the study for at least 2 years, greater severe life stress was associated with a fourfold increase in the odds of experiencing HIV disease progression. Among these same participants, Leserman et al.[51] found that greater cumulative life stress was associated with faster progression to AIDS (i.e. helper T cell count <200 cells/ml) or development of an AIDS-indicator condition. Specifically, men with the greatest stress and the lowest perceived social support had a two- to threefold increase in the probability of developing AIDS at 66-month follow-up compared with men with low stress/high social support. Adding to this research, Leserman et al.[52] found that faster progression to AIDS was associated not only with greater cumulative life stress and lower cumulative social support satisfaction, but also with greater use of denial coping and higher serum cortisol. Importantly, higher serum cortisol has been linked to increased risk for mortality among HIV+ men.[53]

High life stress has also been associated with the status and progression of specific conditions commonly experienced by HIV+ individuals, particularly those initiated by viruses. Two such viruses are herpes simplex virus (HSV) and human papillomavirus (HPV). HIV+ individuals have high rates of HSV-2 seropositivity and genital herpes recurrences. Although HSV-2 infection is generally a benign medical condition in immunocompetent individuals, co-infection with HSV and HIV is associated with significant risk for HSV-related morbidity and mortality. HPV infection, on the other hand, is a common sexually transmitted virus associated with the development and progression of cervical dysplasia and carcinoma.[54] Consistent with other research noting the relationship between life stress, viral reactivation, and risk for HIV disease progression, greater impact of negative life events has been associated with recurrence of genital herpes[55] and increased risk for the progression or persistence of HPV-induced cervical dysplasia[56] in HIV+ Black women.

Overall, these findings suggest that stress predicts HIV disease progression defined not only as movement between CDC categories (asymptomatic→symptomatic→AIDS), but also in the progression of specific clinical conditions. This is particularly impressive given the wide variability in the measurement and operationalization of stress. However, despite this evidence, it is important to note that some early published research failed to uncover a relationship between stress and HIV disease progression. For instance, Kessler et al.[57] reported that the number of life stressors experienced in the previous 6 months failed to predict a 25% decrease in CD4% or the incidence of fever or thrush in HIV+ men. However, problems associated with the measurement and operationalization of stress and disease progression may have confounded a possible relationship between these factors. In general, studies that have successfully uncovered relationships between stress and disease progression have used interview-based measures that attempt to capture the chronicity or severity of life stress, for instance, by assessing the negative impact of life stress or cumulative life stress across a follow-up period. In addition, using CD4% as a measure of HIV disease progression may be inadequate, because CD4% can be significantly affected by fluctuations in other lymphocyte subsets. Therefore it may be most clinically relevant to follow CD4+ CD3+ cell counts longitudinally. Furthermore, as suggested by Nott et al.[42] HIV disease progression should be operationalized by the rate of decline in CD4+ CD3+ cell count rather than by single assessments of cell counts over time.

7.4.2 Cognitive factors

Life stress in and of itself is unlikely to have a direct effect on immunity and health outcome in HIV+ individuals. Rather, the relationship between life stress, immunity, and health outcome is probably moderated by other psychosocial factors, such as cognitive appraisals and coping. More specifically, stress and coping models of health and well-being, as well as cognitive models, emphasize the influence of cognitions on coping, mood, health behaviours, and indices of physical health status.[58–60] Aspects of cognitive functioning that have been related to immunity, neuroendocrine functioning, and disease progression in HIV+ individuals, specifically, include cognitive appraisals of stressful situations and the intrusion and avoidance of HIV-related cognitions.

Both primary and secondary appraisals of stressful events have emerged as significant predictors of biological markers and disease progression in HIV+ individuals.

Primary appraisals are defined as perceptions of the impact of a stressor on one's personal well-being (e.g. 'Is this situation good or bad for me?'). Negative HIV-specific expectancies (e.g. perceptions of lacking control over one's disease progression) are one type of primary appraisal. Several studies have found that negative HIV-specific expectancies predict earlier onset of significant HIV-related symptoms among bereaved HIV+ men who are asymptomatic[61] and decreased survival time among HIV+ men with AIDS.[62] In related research, Segerstrom et al.[63] found that attributing negative life events to internal characterological factors (e.g. mood state, personality, health status, social status) predicted a faster rate of helper T cell decline among HIV+ gay men.

Research also suggests that certain types of appraisals, such as constructing meaning from the experience of difficult life events, may have beneficial effects on immune status and survival time in HIV+ individuals. For instance, Bower et al.[64] demonstrated that recently bereaved HIV+ men who engaged in the cognitive processing of their loss were more likely to report constructing meaning from the experience; men who constructed meaning had a less rapid decline in helper T cell counts and lower AIDS-related mortality rates.

Secondary cognitive appraisals are perceptions about one's ability to cope with a specific stressor (e.g. 'Do I have the resources necessary to get through this?'). To date, most of the research on secondary appraisals in HIV infection has examined relations between coping self-efficacy (i.e. beliefs about one's ability to cope successfully with a stressor) and health-related behaviours (e.g. antiretroviral adherence or condom use).[65] Few studies have examined whether coping self-efficacy predicts biological or health outcomes. Research by Benight et al.[66] suggests that this may be a promising area of research. They found that greater coping self-efficacy was associated with lower distress, fewer PTSD symptoms, and lower norepinephrine-to-cortisol ratios in HIV+ gay men following Hurricane Andrew, a severe environmental disaster.

Significant relationships have also emerged between patterns of cognitive processing following stressful life events and immunity and neuroendocrine functioning in HIV+ individuals. One pattern that has been investigated is the cycle of intrusion and avoidance of HIV-related cognitions that commonly occurs in HIV+ individuals. Notably, this pattern is common in individuals who have experienced a traumatic event, such as an HIV diagnosis, and is associated with the presence of PTSD.[67]

Kimerling et al.[48] demonstrated that greater intrusion and avoidance of trauma-related cognitions was associated with lower CD4-to-CD8 ratios over a 1-year follow-up period. Antoni et al.[68] examined the impact of anticipation of HIV status notification on immunity and neuroendocrine functioning in gay/bisexual men unaware of their HIV status. Men who had persistent intrusive thoughts of being at risk for HIV infection after being notified of HIV seronegativity had persistently higher plasma cortisol levels. In a separate publication drawn from the same study, the relationship between intrusion and avoidance and T-lymphocyte proliferation to pokeweed mitogen (PM), an antigen, was examined. T-lymphocyte proliferation models the immune system's ability to respond to bacteria and viruses, and provides an indication of T-cell anergy. Men ultimately notified of HIV seropositivity who reported increases in avoidance from pre- to post-notification had poorer T-lymphocyte proliferation to PM and a trend towards lower helper T cell percentages Furthermore, increases in intrusive thinking over this time period predicted lower helper T cell percentages.[69] Additional recent research provided evidence that greater intrusive thinking and avoidance is associated with lower cytotoxic/suppressor T-cell counts in HIV+ individuals through greater sleep disruption,[70] which is known to be immunosuppressive.[71]

Taken together, these findings suggest that the frequent pattern of intrusion and avoidance of HIV-related cognitions might be associated with greater cortisol levels and immunosuppression in individuals with HIV. Given that Leserman et al.[53] found that high cortisol was associated with decreased survival time in HIV+ individuals, these findings suggest that this pattern may also be associated with mortality.

7.4.3 Coping

In addition to cognitive appraisals, coping is an important moderator of life stress. Once a life event is experienced and appraised, the selection and implementation of a coping strategy follows. Depending on the 'goodness of fit' of the coping strategy to the characteristics (i.e. controllability or uncontrollability) of the event, the strategy may serve to buffer or exacerbate the effects of the event on subsequent mood, health behaviours, biological outcomes, and clinical health outcomes. Given that negatively appraised life events are regrettably far too common in the lives of HIV+ individuals, the utilization of adaptive and productive methods of coping is essential for the maintenance of both emotional and physical quality of life. Strategies that have been significantly related to immunity, neuroendocrine functioning, and disease progression in HIV+ individuals include the utilization of active coping and denial coping. In addition, perceptions and utilization of social support, utilization of spirituality/religiosity, and emotional expression have been independently examined as specific types of active coping.

7.4.3.1 Active coping

Goodkin et al.[43] examined the relationship between a dispositional, passive coping style as measured by the Millon Behavioral Health Inventory[72] and immune status in a small sample of asymptomatic HIV+ gay men. They found that a passive coping style was significantly correlated with lower total lymphocyte counts and marginally correlated with lower helper T cell counts, specifically.

Similar findings have also been reported for correlation between the utilization of HIV−focused active coping as measured by the COPE[73] and better immune functioning in asymptomatic HIV+ gay men. In particular, Goodkin et al.[74] found that greater utilization of active coping, a combination of problem-focused and emotion-focused coping, was associated with higher NK cell count.

Notably, the use of active coping may also have beneficial effects on disease progression among HIV+ individuals. Mulder et al.[75] found that greater use of HIV-specific active confrontational coping, defined as a style involving seeking social support, active problem solving, and low use of denial, predicted decreased risk for clinical disease progression over a 1-year follow-up period among HIV+ gay men.

In contrast with these findings, Mulder et al.[76] found that active cognitive and behavioural coping was not associated with HIV disease progression; rather, avoidance coping was associated with a lower rate of helper T cell count decline over a 7-year follow-up period. (However, it was not associated with progression to an AIDS-indicator condition.) Although initially counter-intuitive, these findings are congruent with those of Solano et al.,[77] who demonstrated that a 'fighting spirit' was associated with progression to fully symptomatic HIV disease. Given that the participants in both these studies were men in the early stages of HIV infection, these findings may suggest that prolonged sustained attention to 'defeating' HIV with little or no focus on other aspects of living may be associated with deleterious outcomes for asymptomatic individuals with HIV.

7.4.3.2 Denial

In contrast with the potential immune and health benefits associated with active coping, the use of denial coping may be a risk factor for immunosuppression and poorer health status among HIV+ individuals. Solano et al.[77] found that denial/repression coping was associated with progression to fully symptomatic HIV disease. In an elegant longitudinal design, Leserman et al.[52] found that denial coping significantly predicted faster progression to AIDS up to 7.5-year follow-up in HIV+ gay men. Specifically, they found that for every unit increase in denial coping, the risk of AIDS was doubled.

Likewise, in the aforementioned study on the anticipation of HIV serostatus notification in gay men, less use of denial coping significantly predicted lower proliferative response to phytohaematagglutinin (PHA) at baseline. Although these results may appear counter-intuitive, the authors suggest that transient immunosuppression may have followed the highly stressful decision to enter a study and confront one's HIV status, a decision that would also be associated with low use of denial coping.[68] In related research, Ironson et al.[78] examined the psychosocial predictors of 2-year health status among HIV+ gay men. Men who were unaware of their HIV status underwent psychosocial, immune, and neuroendocrine assessments ('pre-notification') and then randomization to a 10-week cognitive–behavioural stress management (CBSM) intervention, a 10-week exercise intervention, or a control condition. Participants were tested and notified of their HIV status approximately 5 weeks after study entry. Five weeks later, participants were assessed again ('post-notification'). Among men randomized to one of the interventions and notified of HIV seropositivity, increases in denial coping from pre- to post-notification predicted clinical disease progression at 2-year follow-up.

7.4.3.3 Social support

Perceptions and utilization of social support have also emerged as significant predictors of immune and health status among HIV+ individuals. In one of the few studies to demonstrate the beneficial effects of CBSM on both psychosocial and immune functioning in an HIV+ sample, Cruess et al.[79] found that a 10-week CBSM intervention decreased HSV-2 IgG titres among HIV+ gay/bisexual men and intervention-associated increases in perceived receipt of social support partially mediated this relationship.

Along with stress, social support is one of the strongest psychosocial predictors of HIV disease progression. Theorell et al.[80] examined the relationship between availability of social and emotional support in difficult situations and decline in helper T cell counts over a 5-year follow-up period among HIV+ men with haemophilia. Results demonstrated that men with low availability of social support had a significantly more rapid decline in helper T cell counts during the follow-up period. Similarly, lower satisfaction with social support has also emerged as a significant predictor of accelerated progression to AIDS among HIV+ gay men,[51–53] and a larger social support network size has been found to predict a longer survival time in HIV+ men.[81]

Some research indicates that the relationship between social support and disease progression may be moderated by HIV disease stage. Patterson et al.[81] demonstrated that greater informational support was associated with a longer time until the onset of an AIDS indicator condition and longer survival time, but only among symptomatic individuals. Contrary to expectations, they also noted that a larger network size was also associated with a shorter symptom-free interval among asymptomatic individuals. This is similar to the findings of Miller et al.[82] who demonstrated that less loneliness predicted more rapid declines in helper T cell counts among HIV+ men. These findings may indicate that negotiating active and large social support networks may be taxing to individuals in the early stages of HIV infection. Thus the literature demonstrates that facets of social support may have both protective functions and deleterious effects on HIV+ individuals.

Research has also examined the impact of more focused population-specific measures of social support on disease progression among HIV+ individuals. Specifically, Cole et al.[83] investigated rejection sensitivity as a predictor of disease progression at 3-year follow-up among HIV+ gay men. Men who were more sensitive to rejection from strangers and the general public (but not friends and family) because of their gay identity had a significantly more rapid progression to critically low CD4 percentages, an AIDS diagnosis, and HIV-related mortality.

7.4.3.4 Spirituality and religiosity

Research on the health benefits of spirituality and religiosity is in its infancy. One recent meta-analytic review of the empirical evidence suggested that enough compelling evidence exists to suggest that spirituality and religiosity are linked to lower mortality rates.[84] However, very little PNI research has been conducted with this focus. In one of the only published studies to date in this area, Ironson *et al.*[85] examined the hypothesis that long-term survival with HIV was associated with greater spirituality and religiosity by comparing a sample of long-term non-progressors and an HIV+ comparison group in four domains: sense of peace, faith in God, religious behaviours, and compassionate view of others. Long-term survivors had higher scores in each of these domains than individuals in the comparison group. In addition, low urinary cortisol concentration and the desire to help others with HIV mediated the relationship between greater spirituality/religiosity and long-term survival status.

7.4.3.5 Emotional expression and disclosure

Emotional expression and disclosure, two potentially important buffers of stress, have been linked to better immunity and physical health status in various populations, including HIV+ individuals. Eisenberger *et al.*[86] evaluated the relationship between availability of social support, percentage of emotionally expressive words expressed during an HIV coping interview, and helper T cell counts among HIV+ women. Although no relationship emerged between availability of social support and CD4 count, a greater percentage of words expressed denoting emotional inhibition (e.g. 'restrain', 'avoid') was significantly associated with lower CD4 cell counts. O'Cleirigh *et al.*[87] assessed the relationship between emotional expression, depth processing, immune status, and long-term survival status among HIV+ individuals. Long-term survivors of HIV demonstrated significantly greater emotional expression and depth processing in written essays describing their reactions to past traumas than individuals in an HIV+ comparison group. Furthermore, greater depth processing mediated the relationship between greater emotional expression and survival status. Among women only, greater emotional expression was associated with lower HIV viral load, and both greater emotional expression and depth processing were significantly associated with greater helper T cell count.

Two particularly salient gauges of emotional inhibition in HIV+ individuals are concealment of HIV status and, for HIV+ gay men specifically, concealment of expression of gay identity. Being one's 'true self' and expressing emotions openly and honestly can be extraordinarily risky for HIV+ individuals. Many HIV+ individuals chose not to disclose their sexual orientation and/or HIV status to friends and family because they fear that the disclosure will lead to estrangement, retaliation, and even physical violence. Given the numerous studies demonstrating the deleterious health effects of emotional inhibition, research has sought to examine whether concealment of gay identity and HIV status, specifically, are associated with deleterious outcomes.

Cole *et al.*[88] found that HIV+ men who concealed their gay identity, a gauge of emotional inhibition, had a significantly higher incidence of cancer and infectious disease over a 5-year follow-up period. Furthermore, data indicated that there is a dose–response relationship between the degree to which HIV+ men conceal their gay identity and the more rapid progression of HIV infection.[89] Some research also exists to suggest that the degree of social support satisfaction may moderate the relationship between concealment of gay identity and immune status in HIV+ men. Ullrich *et al.*[90] found that concealment of gay identity was associated with lower helper T cell count only among HIV+ men who reported greater social support satisfaction.

Few studies have examined the relationship between disclosure of HIV status and immunity and health status. Sherman *et al.*[91] examined the relationship between these variables in HIV+ children and found that children who had disclosed their HIV status to friends during the course of the 1-year study experienced significantly larger increases in helper T cell percentage than those who had not disclosed their status. Future research in this area is warranted.

7.4.4 Mood

As shown in Figure 7.2, cognitive appraisals and coping are significant determinants of mood states, such as anger, depression, and anxiety. Negative mood states have been widely associated with deleterious immune, neuroendocrine, and health outcomes in healthy and medically ill populations alike. Leserman *et al.*[45] found that depressive symptoms, independent of stress, were predictive of decreases in CTLs and NK cells from study entry to 2-year follow-up in HIV+ gay men. Evans *et al.*[92] were among the first to find that depressive and anxiety symptoms were associated with high HIV viral load, as well as higher counts of activated CTLs, in HIV+ women. Significantly, the presence of a greater CD8 cell response in individuals with high HIV viral load may result in the destruction of effective immune responses and organ injury.[93] Evans *et al.*[92] also found that major depressive disorder was significantly associated with lower NK cell count.

Bereavement, specifically, has been associated with significant increases in immune activation,[94] decreases in lymphocyte proliferation to PHA,[94,95] and decreases in NK cell count[95] among HIV+ individuals. However, some data also suggest that it is depressed mood, rather than bereavement status *per se*, that is associated with lowered immunity among HIV+ individuals.[96]

Overall, there is compelling research to indicate that depressive symptomatology is associated with HIV disease progression. (Studies suggesting that there is no relationship between depressive symptoms and immune status or disease progression among HIV+ individuals include Rabkin *et al.*,[97] Lyketsos *et al.*,[98] Sahs *et al.*,[99] and Vedhara *et al.*[100].) However, it is likely that the relationship is complex and may depend on the assessment of depression (e.g. including or excluding somatic complaints possibly related to HIV disease status, utilization of measures to diagnose major depressive disorder versus utilization of measures of depressive affect), the disease stage of the individuals studied, the operationalization of disease progression, and the length of the follow-up period. In one of the first published studies to examine distress and immune status prospectively in HIV, Burack *et al.*[101] found that elevated scores (i.e. >16) on the Center for Epidemiologic Studies—Depression (CES-D) questionnaire[102] predicted significantly greater declines in helper T cell counts over a 5-year follow-up period. However, elevated depression scores were not predictive of faster progression to an AIDS diagnosis using the 1987 CDC AIDS case definition[103] or of shorter survival time. Congruent with this finding, Vedhara et al.[104] demonstrated that greater emotional distress was associated with faster rate in the decline of helper T cells over a 12-month period in HIV+ men. In one of the few studies to examine the relationship between psychosocial factors and health outcomes in HIV+ women specifically, Ickovics et al.[105] found that chronic depressive affect was associated with a greater decline in CD4 cell count, particularly among women with CD4 counts <500 cell/ml and HIV viral loads >10 000 copies/µl.

Leserman et al.[51] found that depressive symptoms were associated with faster progression to an AIDS diagnosis, as defined by the 1993 CDC case surveillance definition,[5] during a 5.5-year follow-up period; however, they also demonstrated that once the effects of stress and social support on disease progression were accounted for, depressive symptoms failed to emerge as an additional significant predictor of accelerated progression to AIDS.[51,52] However, during a longer follow-up period (9 years), Leserman et al.[53] demonstrated that depressive symptoms predicted faster progression to an AIDS indicator clinical condition but not to a decline in helper T cell count below 200 cells/ml. They also noted that higher scores on the Profile of Mood States (POMS)[106] anger subscale predicted faster progression to an AIDS diagnosis.

Several studies have examined the relationship between HIV-specific distress and disease progression. Kemeny and Dean[107] noted that AIDS-related bereavement was a significant predictor of a more rapid decline in helper T cell count over time among HIV+ men. Further analysis revealed that bereavement-associated depressive reactions involving self-reproach, and not grief reactions per se, accounted for this effect. Greater distress following HIV diagnosis has also been significantly related to greater HIV disease progression over time.[78]

Depressive affect has also been associated with increased risk for mortality among HIV+ individuals.[105,108] Ickovics et al.[105] found that HIV+ women with chronic depressive affect were twice as likely to die as those with limited or no depressive affect. Similarly, Patterson et al.[81] noted that depressive symptoms were predictive of shorter survival among HIV+ men after controlling for baseline HIV symptoms and CD4 cell count.

Research has also demonstrated that CBSM interventions have beneficial effects on mood disturbance,[109–111] immune status,[109] HSV-2 IgG titres,[110] and neuroendocrine functioning[109,111,112] among HIV+ gay/bisexual men. Notably, it has also been found that CBSM-induced improvements in mood are significantly associated with positive changes in immune status, HSV-2 titres, and neuroendocrine functioning. Specifically, decreases in anxiety were found to parallel reductions in 24-h urinary norepinephrine output, while more frequent home relaxation practice was associated with higher cytotoxic/suppressor T-cell counts at follow-up.[109] Furthermore, reductions in mood disturbance/dysphoria paralleled lower HSV-2 titres,[110] alterations in free testosterone,[113] buffered increases in cortisol-to-DHEA-S ratios,[112] and decreases in 24-h urinary cortisol output.[111]

7.4.5 Personality

Dispositional personality characteristics may also behave as powerful stress moderators. Dispositional optimism, a widely investigated personality trait in health psychology research, is defined as the dispositional tendency to possess positive future expectancies. As suggested in Figure 7.2, possessing positive future expectancies in the midst of a severe life stressor may result in positive cognitive appraisals, the utilization of adaptive coping strategies, and ultimately immune and health benefits. In support of this model, dispositional optimism has emerged as a predictor of better immune status, lower herpesvirus titres, and lower risk for disease progression in HIV+ individuals. Byrnes et al.[114] found that a more pessimistic attitude was significantly associated with lower NK cell count and marginally associated with lower cytotoxic/suppressor T-cell percentages among women at risk for cervical cancer due to co-infection with HIV and HPV. Although it was hypothesized that stress would also be associated with lower immune status and functioning, stress did not emerge as a predictor of either NK cell count or CD8%. In addition, Cruess et al.[115] demonstrated that greater dispositional optimism was associated with lower Epstein—Barr virus (EBV) and human herpesvirus-type 6 (HHV-6) antibody titres, and further demonstrated that the relationship between greater optimism and lower EBV titres was partially mediated by less depressive symptomatology.

Tomakowsky et al.[116] evaluated the relationship between dispositional optimism, optimistic explanatory style, HIV symptoms, immune status, and immune decline among HIV+ individuals. Both greater dispositional optimism and optimistic explanatory style were associated with fewer HIV-related symptoms, and a more optimistic explanatory style was associated with lower CD4 count cross-sectionally. However, a more optimistic explanatory style was associated with greater declines in CD4 count during the 2-year follow-up period. The authors suggest that this may indicate that optimism is maladaptive under certain conditions, such as in the face of the persistent uncontrollable life stress commonly experienced by HIV+ individuals.

7.4.6 Health behaviours associated with immunity and health status in HIV

In addition to psychosocial factors, health behaviours such as substance use and medication adherence are also significant predictors of immunity and health status among HIV+ individuals. Substance abuse and dependence are prevalent conditions among HIV+ individuals and have well-documented deleterious effects on immunity and health status. For instance, cigarette smoking increases the risk of developing opportunistic respiratory infections,[117] oropharyngeal candidiasis,[118] and cervical[119] and anal neoplasia[120] among HIV+ individuals. Smoking has also been associated with poorer health-related quality of life.[121] Furthermore, alcohol consumption is associated with impairment in immune and viral responses to antiretroviral treatment among HIV+ individuals.[122] Cocaine use has been associated with impaired immune functioning, enhanced HIV infectivity and replication,[123] and increased risk for AIDS dementia and vasculitis.[124] There is also evidence derived from murine transgenic models of AIDS that cocaine exacerbates HIV-associated cardiac dysfunction and increases risk for mortality.[125]

Highly active antiretroviral therapy (HAART) adherence may be one of the most important health care behaviours for HIV+ individuals. Sociodemographic, disease and treatment, behavioural, and psychosocial factors have emerged as significant predictors of adherence to antiretroviral therapy among HIV+ individuals. With regard to sociodemographic variables, heterosexual orientation,[126] lower income and educational attainment,[28] Black race,[28,29] Latino ethnicity,[126,127] immigrant status,[127] and being female[127] have been associated with non-adherence to antiretroviral therapy.

Disease and treatment variables that predict non-adherence among HIV+ individuals include the experience of medication-related adverse clinical events,[30] treatment failure,[30] greater worries about medication use,[128] greater dose frequency,[28] and fewer adherence aids.[28] In addition, non-adherence has been related to lower HIV-specific quality of life,[128] poorer perceived treatment by clinic staff,[127] and poorer access to health care.[127]

Significantly, psychosocial and behavioural variables that predict biological and health outcomes among HIV+ individuals have also been associated with non-adherence to antiretroviral therapy. In particular, hopelessness,[127,129] loss of motivation,[129] greater anxious and depressive symptomatology,[29,127,130] and greater avoidant coping[129] are predictors of non-adherence to antiretroviral therapy. In contrast, adherence to antiretroviral therapy is significantly associated with greater self-efficacy,[130] greater use of active coping,[29,129] and greater use of problem-focused coping.[129] Relationship factors associated with greater adherence to antiretorivral therapy include greater social desirability,[130] lower need for social support,[130] greater perceived availability of social support,[127] and greater perceived satisfaction with one's partner.[126,129] In addition, drug and alcohol use have also been associated with non-adherence to treatment in HIV+ individuals.[28–30] Taken together, these findings are especially noteworthy because they suggest that psychosocial factors may affect health outcomes in HIV+ individuals through both neuroimmunological and behavioural pathways.

One of the most important priorities in HIV health psychology research today involves examining the efficacy of psychosocial interventions on antiretroviral medication adherence.[31] Some preliminary research suggests that the structured writing and processing of traumatic events may have some impact on adherence. Mann[131] found that among HIV+ women low in optimism, a writing intervention produced a marginally significant increase in self-reported medication adherence. In addition, O'Cleirigh et al.[87] found that HIV+ individuals who demonstrated greater depth processing of past traumas during a structured writing exercise had greater adherence to antiretroviral medication.

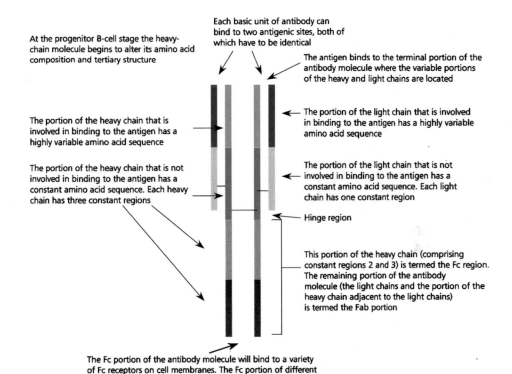

At the progenitor B-cell stage the heavy-chain molecule begins to alter its amino acid composition and tertiary structure

Each basic unit of antibody can bind to two antigenic sites, both of which have to be identical

The antigen binds to the terminal portion of the antibody molecule where the variable portions of the heavy and light chains are located

The portion of the heavy chain that is involved in binding to the antigen has a highly variable amino acid sequence

The portion of the light chain that is involved in binding to the antigen has a highly variable amino acid sequence

The portion of the heavy chain that is not involved in binding to the antigen has a constant amino acid sequence. Each heavy chain has three constant regions

The portion of the light chain that is not involved in binding to the antigen has a constant amino acid sequence. Each light chain has one constant region

Hinge region

This portion of the heavy chain (comprising constant regions 2 and 3) is termed the Fc region. The remaining portion of the antibody molecule (the light chains and the portion of the heavy chain adjacent to the light chains) is termed the Fab portion

The Fc portion of the antibody molecule will bind to a variety of Fc receptors on cell membranes. The Fc portion of different heavy chains will bind to different receptors. For example, mast cells have an Fc receptor for IgE and neutrophils have an Fc receptor for IgG1 and IgG3

Plate 1 The basic structure of the immunoglobulin molecule.

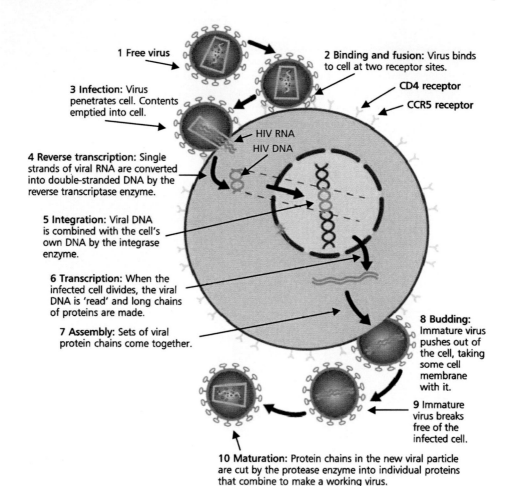

1 Free virus

2 Binding and fusion: Virus binds to cell at two receptor sites.

CD4 receptor

CCR5 receptor

3 Infection: Virus penetrates cell. Contents emptied into cell.

HIV RNA

HIV DNA

4 Reverse transcription: Single strands of viral RNA are converted into double-stranded DNA by the reverse transcriptase enzyme.

5 Integration: Viral DNA is combined with the cell's own DNA by the integrase enzyme.

6 Transcription: When the infected cell divides, the viral DNA is 'read' and long chains of proteins are made.

7 Assembly: Sets of viral protein chains come together.

8 Budding: Immature virus pushes out of the cell, taking some cell membrane with it.

9 Immature virus breaks free of the infected cell.

10 Maturation: Protein chains in the new viral particle are cut by the protease enzyme into individual proteins that combine to make a working virus.

Plate 2 The HIV life-cycle. (Reproduced with permission from New Mexico AIDS InfoNet at http: //www.aids.org/factSheets/415-life-cycle.html)

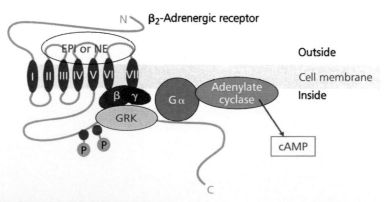

N

β_2-Adrenergic receptor

EPI or NE

Outside

Cell membrane

Inside

I II III IV V VI VII

β γ

Gα

Adenylate cyclase

GRK

cAMP

P P

C

Plate 3 Activity of β_2-adrenergic receptors.

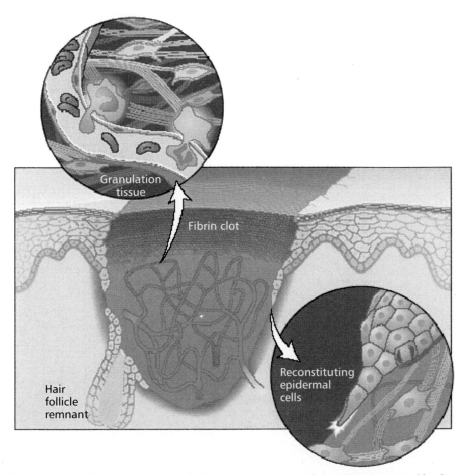

Plate 4 Diagram illustrating the major factors known to play a role in cutaneous wound healing. During clot formation, plasma factors and platelets released from damaged blood vessels form a fibrin clot to temporarily cover the injured area. Within hours after wounding, epithelial cells and remnants of epithelial appendages (e.g. hair follicles) migrate from the wound edge. During the inflammatory phase, inflammatory cells (depicted as blue cells) respond to chemoattractants, escape from the blood vessels through the modulation of integrin expression and secretion of MMPs, and invade the wound site. The presence of cytokines and growth factors secreted by inflammatory cells in the wound further attracts fibroblasts and endothelial cells. The proliferation of these cells and subsequent angiogenesis in the wound result in the formation of the granulation tissue. Remodelling of the wound results in scar formation. (Reproduced with permission from P. Martin (1997) *Science* **276**: 738–46.)

(a)

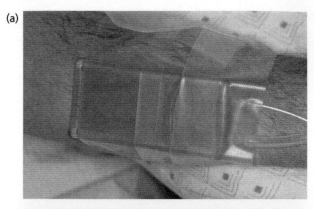

(b)

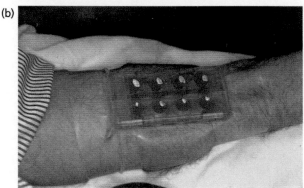

Plate 5 (a) Photograph of the plastic template used to prepare the blister wounds. The template was taped to the surface of the forearm and a vacuum applied until blisters formed approximately1–1.5 h later. This gentle suction separated the junction of the epidermis and dermis, creating eight sterile 8-mm blisters. (b) Photograph of a plastic plate containing eight chambers. Each chamber was able to hold approximately 1 ml of chamber fluid. Using a syringe, the template wells were filled with 0.8–1.0 ml of 70% autologous serum in Hanks' balanced salt solution. The top was sealed with sterile tape. Blister chamber fluid was removed with a syringe for analysis at various time-points after blister induction.

7.5 Directions for future research

The research reviewed here is among the best designed, theory-driven, clinically relevant, and challenging research that has been conducted in the field of PNI to date. Although antiretroviral therapy has improved the quality of life and survival rates of HIV+ individuals, additional PNI research in HIV infection remains absolutely essential for both scientific and humanitarian purposes. HIV provides a unique model in which to examine PNI mechanisms of health outcome and survival in medically ill populations. Perhaps more importantly, given the stressful psychosocial and medical experiences of HIV+ individuals, PNI research in HIV infection may have true clinical and humanitarian significance—a truth that can, at times, be lost in the day-to-day performance of routine research tasks. To promote these two purposes, we outline below some possible future directions for PNI–HIV researchers.

7.5.1 Increased inclusion of women and ethnic minorities in clinical trials

As partially demonstrated by this review, most of the PNI research in HIV infection has been conducted with male and Caucasian participants. Given the current epidemiological trends in HIV infection, the recruitment of HIV+ women and ethnic minorities into PNI research trials is paramount. However, PNI research must go beyond the simple recruitment of these populations. Along with this, PNI research must emphasize the development and utilization of gender- and culture-appropriate research methods.[36]

7.5.2 Greater emphasis on biopsychosocial research among HIV+ individuals in the developing world

Two-thirds of the world's HIV+ population lives in Africa. Health care systems in developing countries, such as those in sub-Saharan Africa, are struggling to meet the needs of millions of HIV+ patients due to inadequate resources and infrastructure and unpredictable antiretroviral supplies. Only an estimated 1% of those in need of antiretrovirals in Africa are receiving them. Many of the world's developing countries affected by HIV/AIDS are struggling with sociopolitical and economic instability and subsequent poverty, forced displacement of residents, sexual violence, and food insecurity—interconnected factors that seriously exacerbate the HIV/AIDS pandemic.[132] Accordingly, future research should examine the biopsychosociocultural mechanisms of health behaviours, health status, and quality of life among HIV+ individuals in the developing world.

7.5.3 Exploration of understudied population-specific psychosocial constructs

Men and women living with HIV are enormously diverse in areas such as race, ethnicity, culture, socioeconomic status, acculturation status, and sexual orientation, to name but a few factors. Future PNI research should be conducted within the context of these factors. One way in which this could be accomplished is for PNI research to continue to examine the impact of population-specific stressors on immune status and health outcomes. Examples include stressors such as racism, sexism, and trauma/violence.

7.5.4 Assessment of HIV-specific immunity, cytokine production, and genital HIV viral load

The enumeration of helper T cells and cytotoxic/suppressor T cells in the peripheral blood has been widely used as a measure of immune status and disease progression in HIV+ individuals. However, it is unclear how valid these cell counts are as markers of the ability to mount an immune response against HIV *per se*. In contrast, HIV-specific immune responses are more valid indicators of the body's ability to fight HIV infection. Research has documented the relationship between HIV disease status and both HIV-specific Th1 CD4 T cells and HIV-specific cytotoxic T cells. In 1987, Walker *et al.*[133] demonstrated the presence of HIV-specific cytotoxic T lymphocytes in HIV+ individuals. Since then, research has demonstrated that HIV+ individuals with non-progressive disease have higher percentages of HIV-specific Th1 CD4 T cells than those with progressive disease.[134] Furthermore, HIV-specific cytotoxic T-cell frequency is inversely associated with HIV plasma viral load.[135] Accordingly, future PNI research may seek to examine the relationship between psychosocial factors, HIV-specific immunity, and disease progression.

Cytokines are components of the immune system that play an integral role in mounting an immune response against HIV. Despite this, few published research studies in PNI and HIV have examined the impact of psychosocial factors on cytokines. Research has already identified negative mood states and poorer social support as correlates of high levels of cytokines that can promote pathological conditions such as cancer.[136,137] Future research should assess the effect of psychosocial factors on cytokine production from Th1- and Th2-type CD4 cells among HIV+ individuals.

Among women, HIV has been isolated in cervicovaginal secretions.[138] This is significant because viral burden in the genital tract is a determinant of transmission. In addition, HIV is capable of replicating in cervicovaginal secretions, and this replication can result in a virus population with significant genotypic differences from that found in plasma.[139] Importantly, HIV viral load obtained from the female genital tract does not correlate with viral load obtained from plasma, suggesting that the kinetics of HIV replication in the blood differ from that in cervicovaginal cells.[140] Nevertheless, to our knowledge there have been no investigations of the effect of psychosocial factors on HIV viral load in the female genital tract. Future research should examine relationships between psychosocial factors and HIV viral load in both the plasma and genital tract.

7.5.5 Examination of psychoneuroimmunologic relations to HIV-specific health outcomes

Most of the PNI research described in this chapter has examined PNI predictors of disease progression operationalized as helper T cell decline, the development of significant

HIV-related symptoms, or the development of an AIDS-indicator condition. Previously, we have demonstrated that psychosocial factors are associated with the status and progression of specific HIV-related conditions, such as the progression/persistence of squamous intraepithelial lesions[56] and the occurrence of genital HSV ulcers.[55] This suggests the possibility that PNI mechanisms may emerge as significant predictors of other HIV-specific disease endpoints. HIV+ individuals are at risk for certain cancers, including cervical carcinoma, rectal/anal carcinoma, non-Hodgkin's lymphoma, and Kaposi's sarcoma.[141] Future research should seek to inform the PNI mechanisms of the development and/or progression of these cancers.

References

1 Centers for Disease Control and Prevention (2001). *HIV/AIDS Surveill Rep* **132**, 1–44.

2 UNAIDS/WHO (2002). *AIDS Epidemic Update-December 2002.* Geneva: UNAIDS/WHO.

3 National Institute of Allergy and Infectious Diseases (2001). *How HIV Causes AIDS.* Bethesda, MD: National Institutes of Health.

4 Cohen DE, Walker BD (2001). Human immunodeficiency virus pathogenesis and prospects for immune control in patients with established infection. *Clin Infect Dis* **32**, 1756–68.

5 Centers for Disease Control and Prevention (1992). 1993 revised classification system for HIV infection and expanded surveillance case definition for AIDS among adolescents and adults. *MMWR Morb Mortal Wkly Rep* **41**, 1–19.

6 Walker BD (2003). Immunopathogenesis and immune response in HIV infection. *Medscape* Electronic Citation.

7 Alimonti JB, Ball TB, Fowke KR (2003). Mechanisms of CD4(+) T lymphocyte cell death in human immunodeficiency virus infection and AIDS. *J Gen Virol* **84**, 1649–61.

8 Clerici M, Galli M, Bosis S, Gervasoni C, Moroni M, Norbiato G (2000). Immunoendocrinologic abnormalities in human immunodeficiency virus infection. *Ann NY Acad Sci* **917**, 956–61.

9 Clerici M, Shearer GM (1994). The Th1–Th2 hypothesis of HIV infection: new insights. *Immunol Today* **15**(12), 575–81.

10 Besedovsky HO, Del Rey A (2001). Cytokines as mediators of central and peripheral immune-neuroendocrine interactions. In Ader R, Felten SY, Cohen N (eds) *Psychoneuroimmunology* (3rd edn). San Diego, CA: Academic Press, 1–17.

11 Kedzierska K, Crowe SM, Turville S, Cunningham AL (2003). The influence of cytokines, chemokines and their receptors on HIV-1 replication in monocytes and macrophages. *Rev Med Virol* **13**, 39–56.

12 Cai Q, Huang XL, Rappocciolo G, Rinaldo CR Jr (1990). Natural killer cell responses in homosexual men with early HIV infection. *J Acquir Immune Defic Syndr* **3**, 669–76.

13 Ader R, Felten DL, Cohen N (eds) (2001). *Psychoneuroimmunology* (3rd edn) San Diego, CA: Academic Press.

14 Kottilil S, Chun TW, Moir S, *et al.* (2003). Innate immunity in human immunodeficiency virus infection: effect of viremia on natural killer cell function. *J Infect Dis* **187**, 1038–45.

15 Ironson G, Balbin E, Solomon G, *et al.* (2001). Relative preservation of natural killer cell cytotoxicity and number in healthy AIDS patients with low CD4 cell counts. *AIDS* **15**, 2065–73.

16 Azar ST, Melby JC (1993). Hypothalamic–pituitary–adrenal function in non-AIDS patients with advanced HIV infection. *Am J Med Sci* **305**, 321–5.

17 Mayo J, Collazos J, Martinez E, Ibarra S (2002). Adrenal function in the human immunodeficiency virus-infected patient. *Arch Int Med* **162**, 1095–8.

18 Collazos J, Mayo J, Martinez E, Ibarra S (2003). Serum cortisol in HIV infected patients with and without highly active antiretroviral therapy. *AIDS* **17**, 123–6.

19 Kumar M, Kumar AM, Waldrop D, Antoni MH, Schneiderman N, Eisdorfer C (2002). The HPA axis in HIV-1 infection. *J Acquir Immune Defic Syndr* **31**(Suppl 2), 89–93.

20 Cole SW, Korin YD, Fahey JL, Zack JA (1998). Norepinephrine accelerates HIV replication via protein kinase A-dependent effects on cytokine production. *J Immunol* **161**, 610–16.

21 Christeff N, Nunez EA, Gougeon ML (2000). Changes in cortisol/DHEA ratio in HIV-infected men are related to immunological and metabolic perturbations leading to malnutrition and lipodystrophy. *Ann NY Acad Sci* **917**, 962–70.

22 Huang JS, Wilkie SJ, Dolan S, *et al.* (2003). Reduced testosterone levels in human immunodeficiency virus-infected women with weight loss and low weight. *Clin Infect Dis* **36**, 499–506.

23 Mylonakis E, Koutkia P, Grinspoon S (2001). Diagnosis and treatment of androgen deficiency in human immunodeficiency virus-infected men and women. *Clin Infect Dis* **33**, 857–64.

24 Yeaman GR, Howell AL, Weldon S, *et al.* (2003). Human immunodeficiency virus receptor and coreceptor expression on human uterine epithelial cells: regulation of expression during the menstrual cycle and implications for human immunodeficiency virus infection. *Immunology* **109**, 137–46.

25 White HD, Crassi KM, Givan AL, *et al.* (1997). CD3+ CD8+ CTL activity within the human female reproductive tract: influence of stage of the menstrual cycle and menopause. *J Immunol* **158**, 3017–27.

26 Money DM, Arikan YY, Remple V, *et al.* (2003). Genital tract and plasma human immunodeficiency virus viral load throughout the menstrual cycle in women who are infected with ovulatory human immunodeficiency virus. *Am J Obstet Gynecol* **188**, 122–8.

27 Department of Health and Human Services (2002). *Guidelines for the Use of Antiretroviral Agents in HIV-Infected Adults and Adolescents.* Bethesda, MD: Department of Health and Human Services.

28 Golin CE, Liu H, Hays RD, *et al.* (2002). A prospective study of predictors of adherence to combination antiretroviral medication. *J Gen Intern Med* **17**, 756–65.

29 Singh N, Squier C, Sivek C, Wagener M, Nguyen MH, Yu VL (1996). Determinants of compliance with antiretroviral therapy in patients with human immunodeficiency virus: prospective assessment with implications for enhancing compliance. *AIDS Care* **8**, 261–9.

30 Ickovics JR, Cameron A, Zackin R, *et al.* (2002). Consequences and determinants of adherence to antiretroviral medication: results from Adult AIDS Clinical Trials Group Protocol 370. *Antivir Ther* **7**, 185–93.

31 Kelly JA, Otto-Salaj LL, Sikkema KJ, Pinkerton SD, Bloom FR (1998). Implications of HIV treatment advances for behavioral research on AIDS: protease inhibitors and new challenges in HIV secondary prevention. *Health Psychol* **17**, 310–19.

32 Kiecolt-Glaser JK, Garner W, Speicher C, Penn GM, Holliday J, Glaser R (1984). Psychosocial modifiers of immunocompetence in medical students. *Psychosom Med* **46**, 7–14.

33 Irwin M, Daniels M, Risch SC, Bloom E, Weiner H (1988). Plasma cortisol and natural killer cell activity during bereavement. *Biol Psychiatry* **24**, 173–8.

34 Cohen S, Tyrrell DA, Smith AP (1991). Psychological stress and susceptibility to the common cold. *N Engl J Med* **325**, 606–12.

35 Glaser R, Pearson GR, Jones JF, *et al.* (1991). Stress-related activation of Epstein–Barr virus. *Brain Behav Immun* **5**, 219–32.

36 Pereira DB (2002). Interventions for mothers during pregnancy and postpartum: behavioral and pharmacological approaches. In Chesney M, Antoni MH (eds) *Innovative Approaches to Health*

Psychology: Prevention and Treatment—Lessons Learned from AIDS. Washington, DC: American Psychological Association Press, 141–66.

37 Nott KH, Vedhara K (1999). Nature and consequences of stressful life events in homosexual HIV-positive men: a review. *AIDS Care* **11**, 235–43.

38 Lichtenstein B, Laska MK, Clair JM (2002). Chronic sorrow in the HIV-positive patient: issues of race, gender, and social support. *AIDS Patient Care STDS* **16**, 27–38.

39 Morrison MF, Petitto JM, Ten Have T, *et al.* (2002). Depressive and anxiety disorders in women with HIV infection. *Am J Psychiatry* **159**, 789–96.

40 Bing EG, Burnam MA, Longshore D, *et al.* (2001). Psychiatric disorders and drug use among human immunodeficiency virus-infected adults in the United States. *Arch Gen Psychiatry*, **58**, 721–8.

41 Antoni MH (2003). Stress management and psychoneuroimmunology in HIV infection. *CNS Spectr* **8**, 40–51.

42 Nott KH, Vedhara K, Spickett GP (1995) Psychology, immunology, and HIV. *Psychoneuroendocrinology* **20**, 451–74.

43 Goodkin K, Fuchs I, Feaster D, Leeka J, Rishel DD (1992). Life stressors and coping style are associated with immune measures in HIV-1 infection–a preliminary report. *Int J Psychiatry Med* **22**, 155–72.

44 Evans DL, Leserman J, Perkins DO, *et al.* (1995). Stress-associated reductions of cytotoxic T lymphocytes and natural killer cells in asymptomatic HIV infection. *Am J Psychiatry* **152**, 543–50.

45 Leserman J, Petitto JM, Perkins DO, Folds JD, Golden RN, Evans DL (1997). Severe stress, depressive symptoms, and changes in lymphocyte subsets in human immunodeficiency virus-infected men. A 2-year follow-up study. *Arch Gen Psychiatry* **54**, 279–85.

46 Howland LC, Gortmaker SL, Mofenson LM, *et al.* (2000). Effects of negative life events on immune suppression in children and youth infected with human immunodeficiency virus type 1. *Pediatrics* **106**, 540–6.

47 Martinez A, Israelski D, Walker C, Koopman C (2002). Posttraumatic stress disorder in women attending human immunodeficiency virus outpatient clinics. *AIDS Patient Care STDS* **16**, 283–91.

48 Kimerling R, Calhoun KS, Forehand R, *et al.* (1999). Traumatic stress in HIV-infected women. *AIDS Educ Prev* **11**, 321–30.

49 Petitto JM, Leserman J, Perkins DO, *et al.* (2000). High versus low basal cortisol secretion in asymptomatic, medication-free HIV-infected men: differential effects of severe life stress on parameters of immune status. *Behav Med* **25**, 143–51.

50 Evans DL, Leserman J, Perkins DO, *et al.* (1997). Severe life stress as a predictor of early disease progression in HIV infection. *Am J Psychiatry* **154**, 630–4.

51 Leserman J, Jackson ED, Petitto JM, *et al.* (1999). Progression to AIDS: The effects of stress, depressive symptoms, and social support. *Psychosom Med* **61**, 397–406.

52 Leserman J, Petitto JM, Golden RN, Gaynes BN, Gu H, Silva SG *et al.* (2000). Impact of stressful life events, depression, social support, coping, and cortisol on progression to AIDS. *Am J Psychiatry* **157**(8), 1221–1228.

53 Leserman J, Petitto JM, Gu H, *et al.* (2002). Progression to AIDS, a clinical AIDS condition and mortality: psychosocial and physiological predictors. *Psychol Med* **32**, 1059–73.

54 International Agency for Research on Cancer (1995). Human papillomaviruses. *IARC Monogr Eval Carcinog Risks Hum* **64**, 1–409.

55 Pereira DB, Antoni MH, Danielson A, *et al.* (2003). Stress as a predictor of symptomatic genital herpes virus recurrence in women with human immunodeficiency virus. *J Psychosom Res* **54**, 237–44.

56 Pereira DB, Antoni MH, Danielson A, *et al.* (2003). Life stress and cervical squamous intraepithelial lesions in women with human papillomavirus and human immunodeficiency virus. *Psychosom Med* **65**, 427–34.

57 Kessler RC, Foster C, Joseph J, *et al.* (1991). Stressful life events and symptom onset in HIV infection. *Am J Psychiatry* **148**, 733–8.

58 Beck AT (1997). The past and future of cognitive therapy. *J Psychother Pract Res* **6**, 276–84.

59 Smith CA, Haynes KN, Lazarus RS, Pope LK (1993). In search of the 'hot' cognitions: attributions, appraisals, and their relation to emotion. *J Pers Soc Psychol* **65**, 916–29.

60 Folkman S, Lazarus RS, Gruen RJ, DeLongis A (1986). Appraisal, coping, health status, and psychological symptoms. *J Pers Soc Psychol* **50**, 571–9.

61 Reed GM, Kemeny ME, Taylor SE, Visscher BR (1999). Negative HIV-specific expectancies and AIDS-related bereavement as predictors of symptom onset in asymptomatic HIV-positive gay men. *Health Psychol* **18**, 354–63.

62 Reed GM, Kemeny ME, Taylor SE, Wang HY, Visscher BR (1994). Realistic acceptance as a predictor of decreased survival time in gay men with AIDS. *Health Psychol* **13**, 299–307.

63 Segerstrom SC, Taylor SE, Kemeny ME, Reed GM, Visscher BR (1996). Causal attributions predict rate of immune decline in HIV-seropositive gay men. *Health Psychol* **15**, 485–93.

64 Bower JE, Kemeny ME, Taylor SE, Fahey JL (1998). Cognitive processing, discovery of meaning, CD4 decline, and AIDS-related mortality among bereaved HIV-seropositive men. *J Consult Clin Psychol* **66**, 979–86.

65 Smith SR, Rublein JC, Marcus C, Brock TP, Chesney MA (2003). A medication self-management program to improve adherence to HIV therapy regimens. *Patient Educ Couns* **50**, 187–99.

66 Benight CC, Antoni MH, Kilbourn K, *et al.* (1997). Coping self-efficacy buffers psychological and physiological disturbances in HIV-infected men following a natural disaster. *Health Psychol* **16**, 248–55.

67 Kelly B, Raphael B, Judd F, *et al.* (1998). Posttraumatic stress disorder in response to HIV infection. *Gen Hosp Psychiatry* **20**, 345–52.

68 Antoni MH, August S, LaPerriere A, *et al.* (1990). Psychological and neuroendocrine measures related to functional immune changes in anticipation of HIV-1 serostatus notification. *Psychosom Med* **52**, 496–510.

69 Lutgendorf S, Antoni M, Ironson G, Klimas N, Fletcher M, Schneiderman N (1997). Cognitive processing style, mood, and immune function following HIV seropositivity notification. *Cognit Ther Res* **21**, 157–84.

70 Cruess DG, Antoni MH, Gonzalez J, *et al.* (2003). Sleep disturbance mediates the association between psychological distress and immune status among HIV-positive men and women on combination antiretroviral therapy. *J Psychosom Res* **54**, 185–9.

71 Savard J, Laroche L, Simard S, Ivers H, Morin CM (2003). Chronic insomnia and immune functioning. *Psychosom Med* **65**, 211–21.

72 Millon T, Green CJ, Meagher RB (1979). The MBHI: A new inventory for the psychodiagnostician in medical settings. *Prof Psychol* **10**, 529–39.

73 Carver C, Sheier M, Weintraub JD (1989). Assessing coping strategies: A theoretically based approach. *J Pers Soc Psychol* **56**, 267–83.

74 Goodkin K, Blaney NT, Feaster D, *et al.* (1992). Active coping style is associated with natural killer cell cytotoxicity in asymptomatic HIV-1 seropositive homosexual men. *J Psychosom Res* **36**, 635–50.

75 Mulder CL, Antoni MH, Duivenvoorden HJ, Kauffmann RH, Goodkin K (1995). Active confrontational coping predicts decreased clinical progression over a one-year period in HIV-infected homosexual men. *J Psychosom Res* **39**, 957–65.

76 Mulder CL, de Vroome EM, van Griensven GJ, Antoni MH, Sandfort TG (1999). Avoidance as a predictor of the biological course of HIV infection over a 7-year period in gay men. *Health Psychol* **18**, 107–13.

77 Solano L, Costa M, Salvati S, *et al.* (1993). Psychosocial factors and clinical evolution in HIV-1 infection: a longitudinal study. *J Psychosom Res* **37**, 39–51.

78 Ironson G, Friedman A, Klimas N, *et al.* (1994). Distress, denial, and low adherence to behavioral interventions predict faster disease progression in gay men infected with human immunodeficiency virus. *Int J Behav Med* **1**, 90–105.

79 Cruess SE, Antoni MH, Cruess DG, *et al.* (2000). Reductions in herpes simplex virus type 2 antibody titers after cognitive behavioral stress management and relationships with neuroendocrine function, relaxation skills, and social support in HIV-positive men. *Psychosom Med* **62**, 828–37.

80 Theorell T, Blomkvist V, Jonsson H, Schulman S, Berntorp E, Stigendal L (1995). Social support and the development of immune function in human immunodeficiency virus infection. *Psychosom Med* **57**, 32–6.

81 Patterson TL, Shaw WS, Semple SJ, *et al.* (1996). Relationship of psychosocial factors to HIV disease progression. *Ann Behav Med* **18**, 30–9.

82 Miller GE, Kemeny ME, Taylor SE, Cole SW, Visscher BR (1997). Social relationships and immune processes in HIV seropositive gay and bisexual men. *Ann Behav Med* **19**, 139–51.

83 Cole SW, Kemeny ME, Taylor SE (1997). Social identity and physical health: accelerated HIV progression in rejection-sensitive gay men. *J Pers Soc Psychol* **72**, 320–35.

84 Powell LH, Shahabi L, Thoresen CE (2003). Religion and spirituality. Linkages to physical health. *Am Psychol* **58**, 36–52.

85 Ironson G, Solomon GF, Balbin EG, *et al.* (2002). The Ironson–Woods Spirituality/Religiousness Index is associated with long survival, health behaviors, less distress, and low cortisol in people with HIV/AIDS. *Ann Behav Med* **24**, 34–48.

86 Eisenberger NI, Kemeny ME, Wyatt GE (2003). Psychological inhibition and CD4 T-cell levels in HIV-seropositive women. *J Psychosom Res* **54**, 213–24.

87 O'Cleirigh C, Ironson G, Antoni M, *et al.* (2003). Emotional expression and depth processing of trauma and their relation to long-term survival in patients with HIV/AIDS. *J Psychosom Res* **54**: 225–35.

88 Cole SW, Kemeny ME, Taylor SE, Visscher B (1996). Elevated physical health risk among gay men who conceal their homosexual identity. *Health Psychol* **15**, 243–51.

89 Cole SW, Kemeny ME, Taylor SE, Visscher B, Fahey JL (1996). Accelerated course of human immunodeficiency virus infection in gay men who conceal their homosexual identity. *Psychosom Med* **58**, 219–31.

90 Ullrich PM, Lutgendorf SK, Stapleton JT (2003). Concealment of homosexual identity, social support and CD4 cell count among HIV-seropositive gay men. *J Psychosom Res* **54**, 205–12.

91 Sherman BF, Bonanno GA, Wiener LS, Battles HB (2000). When children tell their friends they have AIDS: possible consequences for psychological well-being and disease progression. *Psychosom Med* **62**, 238–47.

92 Evans DL, Ten Have TR, Douglas SD, *et al.* (2002). Association of depression with viral load, CD8 T lymphocytes, and natural killer cells in women with HIV infection. *Am J Psychiatry* **159**, 1752–9.

93 Famularo G, Moretti S, Marcellini S, Nucera E, De Simone C (1997). CD8 lymphocytes in HIV infection: helpful and harmful. *J Clin Lab Immunol* **49**, 15–32.

94 Kemeny ME, Weiner H, Duran R, Taylor SE, Visscher B, Fahey JL (1995). Immune system changes after the death of a partner in HIV-positive gay men. *Psychosom Med* **57**, 547–54.

95 Goodkin K, Feaster DJ, Tuttle R, *et al.* (1996). Bereavement is associated with time-dependent decrements in cellular immune function in asymptomatic human immunodeficiency virus type 1-seropositive homosexual men. *Clin Diagn Lab Immunol* **3**, 109–18.

96 Kemeny ME, Weiner H, Taylor SE, Schneider S, Visscher B, Fahey JL (1994). Repeated bereavement, depressed mood, and immune parameters in HIV seropositive and seronegative gay men. *Health Psychol* **13**, 14–24.

97 Rabkin JG, Williams J, Remien RH, Goetz R, Kertzner R, Gorman JM (1991). Depression, distress, lymphocyte subsets, and human immunodeficiency virus symptoms on two occasions in HIV-positive homosexual men. *Arch Gen Psychiatry* **48**, 111–19.

98 Lyketsos CG, Hoover DR, Guccione M, *et al.* (1993). Depressive symptoms as predictors of medical outcomes in HIV infection. Multicenter AIDS cohort study. *JAMA* **270**, 2563–7.

99 Sahs JA, Goetz R, Reddy M, *et al.* (1994). Psychological distress and natural killer cells in gay men with and without HIV infection. *Am J Psychiatry* **151**, 1479–84.

100 Vedhara K, Schifitto G, McDermott M (1999). Disease progression in HIV-positive women with moderate to severe immunosuppression: the role of depression. Dana Consortium on Therapy for HIV Dementia and Related Cognitive Disorders. *Behav Med* **25**, 43–7.

101 Burack JH, Barrett DC, Stall RD, Chesney MA, Ekstrand ML, Coates TJ (1993). Depressive symptoms and CD4 lymphocyte decline among HIV-infected men comment. *JAMA* **270**, 2568–73.

102 Weissman MM, Sholomskas D, Pottenger M, Prusoff BA, Locke BZ (1977). Assessing depressive symptoms in five psychiatric populations: a validation study. *Am J Epidemiol* **106**, 203–14.

103 Centers for Disease Control and Prevention (1987). Revision of the CDC surveillance case definition for acquired immunodeficiency syndrome. Council of State and Territorial Epidemiologists; AIDS Program, Center for Infectious Diseases. *MMWR Morb Mortal Wkly Rep* **36** (Suppl 1), 1S–15S.

104 Vedhara K, Nott KH, Bradbeer CS, *et al.* (1997). Greater emotional distress is associated with accelerated CD4+ cell decline in HIV infection. *J Psychosom Res* **42**, 379–90.

105 Ickovics JR, Hamburger ME, Vlahov D, *et al.* (2001). Mortality, CD4 cell count decline, and depressive symptoms among HIV-seropositive women: longitudinal analysis from the HIV Epidemiology Research Study. *JAMA* **285**, 1466–74.

106 McNair D, Lorr M, Droppleman L (1981). *EITS manual for the Profile of Mood States.* San Diego, CA: EITS.

107 Kemeny ME, Dean L (1995). Effects of AIDS-related bereavement on HIV progression among New York City gay men. *AIDS Educ Prev* **7** (Suppl 5), 36–47.

108 Mayne TJ, Vittinghoff E, Chesney MA, Barrett DC, Coates TJ (1996). Depressive affect and survival among gay and bisexual men infected with HIV. *Arch Int Med* **156**, 2233–8.

109 Antoni MH, Cruess DG, Cruess SE, *et al.* (2000). Cognitive–behavioral stress management intervention effects on anxiety, 24-hour urinary norepinephrine output, and T-cytotoxic/ suppressor cells over time among symptomatic HIV-infected gay men. *J Consult Clin Psychol* **68**, 31–45.

110 Lutgendorf S, Antoni MH, Ironson G, *et al.* (1997). Cognitive-behavioral stress management decreases dysphoric mood and herpes simplex virus-type 2 antibody titers in symptomatic HIV-seropositive gay men. *J Consult Clin Psychol* **65**, 31–43.

111 Antoni MH, Cruess SE, Cruess DG, *et al.* (2000). Cognitive–behavioral stress management reduces distress and 24-hour urinary free cortisol output among symptomatic HIV-infected gay men. *Ann Behav Med* **22**, 29–37.

112 Cruess DG, Antoni MH, Kumar M, *et al.* (1999). Cognitive-behavioral stress management buffers decreases in dehydroepiandrosterone sulfate (DHEA-S) and increases in the

cortisol/DHEA-S ratio and reduces mood disturbance and perceived stress among HIV-seropositive men. *Psychoneuroendocrinology* **24**, 537–49.

113 **Cruess DG, Antoni MH, Schneiderman N, et al.** (2000). Cognitive–behavioral stress management increases free testosterone and decreases psychological distress in HIV-seropositive men. *Health Psychol* **19**, 12–20.

114 **Byrnes DM, Antoni MH, Goodkin K, et al.** (1998). Stressful events, pessimism, and natural killer cell cytotoxicity in HIV+ Black women at risk for cervical cancer. *Psychosom Med* **60**, 714–22.

115 **Cruess S, Antoni M, Kilbourn K, et al.** (2000). Optimism, distress, and immunologic status in HIV-infected gay men following Hurricane Andrew. *Int J Behav Med* **7**, 160–82.

116 **Tomakowsky J, Lumley MA, Markowitz N, Frank C** (2001). Optimistic explanatory style and dispositional optimism in HIV-infected men. *J Psychosom Res* **51**, 577–87.

117 **Miguez-Burbano MJ, Burbano X, Ashkin D, et al.** (2003). Impact of tobacco use on the development of opportunistic respiratory infections in HIV seropositive patients on antiretroviral therapy. *Addict Biol* **8**, 39–43.

118 **Slavinsky J, III, Myers T, Swoboda RK, Leigh JE, Hager S, Fidel PL, Jr** (2002). Th1/Th2 cytokine profiles in saliva of HIV-positive smokers with oropharyngeal candidiasis. *Oral Microbiol Immunol* **17**, 38–43.

119 **Brisson J, Morin C, Fortier M, et al.** (1994). Risk factors for cervical intraepithelial neoplasia: Differences between low- and high-grade lesions. *Am J Epidemiol* **140**, 700–10.

120 **Durante AJ, Williams AB, Da Costa M, Darragh TM, Khoshnood K, Palefsky JM** (2003). Incidence of anal cytological abnormalities in a cohort of human immunodeficiency virus-infected women. *Cancer Epidemiol Biomarkers Prev* **12**, 638–42.

121 **Turner J, Page-Shafer K, Chin DP, et al.** (2001). Adverse impact of cigarette smoking on dimensions of health-related quality of life in persons with HIV infection. *AIDS Patient Care STDS* **15**, 615–24.

122 **Miguez MJ, Shor-Posner G, Morales G, Rodriguez A, Burbano X** (2003). HIV treatment in drug abusers: impact of alcohol use. *Addict Biol* **8**, 33–7.

123 **Baldwin GC, Roth MD, Tashkin DP** (1998). Acute and chronic effects of cocaine on the immune system and the possible link to AIDS. *J Neuroimmunol* **83**, 133–8.

124 **Fiala M, Gan XH, Zhang L, et al.** (1998). Cocaine enhances monocyte migration across the blood-brain barrier. Cocaine's connection to AIDS dementia and vasculitis? *Adv Exp Med Biol* **437**, 199–205.

125 **Sutliff RL, Haase C, Russ R, et al.** (2003). Cocaine increases mortality and cardiac mass in a murine transgenic model of acquired immune deficiency syndrome. *Lab Invest* **83**, 983–9.

126 **Power R, Koopman C, Volk J, et al.** (2003). Social support, substance use, and denial in relationship to antiretroviral treatment adherence among HIV-infected persons. *AIDS Patient Care STDS* **17**, 245–52.

127 **van Servellen G, Chang B, Garcia L, Lombardi E** (2002). Individual and system level factors associated with treatment nonadherence in human immunodeficiency virus-infected men and women. *AIDS Patient Care STDS* **16**, 269–81.

128 **Penedo FJ, Gonzalez JS, Dahn JR, Antoni M, Malow R, Costa P et al.** (2003). Personality, quality of life and HAART adherence among men and women living with HIV/AIDS. *J Psychosom Res* **54**, 271–8.

129 **Singh N, Berman SM, Swindells S, et al.** (1999). Adherence of human immunodeficiency virus-infected patients to antiretroviral therapy. *Clin Infect Dis* **29**, 824–30.

130 **Simoni JM, Frick PA, Lockhart D, Liebovitz D** (2002). Mediators of social support and antiretroviral adherence among an indigent population in New York City. *AIDS Patient Care STDS* **16**, 431–9.

131 **Mann T** (2001). Effects of future writing and optimism on health behaviors in HIV-infected women. *Ann Behav Med* **23**, 26–33.

132 **Joint United Nations Programme on HIV/AIDS** (2002). *Fact Sheet 2002: The impact of HIV/AIDS.* New York: United Nations.

133 **Walker BD, Chakrabarti S, Moss B** *et al.* (1987). HIV-specific cytotoxic T lymphocytes in seropositive individuals. *Nature* **328**, 345–8.

134 **Pitcher CJ, Quittner C, Peterson DM,** *et al.* (1999). HIV-1-specific CD4+ T cells are detectable in most individuals with active HIV-1 infection, but decline with prolonged viral suppression. *Nat Med* **5**, 518–25.

135 **Ogg GS, Jin X, Bonhoeffer S,** *et al.* (1998). Quantitation of HIV-1-specific cytotoxic T lymphocytes and plasma load of viral RNA. *Science* **279**, 2103–6.

136 **Lutgendorf SK, Johnsen EL, Cooper B,** *et al.* (2002). Vascular endothelial growth factor and social support in patients with ovarian carcinoma. *Cancer* **95**, 808–15.

137 **Lutgendorf SK, Garand L, Buckwalter KC, Reimer TT, Hong SY, Lubaroff DM** (1999). Life stress, mood disturbance, and elevated interleukin-6 in healthy older women. *J Gerontol A Biol Sci Med Sci* **54**, M434–9.

138 **Wright TC, Jr., Subbarao S, Ellerbrock TV,** *et al.* (2001). Human immunodeficiency virus 1 expression in the female genital tract in association with cervical inflammation and ulceration. *Am J Obstet Gynecol* **184**, 279–85.

139 **Ellerbrock TV, Lennox JL, Clancy KA,** *et al.* (2001). Cellular replication of human immunodeficiency virus type 1 occurs in vaginal secretions. *J Infect Dis* **184**, 28–36.

140 **Rasheed S, Li Z, Xu D, Kovacs A** (1996). Presence of cell-free human immunodeficiency virus in cervicovaginal secretions is independent of viral load in the blood of human immunodeficiency virus-infected women. *Am J Obstet Gynecol* **175**, 122–9.

141 **Fordyce EJ, Wang Z, Kahn AR,** *et al.* (2000). Risk of cancer among women with AIDS in New York City. *AIDS Public Policy J* **15**, 95–104.

Chapter 8

Psychoneuroimmunology and chronic autoimmune diseases: rheumatoid arthritis

Cobi J. Heijnen and Annemieke Kavelaars

8.1 Introduction

Rheumatoid arthritis (RA) is a chronic inflammatory disease of the joints. Pain, decreased mobility and stiffness are the main clinical problems of patients with RA. It is thought that a response of the immune system to self (autoimmunity) is the cause of the chronic inflammation. Hormones and neurotransmitters can regulate the activity of the immune system. Therefore it is conceivable that the central nervous system and the neuroendocrine system can influence the onset and course of arthritis. In this chapter we review the biological mechanisms that are involved in modulation of the immune response by sex steroids, glucocorticoids, and catecholamines. We present an overview of the evidence that these mechanisms are operative in patients with RA (see Fig. 8.1 for a summary). Glucocorticoids and catecholamines are mediators of the stress response. Because these hormones and neurotransmitters modulate the immune response and play a role in RA, it is likely that stress modulates disease activity and onset. Evidence for a role of stress in disease onset and progression will be summarized at the end of this chapter. RA is an example of a chronic pro-inflammatory autoimmune disease. It is important to realize that the psychoneuroimmunology (PNI) mechanisms that are described in this chapter in the context of RA will also be operative in other pro-inflammatory autoimmune diseases such as multiple sclerosis and Sjögren's disease.

8.2 Rheumatoid arthritis: the biological and clinical context

8.2.1 Rheumatoid arthritis

Rheumatoid arthritis is a chronic inflammatory disease characterized by chronic synovitis mainly of the small joints in the hands and feet. Joint swelling, stiffness, decreased mobility, and joint-space narrowing are the main features of the disease. Synovial hyperplasia (pannus formation) causes the erosions and joint deformities. T cells, B cells, macrophages, and cytokines produced locally by these cells are thought

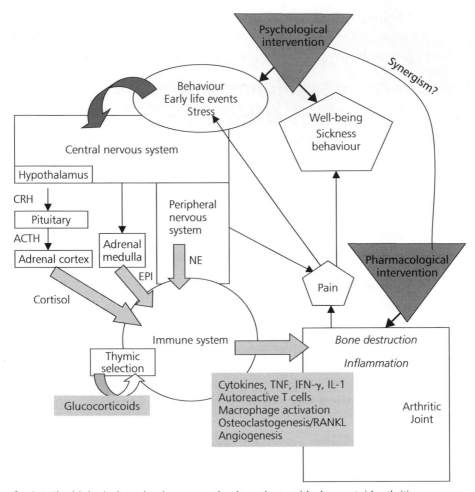

Fig. 8.1 The biological mechanisms operating in patients with rheumatoid arthritis.

to play a major role in the pathogenesis of joint deformation. The ongoing inflammation in the joint and the deformation of the joints are responsible for the pain that is the major complaint of patients with RA. RA is often accompanied by psychological problems, especially depressed mood.[1] The severity of RA is highly variable at onset and during the course of the disease. Some patients present with severe inflammation of the joints, but develop relatively little joint destruction, whereas in others the major problem is the deformation of the joint without severe inflammation.

Rheumatoid arthritis occurs in 0.5–1% of the adult population worldwide, but the incidence is much higher in some populations. The prevalence of RA is extraordinarily high in some groups of Native Americans, with over 5% of individuals affected. Interestingly, the disease already existed in early Native American populations several thousand years ago, whereas in Europe it appeared in the early seventeenth century.[2]

There is a clear sex difference in occurrence of the disease; on average, the female-to-male ratio is 2.5, but in the group of patients aged between 20 and 50 years, there are five females with the disease for every male patient (female-to-male ratio of 5 : 1).[3,4] The current treatment of RA aims at inhibiting the inflammatory response and joint destruction by administering non-steroidal anti-inflammatory drugs, steroids, specific cytokine inhibitors, and even chemotherapy. Bone marrow transplantation is also sometimes applied as a therapeutic strategy for arthritis, especially in children. Orthopaedic and reconstructive surgery can also be an important means of relieving pain and in restoring or maintaining physical function.

8.2.2 Juvenile idiopathic arthritis

Juvenile idiopathic arthritis (JIA) is an inflammatory joint disease of childhood. Three subtypes of the disease are characterized by the clinical parameters at the onset of the disease: oligo- or pauci-articular, polyarticular, and systemic JIA. The abnormalities found in the joints are similar in the three subtypes and resemble the histopathological abnormalities of adult RA. However, the clinical course of the three subtypes is markedly different. Oligo-articular JIA has a good prognosis and, in general, completely remits. In contrast, poly-articular and systemic JIA are usually non-remitting diseases that require aggressive immunosuppressive therapy and are often associated with severe irreversible damage to the joints.

8.2.3 Animal model for arthritis

Adjuvant arthritis in rats is the most widely used animal model with a pathological resemblance to RA. It is induced in rats by a single intradermal immunization with mycobacterial antigens in Freund's adjuvant. The rats develop joint inflammation in the paws and ankles, characterized by swelling and redness, generally starting around day 10 after immunization. The major difference from the human situation is that the inflammatory components of adjuvant arthritis remit spontaneously and completely after 20–30 days. However, joint destruction is completely irreversible, as is found in RA and JIA.

8.2.4 Aetiopathogenesis of RA

Rheumatoid arthritis is a complex disease and as yet no specific cause(s) of the disease has been identified. Theories of the pathogenesis of RA include auto-antibodies and immune complexes, T-cell-dependent and T-cell-independent cytokine production, autoreactive T lymphocytes, production of bone-destructive factors, and aggressive pro-liferation of the synovium. The aetiopathogenesis of RA has been reviewed recently.[2,5,6]

8.2.4.1 Genetic factors

Twin studies have suggested that genetic factors contribute no more than 15% of the risk of developing RA, although there are some alleles that constitute a much higher risk (e.g. HLA-DRB1). Thus both genetic and environmental factors, and their interactions, must accumulate in an individual for the disease to be manifested.

8.2.4.2 Autoimmune factors

The first indication that autoimmunity plays a role in the pathogenesis of RA was the identification of rheumatoid factor in blood, described by Waaler in 1939. Later, rheumatoid factor was characterized as antibodies that bind to the Fc portion of immunoglobulins. Patients who are positive for rheumatoid factor (about 80% of the total patient population) have a more aggressive course of the disease.[2]

During RA, activated CD4+ T cells are present in the synovium (the joint lining). In normal individuals, antigens expressed by infectious microorganisms or foreign substances activate the immune cells and activated T cells are present at the site of infection. The presence of activated T cells at non-infected sites suggests that other processes induce activation. During an autoimmune disease like RA, so-called auto-antigens, which are part of the tissue of the individual and should be ignored by the immune system, can also activate T cells. T lymphocytes are very important in regulating the activity of the other components of the immune system (e.g. B-cell and macrophage activity). Therefore the presence of activated T cells in the synovium strongly suggests that T cells which react with determinants expressed in the joint tissue are the driving force behind the chronic inflammation. However, it is still not clear which auto-antigens induce the inflammatory response that regulates the inflammation and subsequent joint destruction in RA.

In animal models, it has been shown that many different antigenic determinants (e.g. heat shock proteins, collagen, and proteoglycans) can induce arthritis when presented to the animal in the appropriate conditions. In humans, these antigens are recognized by cells or antibodies from RA patients, suggesting a role in the pathogenesis of the disease. Apart from CD4+ T cells, B cells and macrophages also infiltrate the synovium. Synovial cells and macrophages in the synovial lining can produce cytokines, prostaglandins, metalloproteinases and chemokines that can all contribute to the accumulation of inflammatory cells in the joint. Skeletal complications start with focal erosion of cartilage followed by marginal and subchondral bone loss. Joint destruction is characterized by pathological bone resorption due to a disturbed balance in bone remodelling. Extended joint destruction with ankylosis and generalized bone loss are characteristic of late complications.[7] These long-term skeletal complications have serious consequences as they can lead not only to painful joint deformities but also to progressive functional disability and increased mortality rates.[8] Recent successful therapeutic interventions with monoclonal antibodies against TNF-α or with IL-1β inhibitors support the notion that cytokines play a pivotal role in the course of RA. Interestingly, protective cytokines have also been identified. The pro-inflammatory cytokine interferon-gamma (IFN-γ) and the anti-inflammatory cytokine IL-10 have been shown to decrease bone destruction by interfering with osteoclastogenesis.[9] Osteoclasts are involved in the resorption of bone, thereby contributing to joint destruction. An essential factor in osteoclastogenesis is receptor activator of nuclear factor kB ligand (RANKL), which is expressed by various cell types in the synovium. RANKL interacts with its receptor on mononuclear phagocytes and thus can direct the differentiation of these phagocytes to osteoclasts.[10] Another factor that plays an important role in the inflammatory response in the joint is the capacity of the individual to produce angiogenic factors, such as vascular endothelial factor (VEGF), which lead to the expression of blood vessels in the synovium, a process which facilitates the proliferation of the synoviocytes and consequently the synovial hyperplasia. This is also called pannus formation.[11]

8.2.4.3 T-cell selection in the thymus

As mentioned above, auto-antigen-specific T cells are thought to play a major role in initiating and maintaining chronic inflammatory activity in the joints of RA patients. The question arises as to whether aberrant selection of T cells in the thymus contributes to the susceptibility or initiation of autoimmune diseases like arthritis. During differentiation of naive T cells into mature T cells in the thymus, a process of T-cell selection takes place that involves the elimination of those cells that have a high affinity for auto-antigens presented in the thymus. Thus, during this selection process, T cells that recognize auto-antigens, and would therefore give rise to an immune response against self-structures (which can develop into an autoimmune response), are removed. The inadequate selection of T cells in the thymus, in particular a failure to remove T cells that will mount an immune response towards self-antigens, may contribute to the development of autoimmune diseases, including RA.

It has been postulated, based on animal studies, that corticosterone is capable of modifying the window for selection of T cells in the thymus.[12] Therefore, it is possible that changes in corticosterone during the selection process could give rise to inappropriate positive and negative selection of thymocytes, which may contribute to altered susceptibility to autoimmunity. Indeed, in mice with a targeted reduction of glucocorticoid receptors (GRs), expression of specific T-cell receptor Vb genes is found in T cells in the periphery.[13] Interestingly, corticosterone can also be produced locally in the thymus, especially early in life.[14] Therefore the interaction between neuroendocrine substances like corticosterone and the immune system during development of an individual might be of crucial importance for the maintenance of health.

8.3 Theoretical basis for a role for psychoneuroimmunology in rheumatoid arthritis

It has long been known that exogenous administration of pharmacological doses of glucocorticoids can influence the course of arthritis. In addition, gender and pregnancy have major effects on the clinical and epidemiological aspects of RA. Moreover, it has been shown that in RA patients who are paralysed unilaterally (e.g. after stroke), the paralysed side is never inflamed. This clinical observation suggests a role for glucocorticoids, in particular cortisol, the end-product of the hypothalamic–pituitary adrenal axis in humans, for sex steroids, and for the nervous system innervating the joints in determining the onset and/or course of RA.

8.3.1 Glucocorticoids

Glucocorticoid treatment is a potent way of modulating the symptoms of RA, predominantly because of the anti-inflammatory effects of glucocorticoids and their antiproliferative effects on cartilage and bone.[15] Glucocorticoids have long been used as anti-inflammatory drugs, but it is well known that these hormones are also produced endogenously as part of the stress response. Activation of the hypothalamus in response to exposure to a stressor leads to the release of corticotrophin-releasing hormone (CRH), which activates the pituitary to secrete adrenocorticotropic hormone (ACTH). ACTH in turn stimulates the release of endogenous glucocorticoids by the adrenal cortex. In humans, the end-product of the HPA axis is cortisol; in rodents the glucocorticoid corticosterone is produced by the adrenal cortex after stress.

8.3.1.1 Glucocorticoids: cellular mechanism of action

Glucocorticoid receptors and glucocorticoid response elements Glucocorticoids (GCs) exert their biological effects via binding to GRs that are present in the cytosol. Glucocorticoid binding to GRs results in translocation of the GC–GR complex from the cytosol to the nucleus. In the nucleus, the complex can have direct effects on the expression of genes that contain a specific sequence in the promoter, the so-called glucocorticoid response element (GRE). The GC–GR complex can bind to the GRE sequence which will result in a change in the rate of transcription of these genes; thus the production of the product of these genes will be either increased or decreased.[16] Despite the strong anti-inflammatory effects of glucocorticoids, there are not many genes relevant to the immune response that contain such GRE sequences.[16] For example, most cytokines that are downregulated by glucocorticoids do not contain GRE sequences. Therefore it is unlikely that these direct genomic effects of glucocorticoids are the major pathway for the immunomodulatory activity of glucocorticoids.

Interaction GR and transcription factors How can glucocorticoids inhibit cytokine production via non-genomic effects? The production of many of the cytokines involved in RA is controlled by the transcription factor nuclear factor κ binding protein (NF-κB). This transcription factor is present in the cytosol in a complex with the protein inhibitor of NF-κB (I-κB). Upon cellular activation, I-κB is phosphorylated, detaches from NF-κB, and is degraded. NF-κB then migrates to the nucleus where it activates transcription of genes for pro-inflammatory cytokines including TNF-α and IL-6. Interestingly, the GC–GR complex can also bind to NF-κB and will prevent binding of NF-κB to the promoter of pro-inflammatory cytokines. Thus the GC–GR complex can prevent activation of pro-inflammatory cytokine genes by preventing the free NF-κB from binding to the promoter sequences of the cytokine genes.[16]

8.3.1.2 Glucocorticoids and T cell selection in the thymus

As mentioned above, glucocorticoids produced in the thymus can play a role in the selection of thymocytes. At present it is not known whether endogenous glucocorticoids produced outside the thymus (e.g. in response to stress) modulate this process of thymic selection. However, it has been shown that endogenous administration of glucocorticoids can modulate production of corticosterone within the thymus. Treatment of rat pups with the synthetic glucocorticoid dexamethasone on days 1, 2, and 3 after birth results in a transient reduction in endogenous glucocorticoid production by thymic epithelial cells.[17] More importantly, however, this neonatal exposure to pharmacological doses of glucocorticoids has long-term effects on the T-cell receptor (TCR) Vβ repertoire. For example, expression of Vβ20 in splenic CD4 T cells was increased after neonatal administration of glucocorticoids, whereas Vβ2 was decreased at the age of 5 weeks.[17] Thus neonatal changes in the glucocorticoid milieu in the thymus can have long-term consequences for selection of T cells in the thymus and may also modulate susceptibility for autoimmune diseases including arthritis.

8.3.1.3 HPA axis and cortisol

HPA axis activity The elegant pioneering work of Sternberg and colleagues[18,19] has drawn attention to the potential role of endogenous glucocorticoids in the susceptibility to and course of autoimmune inflammatory diseases like arthritis.[18,19] During inflammation, cytokines produced by activated immune cells can signal to the central nervous system via direct and indirect pathways. The cytokine signals to the central nervous system result in activation of the hypothalamic–pituitary–adrenal axis (HPA axis) in a similar way to the stress-induced activation of the HPA axis: cytokines activate the release of CRH from the hypothalamus, resulting in increased plasma ACTH. Increased plasma ACTH levels will induce the release of glucocorticoids by the adrenal glands. As described above, glucocorticoids have immunosuppressive activity and thus can inhibit the inflammatory reaction. Changes in the plasma levels of glucocorticoids have been shown to play an important role in mediating the effects of stress on the immune response. For example, it has been shown that chronic stress is associated with glucocorticoid-dependent increases in susceptibility to infections.[20] In addition, there is evidence that the absence of a glucocorticoid response (after removal of the adrenal glands) during inflammatory processes will result in overactivation of the inflammatory response, increased cytokine production, and even death of the animal.[21] In contrast, short-term elevations in glucocorticoid levels after acute stress are associated with changes in trafficking of immune cells and can actually enhance local inflammatory responses.[22]

HPA axis activity and susceptibility to arthritis in animal models Comparison of various strains of experimental animals has shown that there is an association between blunted HPA axis activity and increased susceptibility to autoimmune diseases including arthritis. For example, Sternberg and colleagues[18,19] have shown that Lewis rats, which are highly susceptible to arthritis, have a blunted reactivity of the HPA axis. In contrast, arthritis-resistant Fisher rats have a hyperactive HPA axis response. Surgical or pharmacological ablation of the glucocorticoid response can render arthritis-resistant Fisher rats susceptible to the disease. These data strongly suggest that endogenous glucocorticoids play an important role in determining susceptibility to arthritis. However, this conclusion should be treated with caution, because more recent studies in other strains of animals have not confirmed a dominant role for HPA axis reactivity in controlling disease susceptibility and progression. For example, Andersson et al.[23] compared the corticosterone response to immune activation and susceptibility to β-glucan-induced arthritis in Dark-Agouti (DA) and MHC-identical PVG.1AV1 rats. Although corticosterone responses are similar in both strains, DA rats develop severe arthritis whereas the arthritis was significantly milder in PVG.1AV1 rats.

Others have explored the possible relationship between differences in HPA axis reactivity and susceptibility to arthritis within a single animal strain. Wistar rats were divided into two groups based on their behaviour in a learned helplessness (LH) paradigm. In this paradigm, rats are first exposed to inescapable foot shock and subsequently to an avoidable stressor. Some of the animals will develop LH, i.e. they do not avoid the escapable stressor upon second exposure. Animals selected as LH+ (i.e. animals developing LH) or LH− (i.e. animals that do not develop LH and avoid the second escapable stressor) differ in their HPA axis reactivity and susceptibility to arthritis. However, LH− animals that have a higher corticosterone response are also more susceptible to arthritis.[24] In another study, inbred Lewis rats were selected based on their activity in an open field. It appeared that rats that showed low activity in the open field were much more susceptible to arthritis with respect to developing bone destruction than rats who expressed the high-activity phenotype. However, there were no differences in HPA axis reactivity between the two groups of rats.[25]

In conclusion, the reactivity of the HPA axis can predict susceptibility to arthritis in specific cases, but the activity of the HPA axis can no longer be regarded as a general predictor for the course of arthritis.

8.3.1.4 HPA axis activity and endogenous glucocorticoids in human RA

It has been shown in patients with RA that blocking endogenous glucocorticoid synthesis by administration of metyrapone induces an increase in disease activity, suggesting that endogenous glucocorticoids also reduce disease activity in humans.

However, similarly to what has been found in animal models regarding the contribution of HPA axis reactivity to the course of arthritis, there is much discussion in the human literature of the role of cortisol and the HPA axis in predicting the severity of RA (reviewed by Harbuz and Jessop[26]). To test the hypothesis that RA is associated with a blunted activity of the HPA axis, a number of different experimental approaches have been used. Initially, total cortisol secretion in urine was determined and showed no differences between patients and controls. Later, the pituitary–adrenal response to infusion of CRH was tested. However, results from these studies were somewhat disappointing because, although some studies showed a small reduction in the cortisol response to CRH in RA patients, many others found no difference between patients and controls.[26] In addition, most studies found no change in the diurnal rhythm of plasma cortisol between RA patients and healthy controls. Surprisingly, many authors still conclude that there is a functional defect of the HPA axis based on the normal plasma levels of cortisol in patients. This conclusion is based on the assumption that in view of the ongoing inflammatory activity and increased levels of circulating cytokines (IL-6), an increase in the response of the HPA axis could be expected that would be represented by an increase in the production of cortisol. Thus, one would expect a higher level of cortisol in RA patients than in healthy individuals, and the fact that this increase is not observed suggests that there is a deficiency of the HPA axis in RA.[27–29] This hypothesis is highly speculative and requires further testing, preferably in animal models initially, to obtain more insight into the effect of chronic elevation of circulating cytokine levels, with possible negative feedback, on HPA axis functioning.

Recently, Harbuz *et al.*[30] used the dexamethasone–CRH suppression test to investigate HPA axis activity in RA patients. In this test, which has been used predominantly to investigate HPA axis functioning in psychiatric disorders, subjects receive a single dose of the synthetic glucocorticoid dexamethasone the evening before the actual test.[31] The next day, CRH was infused and the cortisol response was monitored. In healthy individuals, the dexamethasone treatment will suppress the CRH-induced rise in cortisol. Surprisingly, three out of seven patients escaped from dexamethasone suppression and responded with a cortisol response after CRH challenge in the presence of dexamethasone. However, there was no obvious difference between responders and non-responders with respect to clinical symptoms of the disease. Therefore the clinical relevance of the abnormal response of some patients has still to be elucidated.

In conclusion, the precise role of the HPA axis in the course of RA is as yet unclear and is probably far more complex than initially suggested by the animal literature.

8.3.2 Gender, pregnancy, and sex steroids in RA

It is well known that the incidence of RA is significantly higher in females than in males. Moreover, clinical signs of arthritis are decreased in many RA patients during pregnancy, whereas disease activity is known to increase after delivery.[32] Onset of RA is markedly increased in the early post-partum period; with the likelihood of developing RA during the post-partum period being 10-fold higher than in non-pregnant conditions. It is known that changes in the activity of the HPA axis occur during pregnancy and immediately thereafter, but it is hard to explain the profound effects of pregnancy and gender by these relatively subtle changes in the HPA axis. Therefore it has been proposed that sex steroids may play a major role in determining susceptibility to arthritis and in modulating disease activity, with oestrogen and testosterone as the major candidates. For example, ovariectomy, which leads to a reduction in endogenous oestrogen production, has been shown to reduce susceptibility to arthritis in animal models.[33] Moreover, replacement of oestrogen normalizes arthritis susceptibility in ovariectomized animals. Endogenous differences in testosterone levels may well play an important role in determining susceptibility to arthritis in animal models as well. For example, the arthritis-resistant LH+ rats mentioned earlier differ from their LH− counterparts in plasma testosterone level.[24] In a model of the autoimmune disease systemic lupus erythematosus (SLE), it has been shown that administration of dihydrotestosterone can improve the clinical course.[34]

Little is known about the cellular mechanisms responsible for the effects of oestrogen and testosterone in arthritis. There is evidence that the oestrogen receptor can interact with the transcription factor NF-κB, but this interaction does not inhibit the capacity of NF-κB to regulate cytokine production. However, oestrogen can inhibit degradation of I-κB which in turn will result in the sustained presence of this inhibitory protein and thereby can prevent activation of cytokine genes.[35] Testosterone enhances thymocyte apoptosis and thus may interfere with thymic selection. In addition, there is evidence that testosterone enhances suppressor T cells.[36]

8.3.3 The nervous system in arthritis

The first indications of a role of the sympathetic nervous system in induction and maintaining arthritis came from clinical practice. For example, patients with a hemiparalysis only develop arthritis in the non-paralysed side. In addition, the symptoms of arthritis usually start in the most densely innervated joints (e.g. the fingers). The original studies in animal models supported the hypothesis that innervation of the joints may enhance the symptoms of arthritis since denervation of the joint significantly reduces the severity of adjuvant arthritis.[37] However, these data should be generalized with caution as denervation of immune tissue (draining lymph nodes and spleen) results in earlier onset and increased clinical signs of adjuvant arthritis in rats.[38] Therefore much work has to be done before we have a clear description of the role of the nervous system in RA.

8.3.3.1 Norepinephrine and epinephrine: mechanism of action

Norepinephrine released by nerve terminals in arthritic joints and circulating epinephrine can modulate inflammatory activity in arthritis via binding to adrenergic receptors on immune cells. To obtain a complete picture of the possible pro- and anti-inflammatory consequences of the presence of norepinephrine and epinephrine, it is important to take the receptors involved into account. Virtually all cells in the immune system express β_2-adrenergic receptors, and there is evidence that subpopulations of cells express α_1- and α_2-adrenergic receptors.[39] All adrenergic receptors belong to the family of G-protein-coupled receptors that transduce signals to effector enzymes inside the cell via activation of heterotrimeric G proteins (Fig. 8.2). α_1-Adrenergic receptors couple to G proteins of the Gq subclass which activate phospholipase C, thereby producing a rise in intracellular calcium. In addition, triggering of α_1-adrenergic receptors can activate the important intracellular enzyme mitogen-activated protein kinase. α_2-Adrenergic receptors couple to Gi and signal via inhibition of adenylate cyclase, activation of potassium channels, and inhibition of voltage-gated calcium channels. In the case of α_2-adrenergic receptors, G proteins of the Gs subclass activate adenylate cyclase, which results in the formation of the second messenger cyclic adenosine 3′,5′-monophosphate (cAMP). Increases in the intracellular level of cAMP will result in the activation of protein kinase A (PKA) which in turn activates a number of transcription factors and other regulatory proteins. Kinases can activate proteins by adding a phosphate group (phosphorylation). One important cAMP–PKA-dependent transcription factor is cAMP-responsive element binding protein (CREB). Activation of CREB will result in modulation of the activity of a number of cytokine genes (e.g. inhibition of TNF-α gene expression and enhancement of IL-10 gene expression). However, the ultimate effect of CREB activation on cytokine production will also largely depend on the activity of other transcription factors that interact with it.[40]

Thus it is not possible to generalize the functional effect of triggering of these adrenergic receptors on immune system activity, since much depends on timing of exposure to norepinephrine and/or epinephrine and the specific type of immune cell involved. For example, triggering the β_2-adrenergic receptor on monocytes or

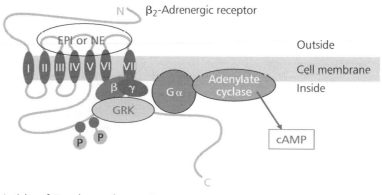

Fig. 8.2 Activity of β_2-adrenergic receptors.

macrophages will inhibit IL-12 production and enhance IL-10 production, thereby reducing IFN-γ production by T cells.[41] Norepinephrine and other β-adrenergic agonists could contribute to reduced disease activity via this mechanism. In contrast, stimulation of $β_2$-adrenergic receptors on naive T helper cells at the time of initiation of the response will lead to the production of Th1 effector cells producing increased amounts of IFN-γ, which could play an enhancing role in the initiation of the autoimmune response.[42]

8.3.3.2 Sympathetic nervous system in arthritis

It has been shown that the response of the sympathetic nervous system to orthostatic stress (i.e. stress on the cardiovascular system induced by the passive change from supine to the upright position) is disturbed in children with JIA. It has also been demonstrated that cardiovascular responses (change in diastolic blood pressure and stroke volume) to orthostatic stress are reduced in JIA patients with active disease.[43] Moreover, patients with active JIA have a higher heart rate at rest and increased levels of the catecholamine metabolite 3-hydroxy-4-phenocyphenylglycol in urine than healthy controls. These data suggest that patients with active JIA have an increased central noradrenergic outflow, leading to increased vasoconstriction and a decreased response to orthostatic stress.[43]

There is also evidence for changes in the activity of the sympathetic nervous system in adults with RA. Cardiovascular stress tests show aberrant results in many RA patients. Moreover, it has been reported that the responsivity of the sympathetic nervous system is decreased early after the onset of RA.[44]

It has recently been shown that the density of sympathetic nerve fibres in the joints of long-term RA patients is significantly reduced,[45] suggesting that the input of sympathetic nerves is decreased during the course of RA. However, it was shown in the same study that the release of norepinephrine from synovial macrophages was increased, suggesting that norepinephrine secretion into the joint was maintained but was independent of neural input. In an animal model of arthritis, it has been shown that treatment with the $β_2$-adrenergic agonist salbutamol at high doses can reduce the clinical signs of arthritis.[46] Although there is evidence that such treatment could alleviate symptoms and reduce pro-inflammatory cytokine production in the human autoimmune disease multiple sclerosis,[46] as yet there are no data regarding possible therapeutic effects of adrenergic agonists in humans with arthritis.

Although norepinephrine is a major neurotransmitter of the sympathetic nervous system, it should not be forgotten that other neurotransmitters (neuropeptides) are co-localized in the nerve endings and released in the joint. For example, endogenous opioids, including enkephalins and endomorphins, are expressed in both neuronal and extra-neuronal tissue in the joints. These opioids have potential immunomodulatory effects, as it has been shown that injection of the mu-opioid agonist morphine can reduce the inflammatory activity in patients with RA.[47] Furthermore, sensory neuropeptides like substance P, which is also a pro-inflammatory peptide, can be released into the joint and may contribute to enhanced inflammation and pain in arthritis. It has been shown in animal studies that capsaicin, which depletes substance P in nerve endings, reduces disease activity.[48] Moreover, local treatment of inflamed joints with a capsaicin smear, although initially producing a transient pain in the skin, finally results in reduced joint pain.[49]

8.3.3.3 A possible role for regulation of adrenergic receptors in RA

Most of the studies of the possible role of the neuroendocrine system in arthritis have focused on the production of mediators by the HPA axis, the gonadal axis, or the sympathetic nervous system. However, for a complete understanding of the effects of mediators from these systems on the course of autoimmune diseases, it is also necessary to take into account the receptors for these mediators that are present in the immune system. This is especially important in view of the evidence that at least some of these receptors function differently in the (activated) immune system of RA patients compared with healthy individuals.

In contrast with the vast literature on β_2-adrenergic receptor expression and function in peripheral blood mononuclear cells (PBMCs), little is known about the expression and function of α-adrenergic receptors. It has been shown in an animal model of acute inflammation in the peritoneum that macrophages express α_2-adrenergic receptors and respond to α_2-adrenergic agonists with changes in pro-inflammatory cytokine production.[50] To our knowledge, there is no information on the function and role of α_2-adrenergic receptors on immune cells in humans.

Role of receptor regulation: functioning of α-adrenergic receptors Some studies describing the role of α_1-adrenergic receptors have been performed. In healthy individuals there are no detectable cells expressing α_1-adrenergic receptor mRNA in the peripheral circulation. However, patients suffering from JIA express mRNA for various subtypes of functional α_1-adrenergic receptors on their PBMCs.[51] Stimulation of PBMCs from JIA patients *in vitro* with a specific α_1-adrenergic receptor agonist results in increased IL-6 production by these cells.[52] In line with the absence of detectable receptors in healthy individuals, no increase in IL-6 production after stimulation of cells from healthy individuals with α_1-agonists was observed. To obtain more insight into the *in vivo* relevance of these observations, JIA patients and healthy individuals were exposed to a noradrenergic stressor and the effect on cytokine production was recorded.[51] An acute physical stressor, the cold pressor test, was used as a noradrenergic stressor. The cold pressor test consists of immersion of one hand in ice water for 2 minutes. Plasma norepinephrine levels and cytokine production by PBMCs were determined before and after the test. Exposure to the cold pressor test resulted in a rapid transient increase in plasma norepinephrine in both JIA patients and healthy controls, and no detectable changes in plasma epinephrine. As expected on the basis of the *in vitro* studies mentioned above, the production of IL-6 by PBMCs from JIA patients was increased on exposure to the stressor.[51] This stress-induced increase in IL-6 production was not observed in the healthy controls. The kinetics of the effect of this stressor on IL-6 were similar to the kinetics of the change in plasma norepinephrine, with maximal effects immediately after exposure to the stressor. Therefore it was concluded that expression of α_1-adrenergic receptor on the PBMCs of JIA patients could result in increased cytokine production after exposure to acute stress, which may contribute to the chronic inflammation in these patients. It would be interesting to investigate whether the α_1-adrenergic-receptor-dependent increase in cytokine production *in vivo* is one of the mechanisms underlying the reported interaction between daily stress and the course of RA.[4]

Role of receptor regulation: functioning of β-adrenergic receptors At the level of the immune system, there is evidence for changes in the responsivity of immune cells to signals provided by catecholamines via β_2-adrenergic receptors. We have shown that PBMCs from patients with RA are more sensitive to signals from β_2-adrenergic agonists. For example, the β_2-adrenergic-agonist-induced decrease in TNF-α production by lipopolysaccharide-stimulated monocytes is more profound in cells from RA patients than from controls.[53] Moreover, exposure of cells from RA patients to a β_2-adrenergic agonist results in increased formation of the second messenger cAMP. This increased response to β_2-adrenergic agonists cannot be attributed to their increased expression on cells from RA patients; to date, only a decreased density of β_2-adrenergic receptors immune cells from RA patients has been described, although other studies have not confirmed this observation.[53,54]

Functioning of receptors can be modulated not only at the level of the number of receptors expressed, but also at the level of receptor type and of receptor (un)coupling. The disease process of RA may give rise to changes in various intracellular signal transduction cascades, which could potentially alter not only the expression but also the function of the receptors. The adrenergic receptors belong to the family of G-protein-coupled receptors (GPCRs). The sensitivity of these receptors, including the adrenergic receptors, is regulated by a family of kinases, designated G-protein-coupled receptor kinases (GRKs) and cofactors called β-arrestins.[55]

In an investigation of the expression of GRK2, a kinase family member that plays a major role in the desensitization of the β_2-adrenergic receptor, we showed that the expression level and activity of this kinase are reduced by about 50% in PBMCs from RA patients.[53] Why is this important? GRK2 is responsible for uncoupling G-protein-coupled receptors, including the β_2-adrenergic receptor, from their intracellular signalling pathways, which turns off receptor signalling. Thus, at low levels of GRK2, signalling via the β_2-adrenergic receptor is less efficiently turned off, and this phenomenon may well result in the observed increased formation of cAMP and increased inhibition of TNF-α production. Interestingly, the reduction in GRK2 can be induced by activation of the inflammatory response. We have shown that induction of arthritis in an animal model results in a marked reduction in the level of GRK2 in splenocytes, in particular in CD4+ T cells and B cells, suggesting that the reduction in GRK2 level is a consequence of the disease.[53] At present it is impossible to predict whether the decrease in GRK2 expression during RA should be viewed as an adaptation or a maladaptation. However, it should be noted that the response of cells not only to β_2-adrenergic agonists, but possibly also to other GPCR ligands including other neurotransmitters or neuropeptides and also chemokines and chemoattractants, could be altered when GRK2 is decreased in RA.[56] The GPCR family is extremely large, encompassing about 1% of the total mammalian genome. Given that the regulation of these GPCRs by kinases is altered during inflammatory diseases like RA, these kinases are an important target for novel therapeutic strategies.

8.4 Empirical evidence

8.4.1 Evidence for a role of behaviour and stress in animal studies of arthritis

Individual differences in behaviour are driven by genetic (nature) as well as environmental (nurture) factors. These behavioural differences will be associated with a specific neuroendocrine pattern that drives the behaviour and/or is the consequence of the behavioural trait. Given that the neuroendocrine system influences the immune system, the individual differences in behaviour may also determine disease susceptibility. Of particular interest in this respect is the model of pharmacogenetically selected apomorphin-susceptible and apomorphin-unsusceptible rats.[57] These two lines of rats have been selected on the basis of their gnawing behaviour after administration of the dopaminergic agonist apomorphin. The two lines show clear differences in behaviour: apomorphin-susceptible rats showing a reduced activity in an open field compared with their apomorphin-unsusceptible counterparts. The selective breeding for the sensitivity for dopamine, which is associated with differences in behaviour, has also led to a clear difference in susceptibility to pro-inflammatory auto-immune diseases like arthritis and experimental autoimmune encephalomyelitis, which is the animal model for multiple sclerosis in humans.[57] As mentioned above, both genetic and environmental factors shape the behaviour of an individual. Interestingly, the differences in behaviour that occur independently of differences in genetic background are also associated with disease outcome. For example, even in an inbred strain of rats, individual differences such as behaviour in an open field are correlated with susceptibility to arthritis. The discriminating factor was shown to be the intensity of bone destruction and not the inflammatory component of the arthritis. The difference in bone destruction was associated with a difference in RANKL expression and the capacity of the animal to form blood vessels in the synovium, also called the angiogenic capacity, which are the main causative factors in bone destruction.[25] Chover-Gonzalez et al.,[24] using the learned helplessness paradigm, also demonstrated that learned helpless rats develop more severe arthritis than the less helpless rats in this paradigm. The neuroendocrine differences associated with the differences in behaviour and disease outcome are not known yet. However, as already stated above, it is clear that the HPA axis is not the dominant system determining the outcome of the pro-inflammatory disease outcome; other systems, such as dopamine and other catecholamines, are also important in tuning the immune system and consequently the severity of disease.

8.4.2 Empirical evidence for a role for psychological factors in RA in humans

The first speculations about a possible relation between stress factors and the onset and course of RA date back to the end of the nineteenth century, and since then there have been many studies investigating this relationship. The main mediators of the stress response (glucocorticoids and catecholamines) are also potent immunomodulators (as summarized above). Therefore it is highly likely that exposure of individuals to acute or chronic stress with concomitant changes in the levels of glucocorticoids and catecholamines will have consequences for the onset and course of the disease. Nevertheless, it is not easy to delineate the exact role of exposure to stress in contributing to the onset and progression of RA. First, humans are exposed to a large variety of stress factors; some of these will be related to the disease, but most will be related to the level of environmental pressure to which the individual is exposed. In this respect it is important to distinguish major life events (e.g. loss of a spouse, severe illness of a relative) and what are often referred to as 'daily hassles', i.e. the daily events that can annoy or irritate a person. Secondly, it is very important to take into account the personality and coping style of the individuals studied. The same stressor can be a major problem for one individual, but only minimally affect another person. Thirdly, it has been shown in numerous studies of patients and healthy individuals that there are a number of factors in the environment of individuals that contribute to the ultimate effect of a particular stressor, with social support as a central modulator of the impact of stress on the individual. Therefore we have to take into account the number and type of stressors to which the individual is exposed, the characteristics of the individual (e.g. personality), and the characteristics of the individual's environment (e.g. social support).

8.4.3 Does stress accelerate or induce the onset of RA?

This is a very difficult question to address, especially since the only reliable way to investigate the effects of stress on onset of a disease is in a prospective study. To date no such studies have been performed to investigate the hypothesis that the onset of RA is preceded by a major life event. Therefore we have to rely on retrospective studies that are mostly based on questionnaires asking about life events prior to the onset of arthritis. In those studies, the incidence of life events in RA patients prior to onset of arthritis is compared with the incidence of such events in age- and sex-matched healthy individuals or in a group with another type of disease. A number of such studies have been performed and the results are mixed (reviewed by Herrmann *et al.*[58]). Some studies clearly support the idea that a major life event is experienced preceding the onset of RA. For example, it has been reported in a retrospective study that stress levels at the onset of disease were significantly higher in RA patients than in patients with osteoarthritis, a non-inflammatory joint disease.[59] However, there are just as many studies that did not find evidence for a role of stress in the onset of RA. For example, a case–control study of 55 patients with RA revealed no evidence for a role of exposure to stressful life events or the impact of stressful life events in the development of RA.[60]

8.4.4 Can stress modulate the course of RA?

To answer this question, we must take into account the effects of major life events and daily hassles on the course of the disease. However, it is also important to realize that the disease itself will act as a stressor not only because pain and disability are major stressors, but also because cytokines that are produced during the inflammatory process can activate the HPA axis. In addition, it has been shown, at least in animal models, that increased levels of cytokines can lead to behavioural changes that are characterized as 'sickness behaviour'.[61] This behavioural model includes reduced social exploration, reduced food intake, altered sleep patterns, and reduced sexual activity. More recently, it has been shown in humans that chronic increases in cytokine levels can also have behavioural consequences. For example, treatment of melanoma patients with the cytokine IFN-α has been shown to induce changes in mood, fatigue, and changes in cognitive function.[62,63] Therefore it is not surprising that behavioural changes occur in patients with RA in response to changes in disease activity. The most common psychological problem in RA patients is a depressed mood.[1] Sleep disturbances and fatigue are also often reported. These psychological disturbances are mostly viewed as consequences of the disease. The occurrence of depression in patients with chronic inflammatory diseases has been attributed to the effects of cytokines on the central nervous system as part of the sickness behaviour associated with an inflammatory process. However, we cannot exclude the possibility that these psychological disturbances also contribute to the pathological process, and could turn it into a vicious circle. Moreover, it may well be possible that patients who are more prone to developing depression during the disease also have a less favourable course of the disease.[64,65] It has been suggested that depression may influence pain. The feeling of helplessness that is associated with depression is thought to increase pain. In addition, increased negative mood in response to stress has been shown to increase pain sensitivity.[65,66]

Nevertheless, a large number of prospective studies have shown that there is a relationship between daily life stress (or daily hassles) and the severity of symptoms (inflammatory symptoms or pain). For example, long-term daily stress (including negative spouse behaviour, depression at beginning of the study) have been associated with adverse disease outcome and more pain.[67] In a longitudinal study, Feigenbaum et al.[68] showed that high daily stress levels at the beginning of a 5-year follow-up period were associated with poorer outcome and more joint damage at the end of the study. Overall, we can conclude that most studies support the hypothesis that a high level of daily hassles (or minor daily stress) is associated with poorer outcome, more pain, and more inflammation. Only a few studies have failed to confirm this notion; for example, Dekkers et al.[69] reported no correlation between life events and disease activity in a group of 54 patients with recently diagnosed RA. Finally, there is also evidence that reduction of daily stress can have a favourable effect on the course of arthritis; patients who report more social support also tend to have a milder course of the disease.[64,67,70]

Interestingly, the factors that are recognized as important for the course of RA (daily hassles as a negative factor and social support as a positive factor) have also been described as important factors contributing to other rheumatic diseases (e.g. SLE and JIA)[58,71]

8.5 Future directions

8.5.1 Translation of animal studies to human research

One of the interesting issues is whether our findings on behaviour and disease in animal models can be translated to the human situation. As shown above, there is not an overwhelming amount of data proving that behaviour and stress are indeed involved in severity and onset of disease. However, the concept that the mind can affect vulnerability to disease and the course of illness and disease has been proposed since the earliest days of medicine, although the evidence supporting these ideas are still controversial.

In animal studies, much attention has focused on stable behavioural characteristics, implying that stable characteristics, including the associated neuroendocrine characteristics, can really 'tune' the immune system and other physiological systems in the body. However, human research showing clear associations between stable behavioural traits and disease are relatively scarce and are not convincing. In arthritis, most studies have focused on the role of personality traits in the patients' perceptions of their symptoms. Some studies show that personality traits are related to self-reported pain and well-being.[72] These data are interesting in the light of perception of pain and behaviour, but cannot be regarded as an exact readout of disease severity. The perception of pain will probably not only include inflammation and joint destruction, but will also (perhaps for the greater part) be associated with the degree of sensitization of central and peripheral neuronal circuits.However, a relation between personality traits and neuroendocrine patterns and joint inflammation and/or destruction is still completely lacking in human studies. In view of the 'seeming controversy or scientific gap' between animal and human studies in this respect, one might ask whether a non-optimal methodology has been used to study this problem in humans. However, a more likely explanation could be that humans have evolved so differently that this 'primary' behaviour, as observed in animals, might be modulated or even overruled by the development of human cognition. If so, perhaps behavioural studies in very young children would be an interesting approach to studying the relation between stable behavioural traits, immune system, neuroendocrine system and disease. In neurodevelopmental research, validated tests have been described in young children, which have a parallel test in laboratory animals like operant discrimination learning, visual habituation, and visual recognition memory.

8.5.2 Contribution of PNI to therapy to arthritis

8.5.2.1 Glucocorticoids

As mentioned before, glucocorticoids are widely used as immunosuppressants in the treatment of RA. Most pharmacological dosages used are well above the plasma cortisol levels that would normally result in physiological effects of glucocorticoids and therefore are not related to the PNI issues discussed here.

8.5.2.2 Neuroendocrine regulation of tolerance induction

It has been suggested that, as an alternative to systemic immunosuppresssion, induction of tolerance for auto-antigens could serve as a specific immunoregulatory therapy for arthritis. The idea is that oral feeding of antigens that resemble or are identical to auto-antigens involved in arthritis could educate the immune system so that it learns not to respond to these antigens any more. The gut immune system has the capacity to learn not to respond to non-harmful food antigens so that the immune system does not mount an immune response towards every novel antigen encountered via food. Indeed, animal studies have shown that feeding heat shock protein prior to the induction of autoimmune arthritis can prevent the development of arthritis later on.[73] However, it has also been shown that it is much more difficult to treat ongoing autoimmune disease in animal models, and for such a therapeutic approach to be clinically useful it is necessary that it can be used in patients who already have the disease. Consequently, we have investigated the possibility of using immunomodulatory mediators of the neuroendocrine system to enhance induction of tolerance for auto-antigen so that the immune system no longer responds to these auto-antigens during arthritis. We explored the use of the β_2-adrenergic agonist salbutamol for this purpose. Adjuvant arthritis was induced in Lewis rats and after appearance of the first clinical signs animals were treated every other day by orally administering heat shock protein combined with the β_2-adrenergic agonist salbutamol. We showed that co-administration of heat shock protein and salbutamol significantly reduced the symptoms of arthritis, whereas either salbutamol alone or HSP alone had no or only marginal effects on disease severity.[74]

Although this is only a first step, it may be worthwhile to further explore the possibility of using neuroendocrine mediators to enhance immunomodulatory therapies (especially in the gut) in autoimmune diseases like RA.

8.5.2.3 Psychological intervention

In view of the data indicating a role of daily life stress and psychological factors in the course of arthritis, it is likely that psychotherapeutic treatment could increase the quality of life of RA patients. In addition, one could imagine that psychotherapy may enhance the efficacy of pharmacological treatment of RA. Relaxation techniques, cognitive behavioural therapy aimed at increasing coping skills, and stress management training have all been reported to decrease pain and to increase mood, well-being and physical activity of the patients [58].Thus, there is some evidence that psychological interventions can ameliorate the clinical course of RA and we propose that a combination of conventional therapy and psychological intervention may lead to synergy.

In animal experiments it has been demonstrated beyond doubt that stable behavioural traits are associated with the severity of and the susceptibility to arthritis. In view of the evolutionary aspects, one has to assume that these mechanisms must operate in humans as well. With respect to the design of new experiments that will better define the relation between mind and body, researchers in the field of PNI will have to focus their future studies more on 'primary' behavioural parameters, as have been used in animal studies, than on the more complex classical psychological approaches of self reports and questionnaires.

References

1 Hawley DJ, Wolfe F (1988). Anxiety and depression in patients with rheumatoid arthritis: a prospective study of 400 patients. *J Rheumatol* **15**, 932–41.

2 Firestein GS (2003). Evolving concepts of rheumatoid arthritis. *Nature* **423**, 356–61.

3 Masi AT, Feigenbaum SL, Chatterton RT (1995). Hormonal and pregnancy relationships to rheumatoid arthritis. Convergent effects with immunologic and microvascular systems. *Semin Arthritis Rheum* **25**, 1–27.

4 Masi AT (1994). Incidence of rheumatoid arthritis: do the observed age-sex interaction patterns support a role of androgenic-anabolic steroid deficiency in its pathogenesis? *Br J Rheumatol* **33**, 697–9.

5 Klinman D (2003). Does activation of the innate immune system contribute to the development of rheumatoid arthritis? *Arthritis Rheum* **48**, 590–3.

6 Cope AP (2003). Exploring the reciprocal relationship between immunity and inflammation in chronic inflammatory arthritis. *Rheumatology* **42**, 716–31.

7 Feldmann M, Brennan FM, Maini RN (1996). Rheumatoid arthritis. *Cell* **85**, 307–10.

8 Pincus T, Callahan LF (1993). The 'side effects' of rheumatoid arthritis: joint destruction, disability and early mortality. *Br J Rheumatol* **32** (Suppl 1), 28–37.

9 Moore KW, de Waal MR, Coffman RL, and O'Garra A (2001). Interleukin-10 and the interleukin-10 receptor. *Annu Rev Immunol* **19**, 683–765.

10 Kong YY, Feige U, Sarosi I, *et al.* (1999). Activated T cells regulate bone loss and joint destruction in adjuvant arthritis through osteoprotegerin ligand. *Nature* **402**, 304–9.

11 Harada MK, Mitsuyama H, Yoshida S, *et al.* (1998). Vascular endothelial growth factor in patients with rheumatoid arthritis. *Scand J Rheumatol* **27**, 377–80.

12 Vacchio MS, Ashwell JD (1997). Thymus-derived glucocorticoids regulate antigen-specific positive selection. *J Exp Med* **185**, 2033–8.

13 King LB, Vacchio MS, Dixon K, *et al.* (1995). A targeted glucocorticoid receptor antisense transgene increases thymocyte apoptosis and alters thymocyte development. *Immunity* **3**, 647–56.

14 Ashwell JD, King LB, Vacchio MS (1996). Cross-talk between the T cell antigen receptor and the glucocorticoid receptor regulates thymocyte development. *Stem Cells* **14**, 490–500.

15 Eggert M, Schulz M, Neeck G (2001). Molecular mechanisms of glucocorticoid action in rheumatic autoimmune diseases. *J Steroid Biochem Mol Biol* **77**, 185–91.

16 McKay LI and Cidlowsky JA (2000). Molecular control of immune/inflammatory responses: interactions between nuclear factor-kappa B and steroid receptor-signaling pathways. *Endocr Rev* **20**, 435–59.

17 Bakker JM, Kavelaars A, Kamphuis PJ, *et al.* (2001). Neonatal dexamethasone treatment induces long-lasting changes in T-cell receptor vbeta repertoire in rats. *J Neuroimmunol* **112**, 47–54.

18 Sternberg EM, Hill JM, Chrousos GP, *et al.* (1989). Inflammatory mediator-induced hypothalamic–pituitary–adrenal axis activation is defective in streptococcal cell wall arthritis-susceptible Lewis rat. *Proc Natl Acad Sci USA* **86**, 2374–8.

19 Sternberg EM, Young WS, Bernardini R, *et al.* (1989). A central nervous system defect in biosynthesis of corticotropin releasing hormone is associated with susceptibility to streptococcal cell wall-induced arthritis in Lewis rats. *Proc Natl Acad Sci USA* **86**, 4771–5.

20 Sheridan JF, Stark JL, Avitsur R, Padgett DA (2000). Social disruption, immunity, and susceptibility to viral infection. Role of glucocorticoid insensitivity and NGF. *Ann NY Acad Sci* **917**, 894–905.

21 MacPhee IA, Antoni FA, Mason DW (1989). Spontaneous recovery of rats from experimental allergic encephalomyelitis is dependent on regulation of the immune system by endogenous adrenal corticosteroids. *J Exp Med* **169**, 431–45.

22 Dhabhar FS (2002). Stress-induced augmentation of immune function–the role of stress hormones, leukocyte trafficking, and cytokines. *Brain Behav Immun* **16**, 785–98.

23 Andersson IM, Lorentzen JC, Ericsson-Dahlstrand A (2000). Analysis of adrenocortical secretory responses during acute an prolonged immune stimulation in inflammation-susceptible and -resistant rat strains. *J Neuroendocrinol* **12**, 1096–1104.

24 Chover-Gonzalez AJ, Jessop DS, Tejedor-Real P, Gibert-Rahola J, Harbuz MS (2000). Onset and severity of inflammation in rats exposed to the learned helplessness paradigm. *Rheumatology* **39**, 764–71.

25 Sajti E, van Meeteren N, Kavelaars A, van der Net J, Gispen WH, Heijnen CJ (2004). Individual differences in behavior of inbred Lewis rats are associated with severity of joint destruction in adjuvant-induced arthritis. *Brain Behav Immun* **18**: 505–14.

26 Harbuz MS, Jessop DS (1999). Is there a defect in cortisol production in rheumatoid arthritis? *Rheumatology* **38**, 298–302.

27 Straub RH, Cutolo M (2001). Involvement of the hypothalamic–pituitary–adrenal/gonadal axis and the peripheral nervous system in rheumatoid arthritis: viewpoint based on a systemic pathogenetic role. *Arthritis Rheum* **44**, 493–507.

28 Chikanza IC, Petrou P, Kingsley G, Chrousos G, and Panayi GS (1992). Defective hypothalamic response to immune and inflammatory stimuli in patients with rheumatoid arthritis. *Arthritis Rheum* **35**, 1281–8.

29 Crofford LJ, Kalogeras KT, Mastorakos G, *et al.* (1997). Circadian relationships between interleukin (IL)-6 and hypothalamic–pituitary–adrenal axis hormones: failure of IL-6 to cause sustained hypercortisolism in patients with early untreated rheumatoid arthritis. *J Clin Endocrinol Metab* **82**, 1279–83.

30 Harbuz MS, Korendowych E, Jessop DS, Crown AL, Lipdfan SL, Kirwan JR (2003). Hypothalamo–pituitary–adrenal axis dysregulation in patients with rheumatoid arthritis after the dexamethasone/corticotrophin releasing factor test. *J Endocrinol* **178**, 55–60.

31 von Bardeleben U, Holsboer F (1991). Effect of age on the cortisol response to human corticotropin-releasing hormone in depressed patients pretreated with dexamethasone. *Biol Psychiatry* **29**, 1042–1050.

32 Kanik KS, Wilder RL (2000). Hormonal alterations in rheumatoid arthritis, including the effects of pregnancy. *Rheum Dis Clin North Am* **26**, 805–23.

33 Allen JB, Blatter D, Calandra GB, Wilder RL (1983). Sex hormonal effects on the severity of streptococcal cell wall-induced polyarthritis in the rat. *Arthritis Rheum* **26**, 560–3.

34 Roubinian JR, Talal N, Greenspan JS, Goodman JR, Siiteri PK (1978). Effect of castration and sex hormone treatment on survival, anti-nucleic acid antibodies and glomerulonephritis in NZB/NZW F1 mice. *J Exp Med* **147**, 1568–83.

35 Cutolo M, Wilder RL (2000). Different roles for androgens and estrogens in the susceptibility to autoimmune rheumatic diseases. *Rheum Dis Clin North Am* **26**, 825–39.

36 Tanriverdi F, Silveira LF, MacColl GS, Bouloux PM (2003). The hypothalamic–pituitary–gonadal axis: immune function and autoimmunity. *J Endocrinol* **176**, 293–304.

37 Levine JD, Dardick SJ, Roizen MF, Helms C, Basbaum AI (1986). Contribution of sensory afferents and sympathetic efferents to joint injury in experimental arthritis. *J Neurosci* **6**, 3423–3429.

38 Lorton D, Lubahn C, Klein N, Schaller J, Bellinger DL (1999). Dual role for noradrenergic innervation of lymphoid tissue and arthritic joints in adjuvant-induced arthritis. *Brain Behav Immun* **13**, 15–334.

39 Kavelaars A (2002). Regulated expression of alpha-1 adrenergic receptors in the immune system. *Brain Behav Immun*, in press.

40 Platzer C, Fritsch E, Elsner T, Lehmann MH, Volk HD, Prosch S (1999). Cyclic adenosine monophosphate-responsive elements are involved in the transcriptional activation of the human IL-10 gene in monocytic cells. *Eur J Immunol* **29**, 3098–104.

41 Panina-Bordignon P, Mazzeo D, Di Lucia P, D'Ambrosio D, Lang R, Fabbri L (1997). β2-agonists prevent Th1 development by selective inhibition of interleukin-12. *J Clin Invest* **100**, 1513–19.

42 Swanson MA, Lee WT, Sanders VM (2001). IFN-gamma production by Th1 cells generated from naive CD4+ T cells exposed to norepinephrine. *J Immunol* **166**, 232–40.

43 Kuis W, de Jong-de Vos van Steenwijk CC, Sinnema G *et al.* (1996). The autonomic nervous system and the immune system in juvenile chronic rheumatoid arthritis: an interdisciplinary study. *Brain Behav Immun* **10**, 387–98.

44 Geenen R, Godaert GL, Jacobs JW, Peters ML, Bijlsma JW (1996). Diminished autonomic nervous system responsiveness in rheumatoid arthritis of recent onset. *J Rheumatol* **23**, 258–64.

45 Miller LE, Justen HP, Scholmerich J, Straub RH (2000). The loss of sympathetic nerve fibers in the synovial tissue of patients with rheumatoid arthritis is accompanied by increased norepinephrine release from synovial macrophages. *FASEB J* **14**, 2097–107.

46 Malfait AM, Malik AS, Marinova-Mutafchieva L, Butler DM, Maini RN, Feldmann M (1999). The beta2-adrenergic agonist salbutamol is a potent suppressor of established collagen-induced arthritis: mechanisms of action. *J Immunol* **162**, 6278–83.

47 Stein A, Yassouridis A, Szopko C, Helmke K, Stein C (1999). Intraarticular morphine versus dexamethasone in chronic arthritis. *Pain* **83**, 525–32.

48 Hood VC, Cruwys SC, Urban L, Kidd BL (2001). The neurogenic contribution to synovial leucocyte infiltration and other outcome measures in a guinea pig model of arthritis. *Neurosci Lett* **299**, 201–4.

49 Deal CL, Schnitzer TJ, Lipstein E, *et al.* (1991). Treatment of arthritis with topical capsaicin: a double-blind trial. *Clin Ther* **13**, 383–95.

50 Spengler RN, Allen RM, Remick RM, Strieter RM, Kunkel SL (1990). Stimulation of α-adrenergic receptor augments the productionof macrophage-derived tumor necrosis factor. *J Immunol* **145**, 1430–4.

51 Rouppe van der Voort C, Heijnen CJ, Wulffraat N, Kuis W, Kavelaars A (2000). Stress-induced increase in IL-6 production by leukocytes of patients with the chronic inflammatory disease juvenile rheumatoid arthritis, a putative role for α1-adrenergic receptors. *J Neuroimmunol* **110**, 223–9.

52 Heijnen CJ, Rouppe van der Voort C, Wulffraat N, van der Net J, Kuis W, Kavelaars A (1996). Functional α1-adrenergic receptors on leukocytes of patients with polyarticular juvenile rheumatoid arthritis. *J Neuroimmunol* **71**, 223–6.

53 Lombardi MS, Kavelaars A, Schedlowski M, *et al.* (1999). Decreased expression and activity of G protein-coupled receptor kinases by peripheral blood mononuclear cells of patients with rheumatoid arthritis. *FASEB J* **13**, 715–25.

54 Baerwald C, Grafee C, Von Wichert P, Krause A (1992). Decreased density of β-adrenergic receptors on peripheral blood mononuclear cells in patients with rheumatoid arthritis. *J Rheumatol* **19**, 204–10.

55 Pitcher JA, Freedman NJ, Lefkowitz RJ (1998). G protein-coupled receptor kinases. *Annu Rev Biochem* **67**, 653–692.

56 Lombardi MS, Kavelaars A, Heijnen CJ (2002). Role and modulation of G protein-coupled receptor signalling in inflammatory processes. *Crit Rev Immunol* **22**, 141–63.

57 Kavelaars A, Heijnen CJ, Ellenbroek B, van Loveren H, Cools AR (1997). Apomorphine-susceptible and apo-morphine-unsusceptible Wistar rats differ in their susceptibility for inflammatory and infectious diseases: a study on rats with groupific differences in structure reactivity of hypothalamic–pituitary–adrenal axis. *J Neurosci* **17**, 2580–4.

58 Herrmann M, Scholmerich J, Straub RH (2000). Stress and rheumatic diseases. *Rheum Dis Clin North Am* **26**, 737–63, viii.

59 Latman NS, Walls R (1996). Personality and stress: an exploratory comparison of rheumatoid arthritis and osteoarthritis. *Arch Phys Med Rehabil* **77**, 796–800.

60 Carette S, Surtees PG, Wainwright NW, Khaw KT, Symmons DP, Silman AJ (2000). The role of life events and childhood experiences in the development of rheumatoid arthritis. *J Rheumatol* **27**, 2123–30.

61 Kelley KW, Bluthe RM, Dantzer R, *et al.* (2003). Cytokine-induced sickness behavior. *Brain Behav Immun* **17** (Suppl 1), S112–18.

62 Capuron L, Ravaud A, Dantzer R (2000). Early depressive symptoms in cancer patients receiving interleukin 2 and/or interferon alfa-2b therapy. *J Clin Oncol* **18**, 2143–51.

63 Capuron L, Ravaud A, Dantzer R (2001). Timing and specificity of the cognitive changes induced by interleukin-2 and interferon-alpha treatments in cancer patients. *Psychosom Med* **63**, 376–86.

64 Evers AW, Kraaimaat FW, Geenen R, Jacobs JW, Bijlsma JW (2002). Longterm predictors of anxiety and depressed mood in early rheumatoid arthritis: a 3 and 5 year followup. *J Rheumatol* **29**, 2327–36.

65 Zautra AJ, Smith BW (2001). Depression and reactivity to stress in older women with rheumatoid arthritis and osteoarthritis. *Psychosom Med* **63**, 687–96.

66 Smith TW, Peck JR, Ward JR (1990). Helplessness and depression in rheumatoid arthritis. *Health Psychol* **9**, 377–89.

67 Waltz M, Kriegel W van't Pad BP (1998). The social environment and health in rheumatoid arthritis: marital quality predicts individual variability in pain severity. *Arthritis Care Res* **11**, 356–74.

68 Feigenbaum SL, Masi AT, Kaplan SB (1979). Prognosis in rheumatoid arthritis. A longitudinal study of newly diagnosed younger adult patients. *Am J Med*, **66**, 377–84.

69 Dekkers JC, Geenen R, Evers AW, Kraaimaat FW, Bijlsma JW, Godaert GL (2001). Biopsychosocial mediators and moderators of stress–health relationships in patients with recently diagnosed rheumatoid arthritis. *Arthritis Rheum* **45**, 307–16.

70 Ward MM, Leigh JP (1993). Marital status and the progression of functional disability in patients with rheumatoid arthritis. *Arthritis Rheum* **36**, 581–8.

71 Pawlak CR, Witte T, Heiken H, *et al.* (2003). Flares in patients with systemic lupus erythematosus are associated with daily psychological stress. *Psychother Psychosom* **72**, 159–65.

72 Persson LO and Sahlberg D (2002). The influence of negative illness cognitions and neuroticism on subjective symptoms and mood in rheumatoid arthritis. *Ann Rheum Dis* **61**, 1000–6.

73 Yoshino S (1995). Antigen-induced arthritis in rats is suppressed by the inducing antigen administered orally before, but not after immunization. *Cell Immunol* **163**, 55–8.

74 Cobelens P, Kavelaars A, Vroon A, *et al.* (2002). The beta2-adrenergic agonist salbutamol potentiates oral induction of tolerance suppressing adjuvant arthritis and antigen-specific immunity. *J Immunol* **169**, 5028–35.

Chapter 9

Infectious disease and psychoneuroimmunology

Gregory E. Miller and Sheldon Cohen

9.1 Introduction

Infectious disease is the leading cause of mortality in the world today. Of the more than 50 million humans who die each year, almost 17 million (34%) do so because of an infectious disease.[1] The bulk of these deaths occur in developing countries where insanitary living conditions are widespread, and there is limited access to proper nutrition, vaccination programmes, and effective antibiotics. However, infectious diseases continue to exert a major toll in countries where these safeguards are in place. In the United States, respiratory infections such as pneumonia and influenza are the seventh leading cause of death, and are responsible for more than 50 million missed days of work each year at a cost of more than a billion dollars in lost productivity.[2,3]

Interest in the hypothesis that stressful experiences contribute to morbidity and mortality in the domain of infectious disease has grown steadily in recent decades. In this chapter we provide a selective overview of research in this area. We begin with studies linking stressful experience to acute infection. These are cases in which the immune system eradicates invading pathogens (sometimes with the help of antibiotics) and returns the host to good health after a period of illness. Later in the chapter we turn our attention to the role of stress in chronic and latent infections. These are instances where the immune system does not completely eradicate a pathogen from the body, but instead reaches an equilibrium with it that allows the microbe to linger for months, years, or even a lifetime, intermittently triggering bouts of illness.

9.2 The biological/clinical context

Most infectious diseases arise when a disease-causing organism, or pathogen, gains access to the body via the skin or the respiratory, gastrointestinal, or genitourinary tracts.[4] The most common disease-causing organisms are viruses and bacteria; however, prions, fungi, protozoa, mycoplasma, and a host of other pathogens can be involved. Once a pathogen gains access to the body, it attaches to host tissue and begins reproducing. A person is considered infected when the pathogen is successfully multiplying within the body. Established infections have the potential to inflict various kinds of damage to the organism. Viruses enter host cells and co-opt their genetic machinery, disrupting the cell's ability to carry out normal functions. Bacteria secrete toxins that kill host cells, and degrade tissue by depriving it of nutrients.[5]

Pathogen replication triggers the immune system to mount a defensive response. White blood cells gather at the site of infection and attempt to eliminate the pathogen, rid the body of cells that have been invaded by it, and repair any tissue damage that has arisen in the process. The early phase of the immune response involves cells known as neutrophils and macrophages, which combat the infection by releasing bactericidal substances and engulfing pathogens, respectively. Later in the process other classes of white blood cells become involved. Cytotoxic T lymphocytes prevent further infection by killing host cells that have been colonized by the pathogen; B lymphocytes secrete antibodies to neutralize the pathogen and mark it for destruction. The entire process is directed by molecules called inflammatory cytokines, which are soluble molecules synthesized and released by white blood cells. They direct white blood cells towards sites of infection, induce them to proliferate and differentiate, and activate mechanisms involved in pathogen destruction. The most critical inflammatory cytokines are IL-1β, IL-6, and tumour necrosis factor-α (TNF-α).[4,6,7]

While the goal of the immune response is to eliminate invading pathogens from the body, the process of doing so often results in the host experiencing a constellation of symptoms that define clinical illness. To a large extent the symptom profile depends on the invading pathogen and the tissue it has colonized. Respiratory viruses associated with the common cold tend to elicit congestion, a sore throat, a runny nose, and coughing; bacterial infections of the central nervous system can produce vomiting, headache, stiffness, and even seizures. Apart from these disease-specific indicators, infections generally elicit non-specific symptoms including fever, malaise, sleepiness, anorexia, anhedonia, and withdrawal from activities. This non-specific cluster of symptoms has recently been defined as 'sickness behaviour'. It occurs when inflammatory cytokines, generated as part of the immune response, act on tissues of the central nervous system. While it is not clear how these molecules enter the central nervous system, or what structures they affect once there, research suggests that cytokines are a primary trigger of most non-specific symptoms of infectious disease. (They also elicit many symptoms of common respiratory infections, such as mucus production, runny nose, and nasal congestion.)

Researchers believe that sickness behaviour represents an evolved strategy designed to maximize the chances of survival after infection.[8-10] When an organism has been infected with a pathogen, its chances of survival depend on its capacity to mount a vigorous defence, and avoid contact with pathogens and predators that might capitalize on its vulnerability. To mount a vigorous defence against infection, organisms must initiate a febrile response, which retards the reproductive capacity of pathogens, and mobilize their immune systems to fight. However, mounting these defensive responses poses significant metabolic demands. For example, to raise its core body temperature by 1°C, an organism needs to increase its metabolism by 12%.[5] By spending more time sleeping and withdrawing from activities, the organism conserves energy for this metabolically demanding process,[8] and avoids contact with pathogens and predators that might capitalize on its vulnerability. When understood from this perspective, non-specific illness symptoms represent an adaptive response to infection, rather than a pathological consequence of microbial invasion.[11]

As stated, there are conditions under which the immune system eradicates the invading pathogen, as occurs with acute infectious agents, and conditions under which the invading pathogens and the immune system reach a state of equilibrium that can last for years, decades, or even a lifetime,[4] as is the case with chronic infectious diseases. With regard to chronic diseases, the pathogen typically continues multiplying slowly within the body, intermittently triggering symptoms of clinical illness. There are a number of common infections that can run a chronic course in this way. In developed nations the most common are bacterial in origin (e.g. syphilis, chlamydia, tuberculosis, urinary tract infections); however, in parts of the world with limited access to sanitation, nutrition, and antibiotics, parasites are often the culprits (e.g. hookworm, malaria, giardia).[1]

A variant of chronic infection occurs when a viral pathogen reaches equilibrium with its host immune system after integrating its genetic material into host cells. In this case the virus establishes a latent infection, meaning that it ceases replication and thus does not elicit illness symptoms. This latent (or clinically silent) period can last for years, decades, or a lifetime. However, since the virus is part of the host genome, it can be reactivated (i.e. begin replication) at any time and trigger episodes of symptomatic clinical illness. There are a number of viruses that can latently infect people. They include human immunodeficiency virus (HIV), which causes AIDS, herpes simplex virus 1 (HSV-1), which causes cold sores, herpes simplex virus 2 (HSV-2), which causes genital lesions, Epstein–Barr virus (EBV), which causes infectious mononucleosis, and cytomegalovirus (CMV), which causes conjunctivitis and other conditions.

9.3 Theoretical basis for a role for psychoneuroimmunology

While the preceding descriptions provide an overview of the typical responses involved in acute and chronic infections, not all individuals develop clinical illness after exposure to a disease-causing organism. In fact, only a subset do, and the severity and duration of illness symptoms vary considerably among them.[4,6,12] As a result, much effort has been devoted to identifying factors that contribute to individual differences in susceptibility to clinical illness. One factor that has received increasing attention recently is stressful experience. But how could a nebulous feeling such as stress 'get inside the body' to influence the development and progression of infectious disease?

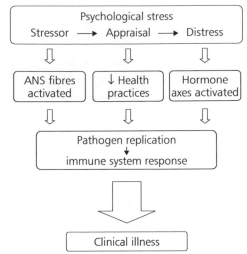

Fig. 9.1 Model depicting proposed relations between stress, mediating pathways, and infectious disease. ANS, autonomic nervous system.

The model shown in Figure 9.1 provides an answer to this question. It begins with the notion that people appraise potentially stressful circumstances along dimensions of threat and manageability.[13] To the extent that they are evaluated as posing a threat and exceeding coping resources, these stressors elicit a psychological stress response that consists of negative emotional and cognitive states (sadness, anxiety, helplessness, etc.). These states set into motion a series of biological and behavioural adaptations that ultimately heighten disease susceptibility. For example, distressed individuals may cope with their difficulties by using tobacco or alcohol, avoiding exercise routines, consuming junk food, or reducing their sleep. These behavioural alterations modify the functions of the immune system in a way that could interfere with its capacity to eliminate or contain invading pathogens.[12,14,15] Distressed individuals also show activation of the sympathetic division of the autonomic nervous system. Sympathetic fibres descend from the central nervous system into lymphoid organs (spleen, thymus, lymph nodes) where most battles between invading pathogens and the immune system are waged.[16] When activated by distress, these fibres release neurohormones such as norepinephrine that can directly facilitate the growth of pathogens[17–19] as well as bind to receptors on white blood cells and influence their function.[16,20] Distress can also activate the body's hormonal response systems (the hypothalamic–pituitary–adrenal axis, the sympathetic adrenal–medullary axis, and the hypothalamic–pituitary–ovarian axis) and trigger them to release hormonal products such as cortisol, epinephrine, substance P, oestradiol, testosterone, etc.[21] High levels of these hormones could increase disease susceptibility by directly facilitating pathogen replication or reactivation (as in the case of latent infections), or by altering the nature of the immune system's response to infection.[17–19] Although most research has assumed that stress hormones diminish the immune response and thereby enable pathogens to spread more easily,[12,22] recent evidence suggests that they may also upregulate the immune response so that it produces greater volumes of the inflammatory cytokines that mediate illness symptoms. This could occur because stressors 'prime' the immune system to respond more aggressively to challenge,[23,24] or because they diminish its sensitivity to hormonal signals such as cortisol that normally terminate inflammation.[25]

We shall now examine the evidence for the role of stressful experiences in modulating responses to acute and chronic infections.

9.4 The empirical evidence

9.4.1 Stressful experience and acute infection

To what extent has this model been borne out by empirical research? Research on stressful experience and acute infection dates back to the 1950s. Although a number of different conditions have been studied during this period, we will focus on upper respiratory illnesses such as colds and influenza, since they are the most common forms of acute infection and have been the most widely researched. The first wave of studies in this area found reliable associations between the presence of stressful experience and higher rates of self-reported respiratory infections.[12] However, the interpretation of these findings was complicated to some extent by evidence that distress can bias cognitive processes underlying symptom perception and labelling.[26–30] In other words, distress may have led subjects in these studies to exaggerate the severity of their illness, or misattribute symptoms of other conditions to infectious disease, rather than affecting the development or progression of respiratory infection.[12] More convincing evidence was obtained from later studies that provided biological verification of illness. Prospective investigations found that high levels of family stress, for instance, were associated with a greater incidence of verified upper respiratory infection.[31,32]

However, the most convincing evidence that stressful experience heightens vulnerability to infectious disease has come from studies that utilize the viral challenge paradigm.[12] In this paradigm volunteers are carefully assessed for stressful experiences and then exposed to a pathogen that causes upper respiratory infection. Since only a subset of the volunteers develop a clinical illness, researchers can examine whether stress levels before exposure predict who resists disease. This paradigm is unique in four ways. First, because stress levels are assessed before pathogen exposure, reverse causality is not a plausible explanation for stress-related differences in disease susceptibility. Secondly, because volunteers are exposed to a controlled dose of pathogen and then quarantined, the findings cannot be attributed to stress-related differences in exposure to infectious agents (e.g. stressed persons may seek out social support and, by doing so, expose themselves to pathogens.) Thirdly, because the challenge pathogen is chosen by the investigator, previous exposure to it can be measured through virus-specific antibody and controlled in statistical analyses. This procedure rules out the possibility that any stressor-related disparities in clinical illness are due to stressed persons having a differential exposure history (and thus a different immune response). Finally, closely monitoring volunteers throughout the course of the study allows the assessment of behavioural and biological pathways that might link stressful experience and disease susceptibility.

Viral challenge studies initially yielded mixed findings concerning stress and respiratory infection.[33–36] However, recent studies utilizing larger samples and more sophisticated methods have yielded robust evidence that stressors heighten disease susceptibility.[37–40] To illustrate these findings, we describe our own programme of research.

9.4.1.1 The British Common Cold Study

Research methods

Subjects and protocol Our initial study was carried out at the British Medical Research Council's Common Cold Unit between 1986 and 1989.[37] The subjects were 154 men and 266 women between the ages of 18 and 54 years who had volunteered for the study and were judged to be in good health following a physical examination.

The temporal sequence of the trial is summarized in Table 9.1. For 2 days before and 7 days after exposure to the virus, volunteers were quarantined in large apartments. During the first 2 days, they were given a thorough medical examination, had blood drawn to measure their previous exposure (through antibody) to the virus they were to

Table 9.1 Temporal sequence of a trial

During 2 days preceding exposure to virus
    Physical examination
    Blood for pre-existing immunity (antibody) to virus
    Psychological stress questionnaires
    Health practices questionnaire
    Demographics
    Baseline nasal secretions for virus cultures
    Baseline signs and symptoms of respiratory illness

Beginning of day 3
    Inoculation with virus

Days 1–6 after exposure
    Nasal secretions for virus culture
    Signs and symptoms of respiratory symptoms

4 weeks after virus challenge
    Blood for antibody to virus

be exposed to, and completed psychological stress and health practice questionnaires. Subsequently, they were exposed via nasal drops to a low infectious dose of one of five viruses that cause the common cold: rhinovirus types 2, 9, and 14, respiratory syncytial virus, and coronavirus type 229E. An additional 26 volunteers received saline.

Starting 2 days before viral exposure and continuing until 6 days after exposure, volunteers were examined daily by a clinician using a standard respiratory symptom protocol. Examples of items on the protocol include sneezing, watering of eyes, nasal stuffiness, sore throat, hoarseness, and cough. Objective signs of illness were also collected on daily basis. These included a count of the number of tissues used daily by the volunteer, the weight of their nasal secretions, and body temperature assessed twice each day. Samples of nasal secretions were also collected daily to assess whether volunteers were infected by the experimental virus. Approximately 28 days after challenge a second blood sample was collected to assess changes in viral-specific antibody. All investigators were blind to volunteers' psychological status and to whether they received virus or saline.

Psychological stress Recall that when demands outstrip an individual's ability to cope, a stress response consisting of negative emotional and cognitive states is triggered. To capture this process, we asked volunteers to complete questionnaires assessing the number of major stressful life events they judged as having a negative impact, the perception that current demands exceeded their ability to cope, and their current negative affect. The major stressful life events scale consisted of events that might happen in the life of the respondent or close others. The Perceived Stress Scale[41] was used to assess the degree to which situations in life were perceived as unpredictable, uncontrollable, and unmanageable. The negative affect scale assessed the extent to which subjects experienced a set of 15 negative emotions. We also created an index of psychological stress that was based on all three of the scales.

Infections and clinical illness Infection is the multiplication of an invading micro-organism. Clinical disease occurs when infection is followed by the development of symptomatology characteristic of the disease. We determined infection status directly by culturing nasal secretion samples for viral proteins or indirectly through establishing significant increases in viral-specific antibody from before until 4 weeks after exposure. Eighty-two per cent of the volunteers receiving virus were classified as infected using these criteria. Cold status was determined by having a clinician judge the severity of each volunteer's cold at the end of the trial. Clinical colds were defined as a positive diagnosis in the presence of verified infection. Thirty-eight per cent developed colds. None of the 26 saline controls developed colds.

Health practice measures We also examined whether health practices operated as a pathway through which stress contributed to disease. Health practice measures were assessed before viral exposure, and included smoking status, alcohol consumption, exercise frequency, subjective sleep quality, and diet.

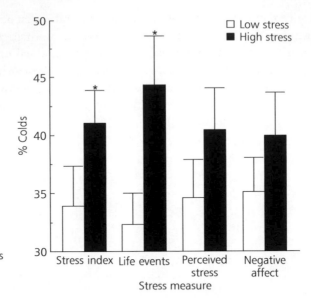

Fig. 9.2 Stress increases susceptibility to upper respiratory infection.

Major findings All our statistical analyses controlled for (included as covariates) a set of variables that could provide alternative explanations for a relation between stress and illness. These variables include age, gender, education, weight, allergic status, season of the year when the trial was conducted, the number of others with whom the subject was housed during the trial, whether housemates were infected or not, type of virus the subject was infected with, and whether the volunteer had previous exposure to the virus.

Figure 9.2 depicts the study's major finding: subjects with more stress had higher rates of clinical illness, irrespective of whether stress was measured as life events, perceived stress, negative affect, or the stress index. Moreover, the association between stress and colds was consistent across the five viruses. These findings suggest that the relation between stress and upper respiratory illness is not dependent on the pathogenesis of any specific virus and probably results from a more generalized dysregulation of the immune response.

To determine whether these effects might be attributable to relations between stress and health practices, we ran an additional set of analyses including smoking rate, drinking rate, diet, exercise, and sleep quality in the equations (as additional covariates). This procedure tests whether stress is associated with greater susceptibility after the possible effects of these variables are subtracted. The addition of health practices did not significantly alter the results, suggesting that these behaviours were not operating as mediational pathways.

9.4.1.2 The Pittsburgh Common Cold Study

Although The British Common Cold Study yielded compelling evidence for a relationship between stress and susceptibility to upper respiratory infection, it provided little information about the nature of stressors that heighten risk for illness. The objective of our second study was to gather more information about this issue. We were interested in answering questions such as the following. Do acutely stressful events have the same impact on susceptibility as more chronic, ongoing stressors? Do certain classes of stressors have a more potent impact than others? Does illness risk vary with the duration of a stressor? We also were interested in studying a broader array of behavioural and biological mediators to discern the mechanisms through which stress might 'get inside the body'.

Research methods

Subjects and protocol This study was carried out in Pittsburgh, PA, between 1993 and 1996.[38] The design was similar to the British Cold Study in that stress and mediators were assessed before volunteers were exposed to a cold virus. As before, following viral exposure, volunteers were monitored in quarantine for the development of a clinical illness. However, there were some important changes including the following: (a) the use of a stressful life events interview that provided detailed information on the durations and types of stressful events that were reported; (b) the addition of tests for endocrine and immune pathways that might link stress to disease susceptibility; (c) objective signs of illness were used instead of physician judgements for a diagnosis of a clinical illness.

Briefly, 276 adults (125 men and 151 women) between the ages of 18 and 55 participated. All volunteers were judged to be in good health after eligibility screening. Stressors and selected health practices (smoking, alcohol consumption, exercise, sleep quality, diet) were also assessed at the screening. Eligible subjects returned to the hospital 4 and 5 weeks after screening to have blood drawn for assessment of a marker of immune function–natural killer (NK) cell activity. Volunteers returned once more after initial screening but before being exposed to the virus to complete a stressful life events interview.

Subjects were quarantined within a week following the second blood draw. Baseline assessment of self-reported respiratory symptoms and two objective indicators of illness (nasal mucociliary clearance and nasal mucus production) were assessed before viral exposure. Urine samples were collected for the assessment of three hormones thought to play a role in stress-induced immune changes: cortisol, epinephrine, and norepinephrine. At the end of the first 24 h of quarantine, volunteers were given nasal drops containing a low infectious dose of one of two types of rhinovirus. Quarantine continued for 5 days after exposure. During this period volunteers were housed individually. Nasal secretion samples for verifying infection by virus culture were collected on each of the 5 days. On each day, volunteers also completed a respiratory symptoms questionnaire and were tested for the two objective markers of illness. Approximately 28 days after challenge, another blood sample was collected to verify infection. All investigators were blinded to the subjects' status on stress, endocrine, health practice, immunity, and pre-challenge antibody measures.

Stress measures A semistructured interview, the Bedford College Life Events and Difficulties Schedule (LEDS), was used to assess life events. LEDS uses strict criteria for whether or not an event occurs, classifies each event on the basis of severity of threat and emotional significance, and makes a distinction between acute events and ongoing chronic difficulties. Raters blind to the individual's subjective response to an event were provided with extensive information regarding each event and the context in which it occurred, and then relied on thorough 'dictionaries' containing previous ratings of hundreds of different events to rate current events. The ratings are based on the likely response of an average person to an event occurring in the context of a particular set of biographical circumstances. We focused on the traditional LEDS outcomes: the occurrence of severe events (<4 weeks duration) and chronic difficulties (>4 weeks duration).

Clinical illness Volunteers were considered to have a cold if they were both infected and met illness criteria. They were classified as infected if the challenge virus was isolated on any of the five post-challenge study days or there was a fourfold increase in serum antibody to the experimental virus. The illness criterion was based on selected objective indicators of illness response after viral exposure: the amount of mucus produced and mucociliary clearance function. Mucus weights were determined by collecting used tissues in sealed plastic bags. After correcting for the weight of the bag and the mucus weight at baseline, the post-challenge weights were summed across the 5 days to create an adjusted total mucus weight score. Nasal mucociliary clearance function refers to the effectiveness of nasal cilia in clearing mucus from the nasal passage toward the throat. Clearance function was assessed as the time required for a dye administered into the nose to reach the throat. Each daily time was adjusted for baseline and the adjusted average time (in minutes) was calculated across the post-challenge days of the trial. To meet illness criteria, subjects had to have a total adjusted mucus weight >10 g or an adjusted average mucociliary nasal clearance time <7 min. By basing the definition of illness entirely on objective indicators, we were able to exclude interpretations of our data based on psychological influences on symptom reporting.

Major findings We used odds ratios (relative risks) to estimate the relative risk of developing a cold. An odds ratio approximates the odds that the cold will occur in one group as compared with another. All odds ratios we report are adjusted for age, gender, ethnicity, education, body mass index, season during which the trial was conducted, type of experimental virus, and pre-challenge antibody.

Impact of acute events and chronic difficulties There were 179 subjects with at least one severe acute life event within 1 year of the study. However, acute events were not associated with developing a cold. There were 75 subjects with a chronic difficulty lasting for 1 month or longer. Those with difficulties were 2.2 times more likely to develop a cold than those without. Moreover, this relation was similar for the two virus

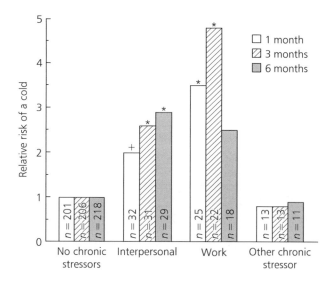

Fig. 9.3 Types of stressors that increase susceptability to upper respiratory infection.

types, for different pre-exposure antibody levels, age, gender, race, education, and body mass, and across the two seasons.

The chronic difficulties were categorized into three domains: interpersonal, work, and other. As is apparent from Figure 9.3, having either work or interpersonal chronic difficulties was associated with greater risk for colds compared with those with no difficulties and with other types of difficulties. We considered the possibility that difficulties at work were in fact interpersonal difficulties as well. To pursue this issue, we rated each of the 30 chronic difficulties for interpersonal content. Only two of the 30 were found to be interpersonal conflicts at work; the rest were attributable to unemployment or underemployment. These findings indicate that chronic interpersonal stressors such as conflicts with friends, family, or spouses, and work problems related to unemployment or underemployment place individuals at greater risk for upper respiratory infection. However, because many types of chronic stressors had a low base rate in our sample, these findings should not be taken to mean that interpersonal or work stressors are the only types of difficulties that heighten illness risk. Instead, our findings suggest that when these stressors occur, they can have potent influences on susceptibility.

Effects of stressor duration We also compared cold rates for persons having stressors of different durations. Subjects were assigned to a group based on their acute or chronic stressor of longest duration. As Figure 9.4 illustrates, there was a linear increase in the risk for illness with increasing duration of the stressor.

Role of health practices Preliminary analyses indicated that those with enduring difficulties were more likely to be smokers, engage in less physical activity, and have poorer sleep efficiency. All these health practices were also associated with susceptibility to

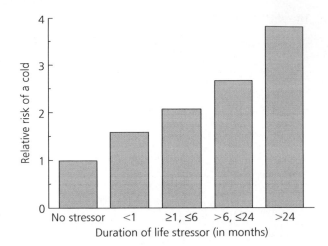

Fig. 9.4 Duration of chronic stressor and susceptibility to upper respiratory infection.

colds, with smokers, those taking less exercise, and those with poor sleep quality all at greater risk. However, these health practices could explain only a small fraction of the relation between chronic stress and susceptibility to infectious illness. Because the health practice measures were all related to susceptibility in the expected manner, we are confident that we assessed this pathway correctly. As a consequence, it seems unlikely that these health practices play a major role in linking stressors with resistance to infectious illness.

Role of endocrine and immune processes Higher levels of the stress hormones epinephrine and norepinephrine were related to a greater cold risk. However, much to our surprise, these hormones were not associated with the presence of acute events or enduring difficulties. Because epinephrine and norepinephrine were assessed during the 24 h before viral exposure, they might have been indicating a stress-type reaction to the beginning of quarantine rather than a basal level of response to volunteers' background environments. In our current work, we are attempting to obtain better background levels by measuring hormones several times during the weeks before volunteers report for quarantine.

Our measure of immune system function, NK cell cytotoxicity, was not associated with enduring difficulties or risk for clinical illness. We chose NK cell activity as our primary marker of immune function for two reasons. First, NK cells are surveillance cells that identify infected cells and kill them. In theory, higher levels of NK cell activity should help limit infection and hence prevent illness. Secondly, there is evidence that chronic stress is associated with a decline in NK activity.[42,43] So why did NK cells not operate as mediators in our study? Measuring immunity in peripheral blood is not always the most appropriate procedure and may be the problem here.[43] In theory, NK activity in the lung might be the essential issue in the case of respiratory infections. It is also possible that NK activity in the blood might make a difference, but that the ability of the immune system to compensate for deficits in single subsystems obscures any relationship.

9.4.1.3 The Pittsburgh Influenza Study

Until now, the major outcome of our work has been whether persons exposed to a virus develop clinical illness. Clinical illness has been defined as a combination of infection and symptoms. Our recent work has moved towards providing a more refined understanding of how stressors influence disease susceptibility. To do this, we need to distinguish between the role stress plays in susceptibility to infection, and the role it plays in expression of illness among infected persons. Our most recent study addressed this issue with a challenge model that allows examination of illness expression among infected persons. Volunteers were exposed to a virus that results in infection in 95% of people without previous exposure. We then examined the extent to which stress predicted illness expression among infected subjects. A major focus of this trial was to test the possibility that stress effects on the regulation of pro-inflammatory cytokines might account for why stress is associated with susceptibility to colds. Psychological stressors have been shown to be reliable activators of the production of pro-inflammatory cytokines such as IL-1β, IL-6, IFN-γ, and TNF-α.[42] Moreover, local increases in the concentrations of one of these cytokines, IL-6, have been linked to greater cold symptomatology among persons with verified upper respiratory infection.[44]

Research methods

Subjects and protocol This study was carried out in Pittsburgh, PA, in 1998.[39] Briefly, 55 adults between the ages of 18 and 55 years participated in the study. All participants were judged to be in good health after medical eligibility screening. Eligible volunteers were quarantined for a total of 8 days. During the first 24 h of quarantine, they had a physical examination, a nasal wash culture for the challenge virus, and provided stressor ratings and baseline symptoms. Nasal secretions were collected and weighed to assess symptoms objectively, and a nasal wash was performed to assess levels of IL-6 in local tissue. At the end of the first 24 h of quarantine, subjects were given nasal drops containing an infectious dose of influenza A/Kawasaki/86 H1N1. Each day for the rest of quarantine, subjects rated the severity of their respiratory symptoms, nasal mucus was collected and weighed to measure symptoms objectively, and nasal washes were performed to verify infection and monitor cytokine levels in local tissue. Approximately 28 days after challenge, a blood sample was collected for serological testing of antibody response to the challenge virus.

Psychological stress The Perceived Stress Scale[41] was used to assess the degree to which life situations were perceived as unpredictable, uncontrollable, and overloading.

Infection status All volunteers included in the statistical analyses were infected with the challenge virus. Infection was verified by isolation of viral particles on any of the seven post-challenge days or through a fourfold increase in virus-specific antibody at the end of the trial.

Cytokine assessment Levels of IL-6 in nasal lavage samples were assessed via enzyme-linked immunosorbent assay (ELISA).

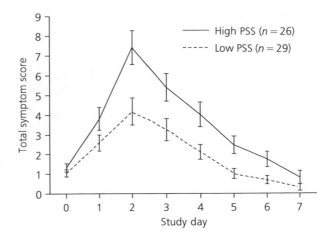

Fig. 9.5 Perceived stress and severity of illness over course of study. PSS, psychological stress score.

Major findings The relation between psychological stress and self-reported symptoms of upper respiratory illness (adjusting for standard controls) is shown in Figure 9.5. Overall, symptoms increased sharply to peak 2 days after inoculation and then decreased to the pre-challenge baseline level by day 7. Total symptom scores after inoculation (controlling for baseline symptoms) increased with increasing levels of psychological stress. An identical pattern of findings emerged for the objective indicator of illness symptoms: mucus weights after inoculation (controlling for baseline) increased with greater levels of psychological stress.

The relation between perceived stress and IL-6 is shown in Figure 9.6. A sharp increase in IL-6 levels occurred over the first 2 days after inoculation and, unlike the pattern for symptoms and mucus weights, remained slightly elevated, not returning to baseline levels during the period of follow-up. These increases were particularly exaggerated among those with high levels of stress; IL-6 levels after inoculation (controlling for baseline) increased with greater psychological stress scores.

Although the correlational nature of these data does not allow for a direct test of whether the documented association between stress and disease expression is mediated by IL-6, we can examine the extent to which such mediation is consistent with the data. After removing (partialling out) the potential contribution of IL-6, the effect sizes of psychological stress on symptoms and on mucus weight were reduced by 58% and 67%, respectively. These results show that our data are consistent with the hypothesis that IL-6 is a primary mediating pathway linking stress and illness severity.

These findings challenge a central assumption in research on stressors, immunity, and infection. Historically, researchers have assumed that stressful experiences heighten vulnerability to infectious disease by diminishing the immune response in a fashion that enables pathogens to spread more easily.[12,22] Rather, our pattern of findings suggests that stressors upregulate the cytokine response to invading pathogens, and by so doing trigger symptoms of clinical illness. In other words, at least in the

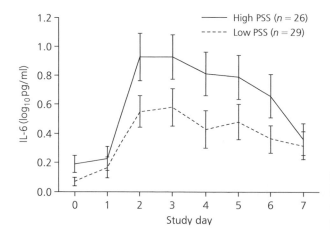

Fig. 9.6 Perceived stress and interleukin-6 expression over course of study. PSS, psychological stress score.

case of pro-inflammatory cytokines, stressors may not 'suppress' the immune response to challenge, but amplify it. A number of hypotheses can be advanced to explain how stressors would upregulate the cytokine response to pathogen challenge. Research in animals has shown that stressors can 'prime' or 'sensitize' white blood cells so that they produce greater volumes of inflammatory cytokines in response to infectious challenge.[23,24] Stressors could also impair the immune system's capacity to turn itself off following challenge. We have recently proposed a glucocorticoid resistance model[25] in which chronic stressors reduce the immune system's sensitivity to hormones that normally terminate inflammation. We have found clear evidence of this process in a recent study.[25] In adults facing a severe chronic stressor, the capacity of glucocorticoids to suppress IL-6 production was significantly diminished. To the extent that this process occurs with more common everyday stressors, it could explain the relations between stress, IL-6, and illness symptoms in our influenza paradigm.

However, it is important to remember that data from this trial are correlational and must be interpreted with care. The pattern of data is also consistent with rises in IL-6 occurring in response to tissue damage associated with illness symptoms or IL-6 responding in concert with other unassayed pro-inflammatory chemicals that might play the causal role here.

9.4.2 Stress and chronic/latent infectious disease

9.4.2.1 Chronic infections

Very little research has examined whether stressful experiences influence vulnerability to chronic infectious disease. Early studies found that individuals who endorsed indicators of stress (life events, perceived stress, negative mood) were more likely to have experienced chronic bacterial infections (tuberculosis, trenchmouth, familial Mediterranean fever).[12,45–48] However, the retrospective nature of these studies, and the lack of emphasis on biological verification of illness, makes it difficult to draw meaningful inferences regarding causality. Stronger evidence derives from a recent cross-sectional study of chronic bacterial vaginosis among low-income women.[49] It found that the ongoing stressor of homelessness was associated with a 6.7-fold increase in risk for verified infection. Another study from this group examined perceived stress in pregnant women, and found that it was associated cross-sectionally with a greater likelihood of bacterial vaginosis.[50] When subjects were split into quartiles on the basis of stress, those in the third and fourth quartiles were 2.3 and 2.2 times more likely to have verified infections compared with women in the bottom quartile. When taken together, these findings are suggestive of a relation between stressful experience and chronic infection. However, further research with better methodology (prospective designs or intervention studies)[51] will be necessary before definitive conclusions can be reached.

9.4.2.2 Latent infections

Interest in the hypothesis that stressful experiences influence vulnerability to latent infectious diseases has grown steadily since the 1970s. This work has primarily centred around three latent viruses: HIV, which causes AIDS, HSV-1, which causes oral herpes, and HSV-2, which causes genital herpes. The role of stress in HIV infection is covered in Chapter 7; here, we will focus our review on studies of oral, genital, and ocular herpes.

Many of the studies in this area have sought to determine whether stressful experiences have the capacity to reactivate latent viruses. There is now sufficient evidence to conclude that this process can occur. Stressors as diverse as academic examinations, marital difficulties, and living near a nuclear power plant have been linked with higher levels of antibody specific to HSV-1, HSV-2, CMV, and EBV.[22,42,52,53] (Antibody production increases with viral replication; thus virus-specific antibody is used as an indirect marker of reactivation.) While these studies illustrate that stressful experiences can trigger a necessary first step in the disease process (viral reactivation), it is important to remember that reactivation may or may not be of sufficient magnitude or duration to elicit symptoms of clinical illness. Thus studies of this nature should be viewed as evidence of potential underlying mechanisms, rather than stressor-triggered episodes of clinical illness.

Oral herpes Early studies examining stressful experiences and clinical episodes of oral herpes yielded mixed results. Some reported that stress was linked to greater risk of illness,[54–57] while others found no relation between the processes.[58] Although a major strength of these studies was the biological and clinical verification of illness, their retrospective and cross-sectional designs make it difficult to sort out the directional relationship between stressors and illness in cases where it emerged. This problem was overcome in a well-designed series of studies by Luborksy and colleagues. In the first study of this series young women entering nursing school completed measures of distress and were then followed for 1 year.[59] The women were asked to report any cold sores that appeared to project staff; a subset then underwent clinical examination and had blood drawn for biological verification of infection. To the extent that they reported being chronically distressed at study entry, women had a greater likelihood of oral herpes lesions in the next year. A follow-up study attempted to replicate and extend these findings using a daily diary paradigm.[60] Student nurses with verified latent HSV-1 infection gave mood ratings daily for a period of 3 weeks; they also underwent examinations each day during which they were monitored for cold sores and evidence of viral replication. Distress was unrelated to outbreaks of oral herpes in both cross-sectional and time-lagged analyses. The final study in this series was a 3-year follow-up of nurses with verified HSV-1 infection and history of herpes episodes.[61] To the extent that they reported being chronically distressed at baseline, nurses again showed a greater risk of developing recurrent oral lesions. Together, findings from these well-designed studies suggest that long-term distress heightens vulnerability to biologically verified outbreaks of oral herpes. Short-term distress, as measured in the second study, does not seem to have the same impact. Apart from the prospective research from this group, there has been one other well-designed study in this area.[62] In this case, 20 patients with a history of oral herpes infection, and the belief that their symptoms were triggered by dirty dishes, were enrolled in an experiment. Half were randomly assigned to view slides of dirty glasses and then exposed to them in person; the other half were exposed to neutral slides and objects. The patients underwent a medical examination 48 h later, and those exposed to the dirty dishes were more likely to exhibit illness symptoms. Although these findings are preliminary, they suggest that activating a persistent source of anxiety may precipitate recurrent infection.

Genital herpes Research on stressful experience and genital herpes has been very active in the past 20 years. Cross-sectional studies have generally reported that indicators of stressful experience, such as life events, distress, and perceived stress, are associated with a greater likelihood of recurrent genital lesions in patients with verified latent HSV-2 infection.[63–65] There have also been negative findings, but these have emerged less often.[66] In an attempt to provide stronger evidence for causal relations between stressors and infection, researchers have conducted a number of prospective investigations in this area. The findings have been generally supportive of a positive relationship, although sometimes inconsistent.

Goldmeier and Johnson[67] studied 58 patients during their first episode of genital herpes. Patients completed measures of distress at study entry, and were followed for 28 weeks to assess recurrent episodes of illness. Greater baseline distress was associated with a higher likelihood of verified recurrence. The reliability of these findings is suspect, however, because the study had a very high attrition rate, especially among patients who remained healthy over follow-up. Moreover, a follow-up study with 57 patients (and better retention) failed to replicate the findings, although when data from the two samples were combined distress was a reliable predictor of disease recurrence.[68]

Hoon *et al.*[69] studied 153 students with verified latent HSV-2 infections and a history of clinical illness. The students completed measures of stressful experiences at baseline (major and minor events and their impacts over past 6 months), and were followed over a period of 6 months during which they returned to the laboratory for examination/verification after noticing new genital lesions. Structural equation modelling revealed that, while stressful experiences were not directly related to the likelihood of recurrence, they were indirectly related through greater overall illness vulnerability (primarily in the form of respiratory infection). These findings suggest that stressors might trigger genital herpes outbreaks by increasing susceptibility to other infections that compete for the immune system resources needed to keep herpes deactivated.

Pereira and colleagues studied a cohort of 34 women with HIV—AIDS who had a history of genital herpes infection. Women completed a life events interview at study entry and were followed for 1 year using chart reviews from the clinic where they received care. To the extent that they reported more negative events in the year prior to the study, women were more likely to experience a recurrent herpes infection during follow-up. This effect was independent of viral activation at baseline, various health practices, and variables related to HIV status.[70]

Given the transient but recurring nature of genital herpes lesions, three recent studies have approached this question with daily diary techniques. Rand *et al.*[71] studied 64 patients with verified HSV-2 infection and a history of clinical illness. Patients completed a diary tracking mood states, social relations, and various stressors each day for a period of 1–3 months. They found no evidence that indices of stress were elevated on any of 6 days preceding lesion outbreaks. Dalvist *et al.*[72] used a similar design in a study of 66 patients with a history of either oral or genital herpes. While patients' mood states were worse in the days preceding herpes onset, these two processes were statistically independent, i.e. no reliable association between them emerged. Interestingly, the best predictor of herpes outbreak was the presence of the common cold.

The most recent study in this area followed 58 women with a history of visible genital herpes recurrences for 6 months.[73] Arguing that previous studies had failed to consider stressor duration, these researchers collected weekly logs from subjects and later classified their stressors into short-term and persistent (>7 days) categories. Measures of depression, anxiety, and anger were also collected weekly, as were symptom checklists for genital herpes and related conditions. In about half the cases of recurrence, subjects reported to a physician for verification of illness. Prospective analyses revealed that persistent stressors were associated with a greater likelihood of recurrence. In other words, to the extent that a subject had a stressor lasting more than 7 days, she was more likely to have a genital herpes outbreak the next week, independent of her illness status during the week that the stressor occurred. Consistent with the authors' expectations, short-term stressors were unrelated to recurrence. Of the mood states, only anxiety predicted likelihood of recurrence; during the month after their greatest anxiety, patients were most likely to have an outbreak.

These findings are generally supportive of a relationship between stressful experience and vulnerability to recurrent genital herpes infections. However, as is the case in oral herpes research, this effect is only evident with persistent stressors; the transient distress captured in diary studies by Rand *et al.*[71] and Dalvist *et al.*[72] is not sufficient to influence vulnerability. Interestingly, there is some indication that persistently stressful experience triggers genital herpes outbreaks by increasing susceptibility to respiratory infections. Presumably this occurs because other infections compete for the immune system resources needed to keep HSV-2 in its latent state.

Ocular herpes One recent study assessed relations between stressful experience and recurrence of ocular herpes infection .[74] Patients (N = 308) with a history of ocular herpes in the past year were enrolled. They completed weekly diaries assessing perceived stress, the presence of chronic stressors, and difficulties in common life domains for up to 15 months. None of the stressor indices was associated with the likelihood of recurrent infection during follow-up. However, subjects exhibited a tendency to retrospectively over-report stress on weeks that infectious symptoms emerged. In other words, when asked to look back and describe their stress levels during the week preceding an outbreak, subjects tended to exaggerate the amount of distress they had experienced. Because over-reporting of this nature can lead to spurious associations between stress and illness, or incorrect conclusions about the direction of their relationship, these findings highlight the importance of conducting prospective studies where stress is measured before symptoms of illness emerge.

9.5 Directions for future research

In this chapter we have briefly discussed the causes of infectious disease, outlined the behavioural and biological pathways through which stressful experiences might contribute to its development and progression, and provided a selective overview of the highest-quality studies in this domain of research. What conclusions can be drawn from this exercise? First, we believe that there is consistent evidence linking stressful experience to heightened vulnerability to acute infectious disease. This evidence is strongest for upper respiratory conditions such as colds and influenza, which are the most common forms of infectious disease and major contributors to morbidity and mortality worldwide. In this domain, stressful experience shows a dose–response relationship with illness vulnerability, such that cold and influenza risk increase in a linear fashion with the duration of the stressor and its perceived severity. While acute events are not sufficient to heighten susceptibility, ongoing chronic stressors do so in a powerful fashion, doubling or tripling a person's risk of developing clinical illness. Secondly, there is suggestive evidence of a relation between stressful experience and chronic infectious diseases such as tuberculosis and trenchmouth. However, further research with better methodology (prospective design and biological verification of illness) will be necessary before any definitive conclusions can be reached in this area.

Finally, findings from a series of well-designed studies suggest that longer-term stressors heighten vulnerability to clinical outbreaks of latent infectious diseases such as oral and genital herpes. As is the case with colds and influenza, more transient forms of stress do not seem to have the same impact.

Collectively, these findings suggest that stressful experiences, especially when they are chronic and ongoing, contribute to the development and progression of a variety of infectious diseases. So what are the next steps for research in this area of psychoneuro-immunology? First, we believe that the search for mediating pathways needs to continue. Although research indicates that stressful experience exacerbates symptoms of influenza by amplifying the inflammatory response, much remains to be learned about how negative feelings and thoughts are transported from the nervous system to the immune system. In the case of latent infectious disease, virtually nothing is known at this point, aside from hints that stress-related respiratory infection may be involved. With a concerted effort towards assessing health practices, endocrine processes, and immune responses in a thorough fashion, researchers can make substantial progress in this area in the next few years.

Secondly, given that nearly all the existing research on stressful experience and infectious disease in humans is correlational, we believe that energy needs to be directed towards experimental investigations that can establish causality. Because deliberately exposing humans to chronic stress would be unethical and unfeasible, this work will most likely need to be carried out using a psychological intervention paradigm, where distressed subjects are assigned to receive a treatment (relaxation, hypnosis, cognitive restructuring) with the idea that it will protect them from illness in the context of a viral challenge. This work will not be easy to implement, however. Researchers have not yet developed a psychological intervention that reliably modifies the immune response,[25] and even when they do, working out the timing of administration relative to pathogen exposure would be tricky. Would distress need to be ameliorated in the days before exposure to reduce illness risk? In the days after? If so, which days? One way to resolve this issue would be to conduct a daily diary study that investigates whether there is a 'critical period' of time when stressors are able to produce a maximal increase disease vulnerability. If such a period was identified, the intervention could be delivered then, presumably maximizing its chances of success. We recently conducted this kind of study using an influenza vaccination paradigm[15]. A cohort of 83 subjects underwent 13 days of ambulatory monitoring before, during, and after vaccination. Subjects reported the extent to which they felt stressed. To the extent that they reported higher levels of stress across the monitoring period, subjects exhibited poorer antibody responses to the vaccine. Stressor ratings on the 2 days before the vaccine, and on the day it was given, were not associated with antibody response. However, the 10 days afterwards seemed to be a window of opportunity during which stressors could shape the long-term antibody response to varying degrees. If this strategy could be extended to a viral challenge paradigm, it would not only simplify the process of designing intervention studies, but would shed light on which stages of host resistance are compromised by stressful experience.

Acknowledgements

The research described in this chapter was supported by National Institute of Allergy and Infectious Disease Grant A123072, National Institute of Mental Health Grant MH50429, Office of Naval Research Contract N00014–88-K-0063, National Institute of Health Grant NCRR/GCRC 5MO1 RR00056 to the University of Pittsburgh General Clinical Research Center, and National Institute of Mental Health Grant MH30915 to the Mental Health Clinical Research Center for Affective Disorders. Supplemental support was provided by the Medical Research Council's Common Cold Unit, the Fetzer Institute and the John D. and Catherine T. MacArthur Foundation. GEM's work on this chapter were supported by a Grant-in-Aid from the American Heart Association (0160367Z), a Young Investigator Award from the National Alliance for Research on Schizophrenia and Depression, and a Career Scholar Award in Clinical Science from the Michael Smith Foundation for Health Research. SC's participation was facilitated by a Senior Scientist Award from the National Institute of Mental Health (MH00721).

References

1 **Murray CJL, Lopez AD** (1997). Mortality by cause for eight regions of the world: global burden of disease study. *Lancet* **349**: 1269–76.

2 **Minino AM, Smith BL** (2001). Deaths: preliminary data for 2000. *Natl Vital Stat Rep* **49**: 1–5.

3 **World Health Organization** (2003). *Influenza Fact Sheet*. Geneva: World Health Organization.

4 **Cotran RS, Kumar V, Collins T** (1999). *Pathologic Basis of Disease* (6th edn). London: W.B. Saunders.

5 **Guyton AC, Hall JE** (1996). *Textbook of Medical Physiology* (9th edn). Philadelphia, PA: W.B. Saunders.

6 **Rabin BS** (1999). *Stress, Immune Function, and Health: The Connection*. New York: John Wiley.

7 **Benjamini E, Sunshine G, Leskowitz S** (1996). *Immunology: A Short Course* (3rd edn). New York: Wiley-Liss.

8 **Maier SF, Watkins LR** (1998). Cytokines for psychologists: implications of bidirectional immune-to-brain communication for understanding behavior, mood, and cognition. *Psychol Rev* **105**: 83–107.

9 **Kent S, Bluthe RM, Kelley KW, Dantzer R** (1992). Sickness behavior as a new target for drug development. *Trends Pharmacol Sci* **13**: 24–28.

10 **Dantzer R** (2001). Cytokine-induced sickness behavior. Where do we stand? *Brain Behav Immun* **15**: 7–24.

11 **Miller GE** (2005). How does stress get inside the body to influence depression? Some answers from the perspective of behavioral immunology. In Barch DM (ed.) *Cognitive and Affective Neuroscience Approaches to Psychopathology*. New York: Oxford University Press.

12 **Cohen S, Williamson GM** (1991). Stress and infectious disease in humans. *Psychol Bull* **109**: 5–24.

13 **Lazarus RS, Folkman S** (1984). *Stress, Appraisal, and Coping*. New York: Springer.

14 Kiecolt-Glaser JK, Glaser R (1988). Methodological issues in behavioral immunology research with humans. *Brain Behav Immun* **2**: 67–78.

15 Miller GE, Cohen S, Pressman S, Barkin A, Rabin B S, Treanor J. Psychological stress and antibody response to influenza vaccination. When is the critical period for stress, and how does it get inside the body? *Psychosom Med* in press.

16 Felten SY, Felten D (1994). Neural—immune interaction. *Prog Brain Res* **100**: 157–62.

17 Cole SW, Jamieson BD, Zack JA (1999). cAMP up-regulates cell surface expression of lymphocyte CXCR4: implications for chemotaxis and HIV-1 infection. *J Immunol* **162**: 1392–1400.

18 Cole SW, Korin YD, Fahey JL, Zack JA (1998). Norepinephrine accelerates HIV replication via protein kinase A-dependent effects on cytokine production. *J Immunol* **161**: 610–16.

19 Lyte M (1993). The role of microbial endocrinology in infectious disease. *J Endocrinol* **137**: 343–5.

20 Blalock JE (1994). The syntax of neuroendocrine–immune communication. *Immunol Today* **15**: 504–11.

21 Weiner H (1992). *Perturbing the Organism: The Biology of Stressful Experience*. Chicago, IL: University of Chicago Press.

22 Glaser R, Rice J, Sheridan JF *et al.* (1987). Stress-related immune suppression: health implications. *Brain Behav Immun* **1**: 7–20.

23 Anisman H, Merali Z, Hayley S (2003). Sensitization associated with stressors and cytokine treatments. *Brain Behav Immun* **17**: 86–93.

24 Johnson JD, O'Connor KA, Deak T, Stark M, Watkins LR, Maier SF (2002). Prior stressor exposure sensitizes LPS-induced cytokine production. *Brain Behav Immun* **16**: 461–76.

25 Miller GE, Cohen S, Ritchey AK (2002). Chronic psychological stress and the regulation of pro-inflammatory cytokines: a glucocorticoid resistance model. *Health Psychol* **21**: 531–41.

26 Salovey P, Birnbaum D (1989). Influence of mood on health-relevant cognition. *J Pers Soc Psychol* **57**: 539–51.

27 Cameron L, Leventhal EA, Leventhal H (1995). Seeking medical care in response to symptoms and life stress. *Psychosom Med* **57**: 37–47.

28 Watson D, Pennebaker JW (1989). Health complaints, stress, and distress: exploring the central role of negative affectivity. *Psychol Rev* **96**: 234–54.

29 Cohen S, Doyle WJ, Skoner DP, Fireman P, Gwaltney JM, Jr, Newsom JT (1995). State and trait negative affect as predictors of objective and subjective symptoms of respiratory viral infections. *J Pers Soc Psychol* **68**: 159–69.

30 Feldman PJ, Cohen S, Doyle W, Skoner D, Gwaltney JM, Jr (1999). The impact of personality on the reporting of unfounded symptoms and illness. *J Pers Soc Psychol* **77**: 370–8.

31 Clover RD, Abell T, Becker LA, Crawford S, Ramsey CN (1989). Family functioning and stress as predictors of influenza B infection. *J Fam Pract* **5**: 535–9.

32 Graham NM, Douglas RM, Ryan P (1986). Stress and acute respiratory infection. *Am J Epidemiol* **124**: 389–401.

33 Broadbent DE, Broadbent MHP, Phillpotts RJ, Wallace J (1984). Some further studies on the prediction of experimental colds in volunteers by psychological factor. *J Psychosom Res* **28**: 511–23.

34 Greene WA, Betts RF, Ochitill HN, Iker HP, Douglas RJ (1978). Psychosocial factors and immunity: preliminary report. *Psychosom Med* **40**: 87.

35 Locke SE, Heisel JS (1977). The influence of stress and emotions and the human immune response. *Biofeedback Self Regul* **2**: 320.

36 Totman R, Kiff J, Reed SE, Craig JW (1980). Predicting experimental colds in volunteers from different measures of recent life stress. *J Psychosom Res* **24**: 155–63.

37 Cohen S, Tyrrell DA, Smith AP (1991). Psychological stress and susceptibility to the common cold. *N Engl J Med* **325**: 606–12.

38 Cohen S, Frank E, Doyle WJ, Skoner DP, Rabin BS, Gwaltney JM, Jr (1998). Types of stressors that increase susceptibility to the common cold in healthy adults. *Health Psychol* **17**: 214–23.

39 Cohen S, Doyle WJ, Skoner DP (1999). Psychological stress, cytokine production, and severity of upper respiratory illness. *Psychosom Med* **61**: 175–80.

40 Stone AA, Bovbjerg DH, Neale JM *et al.* (1992). Development of common cold symptoms following experimental rhinovirus infection is related to prior stressful life events. *Behav Med* **18**: 115–20.

41 Cohen S, Williamson GM (1988). Perceived stress in a probability sample of the United States. In Spacapan S, Oskamp S (eds) *The Social Psychology of Health*. Newbury Park, CA: Sage, 31–67.

42 Segerstrom SC, Miller GE (2004). Psychological stress and the human immune system: a meta-analytic study of 30 years of inquiry. *Psychol Bull* **130(4)**: 601–30.

43 Herbert TB, Cohen S (1993). Stress and immunity in humans: a meta-analytic review. *Psychosom Med* **55**: 364–379.

44 Gentile D, Doyle W, Whiteside T, Fireman P, Hayden FG, Skoner D (1998). Increased interleukin-6 levels in nasal lavage samples following experimental influenza A virus infection. *Clin Diagn Immunol* **5**: 604–8.

45 Imboden JB, Canter A, Cluff LE, Trever RW (1959). Brucellosis. III: Psychologic aspects of delayed convalescence. *Arch Intern Med* **103**: 406–14.

46 Cohen-Cole S, Cogen R, Stevens A, *et al.* (1981). Psychosocial, endocrine, and immune factors in acute necrotizing ulcerative gingivitis. *Psychosom Med* **43**: 91.

47 Hawkins NG, Davies R, Holmes TH (1957). Evidence of psychosocial factors in the development of pulmonary tuberculosis. *Annu Rev Tuberc Pulm Dis* **75**: 768–80.

48 Rahe RJ, Mayer M, Smith M, Kjaer G, Holmes TH (1964). Social stress and illness onset. *J Psychosom Res* **8**: 35–44.

49 Culhane JF, Rauh V, McCollum KF, Elo IT, Hogan V (2002). Exposure to chronic stress and ethnic differences in rates of bacterial vaginosis among pregnant women. *Am J Obstet Gynecol* **187**: 1272–1276.

50 Culhane JF, Rauh V, McCollum KF, Hogan VK, Agnew K, Wadhwa PD (2001). Maternal stress is associated with bacterial vaginosis in human pregnancy. *Matern Child Health J* **5**: 127–34.

51 Miller GE, Cohen S (2001). Psychological interventions and the immune system: a meta-analytic review and critique. *Health Psychol* **20**: 47–63.

52 Kiecolt-Glaser JK, Kennedy S, Malkoff S, Fisher L, Speicher CE, Glaser R (1988). Marital discord and immunity in males. *Psychosom Med* **50**: 213–29.

53 McKinnon W, Weisse CS, Reynolds CP, Bowles CA, Baum A (1989). Chronic stress, leukocyte subpopulations, and humoral response to latent viruses. *Health Psychol* **8**: 389–402.

54 Ship I, Morris AL, Dorucher RT, Burket LW (1960). Recurrent aphthous ulcerations and recurrent herpes labialis in a professional school student population. *Oral Surg* **13**: 1191–1202.

55 Stock C, Guillen-Grima F, de Mendoza JH, Marin-Fernandez B, Aguinaga-Ontoso I, Kramer A (2001). Risk factors of herpes simplex type 1 (IISV-1) infection and lifestyle factors associated with HSV-1 manifestations. *Eur J Epidemiol* **17**: 885–90.

56 Schmidt DD, Zyzanski S, Ellner J, Kumar ML, Arno J (1985). Stress as a precipitating factor in subjects with recurrent herpes labialis. *J Fam Pract* **20**: 359–66.

57 Logan H, Lutgendorf S, Hartwig A, Lilly J, Berberich SL (1998). Immune, stress, and mood markers related to recurrent oral herpes outbreaks. *Oral Surg Oral Med Oral Pathol* **86**: 48–54.

58 Ship I, Brightman VJ, Lastman LL (1967). The patient with herpes labialis: A study of two population samples. *J Am Dent Assoc* **75**: 645–54.

59 Katcher AH, Brightman VJ, Luborsky L, Ship I (1973). Predictors of the incidence of recurrent herpes labialis and systemic illness from psychological measures. *J Dent Res* **52**: 49–58.

60 Luborsky L, Mintz J, Brightman VJ, Katcher AH (1976). Herpes simplex virus and moods: a longitudinal study. *J Psychosom Res* **20**: 543–8.

61 Friedman E, Katcher AH, Brightman VJ (1977). Incidence of recurrent herpes labialis and upper respiratory infection: a prospective study of the influence of biologic, social and psychologic predictors. *Oral Surg Oral Med Oral Pathol* **43**: 873–8.

62 Buske-Kirschbaum A, Geiben A, Wermke C, Pirke KM, Hellhammer D (2001). Preliminary evidence for herpes labialis recurrence following experimentally induced disgust. *Psychother Psychosom* **70**: 86–91.

63 Kemeny ME, Cohen F, Zegans LS, Connant MA (1989). Psychological and immunological predictors of genital herpes recurrence. *Psychosom Med* **51**: 195–208.

64 Longo DJ, Clum GA (1989). Psychosocial factors affecting genital herpes recurrences: linear vs mediating models. *J Psychosom Res* **33**: 161–6.

65 VanderPlate C, Aral S, Madger L (1988). The relationship among genital herpes simplex virus, stress, and social support. *Health Psychol* **7**: 159–68.

66 Silver PS, Auerbach SM, Vishniavsky N, Kaplowitz LG (1986). Psychological factors in recurrent genital herpes infection: stress, coping style, social support, emotional dysfunction, and symptom recurrence. *J Psychosom Res* **30**: 163–71.

67 Goldmeier D, Johnson A (1982). Does psychiatric illness affect the recurrence rate of genital herpes? *Br J Vener Dis* **58**: 40–3.

68 Goldmeier D, Johnson A, Jeffries D, *et al.* (1986). Psychological aspects of recurrences of genital herpes. *J Psychosom Res* **30**: 601–8.

69 Hoon EF, Hoon PW, Rand KH, Johnson JH, Hall NRS, Edwards NB (1991). A psychobehavioral model of genital herpes recurrence. *J Psychosom Res* **35**: 25–36.

70 Pereira DB, Antoni MH, Danielson A *et al.* (2003). Stress as a predictor of symptomatic genital herpes virus recurrence in women with human immunodeficiency virus. *J Psychosom Res* **54**: 237–44.

71 Rand KH, Hoon EF, Massey JK, Johnson JH (1990). Daily stress and recurrence of genital herpes simplex. *Arch Intern Med* **150**: 1889–93.

72 Dalvist J, Wahlin TB, Bartsch E, Forsbeck M (1995). Herpes simplex and mood: a prospective study. *Psychosom Med* **57**: 127–37.

73 Cohen F, Kemeny ME, Kearney KA, Zegans LS, Neuhaus JM, Conant MA (1999). Persistent stress as a predictor of genital herpes recurrence. *Arch Intern Med* **159**: 2430–6.

74 Herpetic Eye Disease Study Group (2000). Psychological stress and other potential triggers for recurrences of herpes simplex virus eye infections. *Arch Opthalmol* **118**: 1617–25.

Chapter 10

Depression and psychoneuroimmunology

Michael R. Irwin and Jason C. Cole

10.1 Introduction

In the most comprehensive analysis of the findings implicating depression to immune changes, Zorrilla *et al.*[1] conducted a meta-analysis of over 180 studies with more than 40 immune measures that examined the relationships between immune alternations with depression. The authors concluded that many enduring immunological findings are related to depression. Given the quantity of evidence implicating depression in immunological variation and the progression of immune-mediated disease and health outcomes, this field has become an area of interest for researchers in psychoneuroimmunology.

This chapter provides a review of the psychoneuroimmunological research being conducted on the relationship between depression and immunity. The chapter begins with a description of the clinical importance of depressive disorders with attention to the effects of depression on mortality risk. Depression is associated with changes in behaviours such as sleep disturbance that also impact immune function. A detailed review of the research conducted on the various immune findings that occur during depression is provided. Immune activation is also found in depression, and we discuss the possible roles of abnormal cytokine expression in inducing mood disturbance and behavioural changes associated with depression. Finally, the chapter concludes with a discussion of the clinical implications of immune changes in depression for several medical disorders.

10.2 Clinical context: depression and mortality risks

10.2.1 Definition of depression

Depression can be defined as a condition that primarily entails a disturbance of mood, and this affective disturbance is often characterized by a mood that is sad, hopeless, discouraged, or simply depressed.[2] The diagnostic definition of a major depressive disorder states that the depressed mood or loss of pleasure (i.e. anhedonia) must last for at least 2 weeks, be accompanied by a series of related symptoms (e.g. vegetative signs, sleep disturbance), and should not be caused by another psychiatric disorder, a general medical condition, or substance use/abuse. The symptoms typically experienced during depression include significant weight change ($\pm 5\%$), sleep disturbance (either insomnia or hypersomnia), psychomotor retardation or agitation, pervasive fatigue, feelings of worthlessness or irrational guilt, mental concentration difficulties, and recurrent suicidal ideation.

Although most studies of immune abnormalities have focused on major depression, there appears to be a dose–response relationship between severity of depression and changes of immunity. Thus, as discussed below, several recent studies have examined the effects of minor depression on immunity. While minor depression is noted as a potential diagnostic category that needs further empirical validation,[3] it is essentially characterized by a disturbance in mood or a loss of pleasure with the presence of two additional symptoms (rather than four for major depressive disorder). Minor depression is also associated with functional impairments and is often viewed as a prodromal state for the occurrence of major depression.[3]

10.2.2 Prevalence of depression

Lifetime prevalence rates of depressive disorders are estimated to be about 15%,[4] with women experiencing a lifetime prevalence of 20% and men showing a prevalence of about 10%. Even higher rates of depression are found in certain populations; primary care out-patients with chronic disease have point prevalence rates ranging from 9% to 20% for all depressive disorders,[5,6] and medical in-patients, who probably experience even greater acute or chronic disease morbidity stress, show even higher rates of 15–36% for all depressive disorders.[7,8]

10.2.3 Clinical course

The clinical course of major depressive disorder varies markedly with age; its onset is protracted in older adults with prodromal and progressive elevation of depressive symptoms, in contrast to the relatively short clinical onset in younger patients.[9] Furthermore, in older adults, depressive symptoms and stress of physical disability can initiate a continuous decline in physical and psychological health. Even with ongoing clinical management, there are often lingering depressive symptoms and an increased risk of relapse in older adults who are experiencing life stress and chronic disease burden.[10] Together, these data are consistent with the view of depressive disorders as chronic and recurrent with residual disability.[11]

10.2.4 Depression and comorbidity: effects on mortality

Despite the aforementioned prevalence of depressive disorders, the impact of major depression on disease outcomes, as well as on the onset and progression of chronic disease, has received little attention. For example, there have been few studies examining whether depression comorbidity exacerbates limitations in functioning, well-being, and health over time, although compelling evidence shows that depression alone produces large declines in health status comparable with other medical disorders.

Depression predicts mortality whether it is considered as a taxonomical disorder (e.g. meeting or not meeting diagnostic criteria) or as a continuum (e.g. scores on a depression measure).[12-14] The findings linking depression to mortality are most robust for patients with cardiovascular disease; patients recovering from myocardial infarction who have depression show about a twofold elevated risk of mortality, even after controlling for the effects of previous cardiovascular severity and extent of cardiac compromise.[15,16] The associations between depression and mortality may also be related to behavioural changes found in depression. Sleep disturbance, a common symptom of depression,[17] is independently related to mortality risk. Dew et al.[18] found that increased sleep latency, increased REM sleep, and decreased sleep efficiency prospectively predicted increased risk of death in older adults after controlling for age, gender, and medical status. In heterogeneous patient populations typical of a hospital setting[13] as well as older adults residing in a nursing home,[14] mortality rates in depressives are nearly twice those of non-depressives with death also related to infectious disease complications (e.g. pneumonia). In sum, depression substantially increases the risk of death, especially by unnatural causes and cardiovascular disease, although the mediating links between depression and morbidity and mortality risks are not known.

10.3 Theoretical basis for a role of psychoneuroimmunology in depression

10.3.1 Multisystem abnormalities in depression: links to immune dysfunction

10.3.1.1 Central modulation of immunity: effects of corticotrophin-releasing hormone

Depressed patients show elevated levels of corticotrophin-releasing hormone (CRH).[19] This key peptide is involved in integrating neural, neuroendocrine, as well as immune responses to stress. Release of this peptide in the brain alters a variety of immune processes including aspects of innate immunity, cellular immunity, and in vivo measures of antibody production.[20,21] Peripheral immune measures also change following lesioning of the brain (e.g. hypothalamus) or in response to the stimulation of certain brain regions which ultimately impact CRH systems. The brain controls immune cells in lymphoid tissue in the same manner that it controls other visceral organs, namely by coordinating autonomic and neuroendocrine pathways; when these pathways are blocked by specific factors that bind to sympathetic or hormone receptors, the effects of CRH on immune function are also blocked.[20,21]

10.3.1.2 Autonomic nervous system

At rest and in response to acute physical and/or psychological challenge, depressed patients show elevated levels of circulating catecholamines and neuropeptide Y,[22] consistent with the notion that depression is associated with activation of the peripheral sympathetic nervous system. The sympathetic nervous system regulates multiple aspects of the immune system, and is thought to mediate changes of immunity in depression. For example, it is known that sympathetic nerve terminals are juxtaposed with immune cells in organs where the immune system cells develop and respond to pathogens (e.g. bone marrow, thymus, spleen, and lymph nodes).[23,24] When sympathetic release of norepinephrine and neuropeptide Y occurs, receptor binding serves as a signal in this 'hard-wired' connection between the brain and the immune system. In addition, sympathetic nerves penetrate into the adrenal gland and cause the release of epinephrine into the bloodstream, which circulates to immune cells as another sympathetic regulatory signal.

Under both laboratory and natural conditions including depression, sympathetic activation has been shown to suppress the activity of diverse populations of immune cells including natural killer (NK) cells and T lymphocytes.[23,24] In contrast, other aspects of the immune response can be enhanced. For example, catecholamines can increase the production of antibodies by B cells and the ability of macrophages to release cytokines and thereby signal the presence of a pathogen. Additional studies indicate that sympathetic activation can also shunt some immune system cells out of circulating blood and into the lymphoid organs (e.g. spleen, lymph nodes, thymus) while recruiting other types of immune cells into circulation (e.g. NK cells). It is thought that sympathetic activation reduces the immune system's ability to destroy pathogens that live inside cells (e.g. viruses) via decreases of the cellular immune response, while enhancing the humoral immune response to pathogens that live outside cells (e.g. bacteria).[24]

10.3.1.3 Neuroendocrine axis

A hallmark of major depression is dysregulation of the hypothalamic–pituitary–adrenal (HPA) axis and the overexpression of cortisol as measured by increases in circulating levels of cortisol, increased rates of cortisol excretion, or a failure to suppress cortisol release in the presence of a synthetic steroid [e.g. dexamethasone suppression test (DST)] . Cortisol exerts diverse effects on a wide variety of physiological systems, and also coordinates the actions of various cells involved in an immune response by altering the production of cytokines or immune messengers.[25] Similar to sympathetic activation, cortisol can suppress the cellular immune response critical to defending the body against viral infections. Cortisol can also prompt some immune cells to move out of circulating blood into lymphoid organs or peripheral tissues such as the skin.[26]

10.4 Empirical evidence

10.4.1 Immunological findings in depression

Converging evidence indicates that depression is associated with alterations of neuroendocrine and autonomic nervous system activity which legitimizes the possibility that depression might also have a physiological role in the regulation of immunity. Below, we detail the extent of immune abnormalities that have been found in association with depression.

10.4.1.1 Enumerative measures

One of the first immunological findings identified in depressed persons were increases in the total number of white blood cells and in the numbers and percentages of neutrophils and lymphocytes.[27–30] Inconsistent findings regarding monocyte counts have been reported, with increases found for depressed persons in some studies[29] while others have found decreases or no difference in the absolute or relative numbers of monocytes.[27,28,31] Cellular enumeration of lymphocyte subsets by the quantification of phenotype-specific cell surface markers has been widely used to evaluate alterations of the immune system in relation to diagnostic depression. Depression is negatively related to the number and percentage of lymphocytes (B cells, T cells, T helper cells and T suppressor/cytotoxic cells).[32] A decrease in the circulating number of cells that express the NK cell phenotype which, in part, is moderated by gender has also been reported; a decline in NK cell numbers is found in male but not female depressed subjects compared with gender-matched controls.[33] However, multiple discrepant findings have also been reported, and in one of the largest study samples of depressed subjects no difference in the number of peripheral blood lymphocytes or T-lymphocyte subsets was found between depressed patients and controls.[34] Indeed, with the recent accumulation of studies, it is questionable as to whether there are consistent changes in the number of circulating B, T, or NK cells in depression.

10.4.1.2 Functional measures

Function of the immune system in depressed subjects has typically been evaluated by assays of non-specific mitogen-induced lymphocyte proliferation, mitogen-stimulated cytokine production, and NK cytotoxicity (see Chapter 3 for a description of these assays). A reliable association between depression and lower proliferative responses to the mitogens phytohaemaglutinin (PHA), concanavalin-A (Con A), and pokeweed (PWM) has been found.[1,32] Some of the first observations evaluating depression and mitogen responses showed reduced proliferation in depressed subjects compared with controls.[35,36] However, subsequent studies failed to replicate these observations, raising questions about the reliability of this immune alteration in depression.[34] Nevertheless, with more than a dozen studies now conducted on lymphocyte proliferation in depression,[34,37–50] it appears that an impairment in the response of lymphocytes to all three non-specific mitogens predominates in studies of depressed subjects.

A reduction of NK activity is also considered to be one of the most reliable and reproducible alterations of *ex vivo* immune function in depression.[51] Irwin *et al.*[28] first reported a decline of NK activity in depressed subjects compared with age- and gender-matched controls, and 10 subsequent independent samples have replicated this observation.[52,53] Several caveats must be considered when reviewing the associations between NK activity, NK numbers, and depression. Compared with controls, decreases in NK counts and NK activity were found in male but not female depressed subjects,[33] and other studies have found no difference of NK activity in depression[34,54] Nevertheless, the meta-analyses of Zorrilla et al.[1] and Herbert and Cohen[32] found that depression is associated with a reliable decrease in NK activity. The factors that might moderate or mediate the effects of depression on NK activity are discussed later in this chapter.

10.4.1.3 Stimulated cytokine production

In contrast with the investigations of lymphocyte proliferation and NK activity, studies of stimulated cytokine production have not yielded consistent findings. In whole-blood assays, Kronfol et al.[55] found increased lipopolysaccharide-stimulated production of IL-1β and IL-6, but no change in the expression of tumour necrosis factor α (TNF-α). Other studies have found no difference in the expression of T cells or IL-2.[56]

10.4.1.4 Viral specific immune measures

Extension of these non-specific measures of immunity to viral-specific immune response has begun to yield promising findings relevant to the increased risk of infectious disease in depression and psychological stress (see Chapter 9). For example, major depression is associated with a functional decline in memory T cells that respond to varicella zoster virus,[57] and this immune response is thought to be a surrogate marker for herpes zoster risk.

10.4.1.5 Assays of *in vivo* responses

Recent evidence further indicates that depression can impact *in vivo* immune responses as measured by delayed-type hypersensitivity (DTH) (antigen specific cell mediated immune response). In animals, administration of an acute stressor leads to a rapid increase in the DTH response[58] which remains elevated for several days following the challenge. In contrast, chronic stress in animals suppresses the DTH response.[58] In depressed patients, suppression of the DTH response to a panel of antigenic challenges has been found.[59] In contrast, Shinkawa et al.[60] found that older depressed patients were more likely to show positive tuberculin responses than non-depressed patients. To our knowledge, no study has investigated whether depression alters immunological response to vaccination, although several studies have revealed that psychological stress is associated with declines of hepatitis B antibody responses as well as antibody response to influenza immunization (see Chapter 9).

10.4.1.6 Immune activation

Most previous studies have suggested that depression results in reductions of non-specific cellular and natural immunity. However, Maes et al.[61] have argued that major depression is associated with immune activation reminiscent of an acute phase response.[29,62] In addition, cytokines such as IL-6 that are typically associated with an inflammatory process are reportedly elevated in depression. Increases in the circulating concentration of the soluble IL-2 receptor that is released with immune activation have also been reported.[63,64] As discussed below, immune activation and the expression of inflammatory cytokines are thought to mediate the link between depression and inflammatory disorders including cardiovascular disease [65] and rheumatoid arthritis.[66] In addition, expression of these pro-inflammatory cytokines may contribute to the constellation of behavioural symptoms known as 'sickness behaviour' and the occurrence of depressive symptoms in certain medical populations.[67]

10.4.1.7 Role of clinical moderating factors

Research on the role that clinical factors, including demographics, exert on the link between depression and immunity is limited. Reportedly, alterations in the immune system during major depressive disorder are not merely biological correlates, but rather conjointly occur with other factors characterizing depressed subjects, such as age, hospitalization stress, and severity of depressive symptoms,[51] which may serve as possible moderators to partially explain the relationship between depression and immunity.[32,52] For example, older adults show declines in cellular immunity, and the presence of comorbid depression, and possibly stress, further magnify age-related immune alterations. The gender of the subject also exerts differential effects on pituitary, adrenal, and immune systems by modulating the sensitivity of target tissues, and women show exaggerated expression of cytokines that lead to inflammation. Such inflammatory responses to stress may place women at increased risk for autoimmune disorders. In contrast, declines in T-cell and NK-cell responses appear to be more prominent in depressed men than in depressed women. With regard to ethnicity, African American ethnicity interacts with a history of alcohol consumption to exacerbate immune abnormalities,[68] although the influence of ethnicity on depression-related changes of immunity is not known. Finally, specific diagnostic comorbidity might moderate immune system functioning in depression. For example, a number of studies have identified sleep in the regulation of some aspects of immune function,[69–71] and depressed individuals with neurovegetative symptoms such as disordered sleep or appetite loss are more likely to show immune changes[72] than those without such symptoms.

10.4.1.8 Treatment of depression

Castanon *et al.*[73] recently reviewed animal research that focused on the immunological effects of antidepressant medications and concluded that antidepressants decrease pro-inflammatory cytokine expression. Although the specific mechanism(s) involved have not yet been identified, antidepressants modify the expression of glucocorticoids and their receptors,[74,75] limit the synthesis of prostaglandin and nitric oxide which contribute to pro-inflammatory effects,[76,77] and act on intracellular messenger pathways with downstream effects on pro-inflammatory cytokines.[78]

Several studies have now investigated the clinical course of depression and changes of immunity in relation to antidepressant medication treatment and symptom resolution. In one longitudinal case–control study, Irwin et al.[79] found that depressed patients showed decreased Hamilton depression scores and increased NK activity from baseline to follow-up. Changes in NK activity were related to changes in severity of depressive symptoms but not to treatment status with antidepressant medications. In another longitudinal follow-up study of young adults with unipolar depression involving 6 weeks of treatment with nortriptyline and alprazolam,[80] clinical improvement in the severity of depressive symptoms was associated with decreased numbers of circulating lymphocytes and decreased responses to PHA and Con A but not to PWM. In addition, decreases in T cells, CD4+, and CD29 were found, although there were no changes in B-cell numbers or CD8+ cells. None of these changes were related to nortriptyline blood levels.[80] In addition, Frank et al.[81] found that in vivo and in vitro treatment with fluoxetine, a selective serotonin-reuptake inhibitor, resulted in enhanced NK activity together with changes in depressive symptoms. Finally, one study found that treatment with psychotropic medications reduced pro-inflammatory cytokine IL-12 expression in hospitalized psychiatric patients (with schizophrenia, depression, or bipolar disorder) compared with controls,[82] consistent with the view held by Kenis and Maes[83] that antidepressants decrease pro-inflammatory cytokine expression.

10.4.2 Mechanisms of immune dysfunction in depression

10.4.2.1 Biological mediators

As discussed above, depression is known to alter two pathways that have effects on immune system functioning, i.e. the sympathetic nervous system and the HPA axis. Moreover, some changes in functioning of these paths have been related to immune abnormalities in depression. With regard to sympathetic activity, Irwin et al.[22] have shown that plasma concentrations of neuropeptide Y are elevated in depressed patients, older individuals, and persons undergoing severe Alzheimer caregiver stress. Furthermore, activation of the sympathetic nervous system and release of catecholamines is associated with a reduction of natural cytotoxicity in chronic life stress.[84] Additional findings also support the hypothesis that elevated sympathetic activity in depression is associated with immune alterations. In depressed patients, excretion of 3-methoxy-4-hydroxy-phenylglycol (MHPG), a metabolite or breakdown product of norepinephrine, has been used as an index of total body noradrenergic turnover, or sympathetic activity. MHPG excretion was inversely related with lymphocyte proliferative responses in depressed patients.[43] In a study of immunity in spinal-cord-injured (SCI) patients, only those patients with high levels of injury (cervical) and loss of sympathetic nervous system integrity were found to have altered lymphocyte function compared with matched normal healthy controls.[85] Similarly, tetraplegic but not paraplegic SCI patients were found to have impaired phagocytic ability compared with matched healthy controls.[86] Together, these data suggest that the autonomic nervous system activity is important in immune function, and that elevated sympathetic tone in patients with depression is inversely correlated with cellular immune function.

The relationship between HPA axis activation and immune alterations in depression has not been compelling. For example, in depressed patients, decreased lymphocyte responses to mitogens are not associated with dexamethasone non-suppression (DST)[35] or with increased excretion rates of urinary free cortisol.[40] Furthermore, in bereavement, which is complicated by depressive symptoms, changes of NK activity are not associated with plasma cortisol levels.[87] Nevertheless, disruption of one's physiological homeostasis is implicated in depression, and neuroendocrine–immune interactions are thought to contribute to this dysregulation. As noted above, major depression is associated with the increased expression of pro-inflammatory cytokines which in turn leads to the progression of the immune response and activation of the HPA axis.[88–91] In a study of 28 in-patients with major depression, Maes et al.[92] found a significant positive correlation between mitogen-induced IL-1β production and post-DST cortisol values which suggested that IL-1β oversecretion may contribute to HPA axis overactivity in depression.

10.4.2.2 Behavioural mechanisms

In addition to the biological mediators of immune changes in depression, there are several behavioural factors associated with depression that might contribute to immune dysfunction. Indeed, as reviewed by Cohen and Miller,[93] examination of health status and behavioural factors is needed in clinical psychoneuroimmunology. For example, alcohol and tobacco have well-recognized effects on immunity. However, there is limited empirical information on the processes by which these substances alter immune function in depressed subjects, despite their high rates of use in such patients. In the following section, four of the more pertinent behavioural factors linking depression and immune dysfunction are discussed: tobacco smoking, alcohol/substance abuse, activity/exercise, and sleep disturbance.

10.4.2.3 Smoking: prevalence and immune effects

Cigarette smoking has long been considered a health risk, with effects on immunity via direct actions or possibly endocrine-mediated mechanisms.[94] Nicotine is reported to affect the HPA axis[95] as well as humoral and cellular immunity.[96] Additionally, specific immunological alterations occur in adult smokers, affecting a variety of parameters. Adult male smokers have been found to exhibit higher white blood cell counts and lower NK activity than non-smoking controls. However, only two studies concerned with immune alterations in depressed subjects have assessed smoking histories.[31,97] While neither study found that smoking histories correlated with immune function in depressed subjects, the lack of a relationship between quantity of cigarettes used and NK activity is not surprising because of the rather restricted range of cigarette use in the depressed subjects, with most reporting moderate (one to two packs per day) consumption. Jung and Irwin[98] reported that depression and smoking status interact to produce greater declines of NK activity than those found in depressed or smoking groups alone. Cigarette use alone, or in combination with depression, might also contribute to the suppression of other non-specific measures of immune function such as mitogen-induced lymphocyte proliferation. Given the effects of cigarette smoking on markers of immune activation,[99] it is also important to address whether smoking status alters the reported relationship between depression and increases in serum levels of IL-6 and acute phase proteins. Importantly, depression appears to interact with cigarette smoking to impact on health, rather than there being a unitary link between depression and cancer. In a 12-year follow-up of 2264 adult men and women, depressed mood was found to interact with cigarette smoking, and depressed mood and cigarette smoking together were associated with a marked increase in the relative risk of cancer[100] compared with the risk associated with smoking or depression status alone.

10.4.2.4 Alcohol dependence: prevalence and immune effects in depression

According to Schuckit,[101] nearly 30% of individuals with depression also suffer from alcohol dependence and over 30% of depressives escalate their drinking during the depressive episode. Whereas alcohol/substance dependence and depression each have a significant negative impact on the immune system, the interaction of alcohol/substance abuse with affective disorders may result in significantly more immune impairment than either condition alone. In a study by Irwin *et al.*,[27] individuals with a dual diagnosis of alcoholism and depression had further decreases of NK activity compared with individuals diagnosed with alcoholism or depression alone. Furthermore, these researchers found that depressed subjects with histories of alcoholism had lower NK activity than depressed subjects without such histories. Alcoholics with secondary depression showed a further decrease in cytotoxicity compared with alcoholics who were not clinically depressed.[27] Strikingly, this result reflects the effects of past consumption of alcohol. Depressed and alcoholic subjects were free from alcohol for a minimum of 2 weeks, and thus the decline of NK activity was not due to a direct pharmacological effect of alcohol. Consequently, in studies of depressed subjects, the influence of alcohol abuse on the immune parameter may not dissipate simply due to a washout period lasting days to weeks. Rather, more systematic assessment of current alcohol use along with dependence histories is needed in future studies of the relation between depression and immunity in order to contend with the compounding effect of variations in alcohol consumption.

10.4.2.5 Activity and exercise: immune consequences in depression

Activity, or a lack thereof, can have negative consequences on the immune system, and some data suggest that older adults with depression may be especially vulnerable to the harmful effects of sedentary lifestyles. Conversely, exercise has been shown to have potent salutary effects on immune measures and has even been found to promote a remission of depressive symptoms in older adults. In the meta-analysis by Herbert and Cohen,[32] melancholic depression correlated with greater impairment of cellular immunity which may be due, at least in part, to an increased predominance of neurovegetative symptoms.[52] Cover and Irwin[72] found that severity of psychomotor retardation uniquely predicted declines of NK activity, similar to the effects of insomnia.

10.4.2.6 Disordered sleep and immunity: relevance to depression

Disordered sleep and loss of sleep are thought to adversely affect resistance to infectious disease, increase cancer risk, and alter inflammatory disease progression. Animal studies show that sleep deprivation impairs influenza viral clearance and increases rates of bacteraemia. In humans, normal sleep is associated with a redistribution of circulating lymphocyte subsets, increases of NK activity, increases of certain cytokines (e.g. IL-2, IL-6), and a relative shift towards Th1 cytokine expression that is independent of circadian processes. Conversely, sleep deprivation suppresses NK activity and IL-2 production, although prolonged sleep loss has been found to enhance measures of innate immunity and pro-inflammatory cytokine expression.

Insomnia is one of the most common complaints of depressed subjects, but its role in moderating and/or mediating immune alterations in depression is relatively unexplored. However, with evidence that subjective insomnia correlates with NK activity in depression, but not with other depressive symptoms including somatization, weight loss, cognitive disturbance, or diurnal variation,[102] the hypothesis has emerged that disordered sleep may be a distinct factor accounting for some of the observed immune alterations found in depression.

In depressed samples who are at risk for disordered sleep, alterations of natural and cellular immune function among depressed patients correlate with disturbances of EEG sleep.[71,72] Recent studies of bereaved subjects have replicated this correlation, and causal statistical analyses have shown that disordered sleep also mediates the relationship between severe life stress and a decline in NK responses.[103] Further studies involving subjects with primary insomnia (e.g. no depression, other psychiatric disorder, and medical disorder) have found that prolonged sleep latency and fragmentation of sleep are associated with nocturnal elevations of sympathetic catecholamines and declines in daytime levels of NK cell responses.[104,105] A more extensive line of research focused on alcohol-dependent patient populations who have profound disturbances of sleep continuity and sleep architecture[106,107] has found that decreases of total sleep time, declines of delta sleep, and increases of REM are associated with increases in the nocturnal and daytime expression of IL-6, possibly with consequences for daytime fatigue.[108] Thus it appears that disordered sleep may be a critical behavioural factor that mediates the relationship between depression and immune alterations.

10.4.3 Immunity and depression onset: cytokine hypothesis

Not only does the brain participate in the regulation of immune responses, but the central nervous system receives information from the periphery that an immune response is occurring, with consequent changes in both electrical and neurochemical activity of the brain. During immunization to a novel protein antigen, the firing rate of neurons within the part of the brain controlling autonomic activity (e.g. ventromedial hypothalamus) increases at the time of peak production of antibody.[109] Cytokines released by immune cells are increasingly implicated as messengers in this bidirectional interaction. The release of IL-1 following activation of macrophages with virus or other stimuli induces alterations of brain activity and changes in the metabolism of central brain chemicals and neurotransmitters such as norepinephrine, serotonin, and dopamine in discrete brain areas.[110] Much recent research has focused on how these cytokines communicate with the brain, given their large molecular size and inability to cross the blood–brain barrier. It is now known that IL-1 and possibly other inflammatory cytokines communicate with the brain by stimulating peripheral nerves such as the vagus which provide information to the brain.[110] In summary, the immune system acts like a sensory organ, conveying information to the brain which ultimately regulates neuroendocrine and autonomic outflow and the course of the immune response.

Immune activation leads to changes of peripheral physiology and behaviours that are similar to a stress response. With peripheral immune activation, pro-inflammatory cytokines are expressed in the central nervous system, CRH is released by the hypothalamus, and there is an induction of a pituitary adrenal response and autonomic activity.[111] Coincident with these physiological changes, animals show reductions in activity, exploration of novel objects, social interactions, food and water intake, and willingness to engage in sexual behaviours.[112] Taken together, this pattern of behavioural changes (i.e. sickness behaviours) is similar to that found in animals exposed to fear or anxiety-arousing stimuli, and can be reproduced by the central or peripheral administration of IL-1. In contrast, central administration of factors that block IL-1 antagonize these effects. These cytokine–brain processes are also implicated in increased sensitivity to pain stimuli that is found following nerve or tissue injury.[113]

Bidirectional actions of cytokines on sleep have also been identified. In animals, cytokines have both somnogenic (e.g. sleep-producing) and inhibitory effects on sleep, depending on the cytokine, plasma level, and circadian phase.[114] Less is known about the sleep-regulatory effects of cytokines in humans. Expression of the Th2 or anti-inflammatory cytokine IL-10 prior to sleep predicts amounts of delta sleep during the nocturnal period.[108] In contrast, peripheral administration of the pro-inflammatory cytokine IL-6 reduces delta sleep, and nocturnal levels of IL-6 and TNF temporally correlate with increases of REM sleep, particularly during the later part of the night.[115]

Translation of these basic observations into the clinical setting has led to the formulation of the cytokine hypothesis of major depression. Briefly, it is thought that physical or psychological stress increases the prevalence of pro-inflammatory cytokines, which in turn results in neurochemical changes (e.g. serotonin, norepinephrine), neuroendocrine abnormalities (e.g. increased HPA activity), and behavioural changes (e.g. vegetative symptoms). This has not yet been confirmed in human studies, as they rely on measurements of cytokines, soluble cytokine receptors, or both, in body fluids and are not necessarily indicative of cytokine activity in the brain. Furthermore, there is contradictory evidence; whereas cytokine abnormalities are often found in mild forms of depression, HPA activation is often not present and vegetative symptoms are not very prominent in such depressed patients.

Nevertheless, human studies have begun to reveal links between peripheral cytokines and behavioural changes. The associations between cytokines and sleep described above have recently been extended to measures of daytime fatigue. In cancer survivors, the occurrence of fatigue is associated with increases of pro-inflammatory cytokines.[116] Moreover, immune activation may contribute to fatigue in patients with chronic fatigue syndrome.[117,118]

Large doses of cytokines, given as immunotherapy for cancer or hepatitis C, frequently induce depression-like symptoms such as depressed mood, anhedonia, fatigue, poor concentration, and disordered sleep which can be treated effectively by giving antidepressant medications.[119,120] Interestingly, the presence of depressive symptoms at the beginning of cytokine therapy predicts cytokine-induced clinical depression.[121] Similar effects are produced following physiological activation of the immune system. For example, the administration of endotoxin (a bacterial product) leads to the release of pro-inflammatory cytokines with consequent effects on depressed mood and anxiety and on verbal and non-verbal memory functions.[122]

Conversely, treatment with antidepressant medications decreases levels of specific cytokines.[123] Sluzewska et al.[124] reported that elevated plasma levels of IL-6 in depressed patients treated with fluoxetine were decreased in six out of 22 patients and, increased levels of IL-1 and IL-2 for depressives were reversed by treatment with imipramine, a tricyclic antidepressant.[123] However, the production of TNF in depressed patients was not altered by meclobemide, a monoamine oxidase inhibitor.[125]

10.5 Directions for future research: clinical implications of immunity in depression

The factors that account for individual differences in the rate and severity of disease progression are not fully understood. However, there is increasing evidence to suggest that behaviour and multisystem physiological changes that occur during depression come together to exacerbate the course of many chronic diseases. In the following sections, several pertinent disease examples are presented in relation to relevant psycho-neuroimmunology processes in depression.

10.5.1 Cardiovascular disease

Atherosclerosis is now thought to be an inflammatory process that involves a series of steps,[126] each of which appears to be impacted by stress and/or depression. Activated macrophages within the vascular system secrete pro-inflammatory cytokines, which in turn lead to expression of adhesion molecules. With recruitment of immune cells to the vascular cell wall or endothelium and the release of inflammatory cytokines, the vascular endothelium expresses adhesion molecules that facilitate further binding of immune cells. Importantly, psychological and physical stressors increase the release of pro-inflammatory cytokines and expression of adhesion molecules that tether ('slow down') and bind immune cells to the vascular endothelium.[127,128] Moreover, it appears that depression is associated with endothelium activation. Acute coronary patients who are depressed show an increased expression of an adhesion molecule that is released following activation of the vascular endothelium (i.e. soluble intracellular adhesion molecule).[65] Importantly, this molecular marker of endothelial activation, as well as IL-6, predicts risk of future myocardial infarction.

10.5.2 Infectious disease risk

Compelling evidence has shown that inescapable stress, a putative animal model of depression, increases susceptibility to some viral diseases via alterations in immune function.[129] In humans, prospective epidemiological studies and experimental viral challenge studies show that individuals reporting more psychological stress have a higher incidence and a greater severity of certain infectious illnesses, such as the common cold.[93] In most studies, immune correlations were not obtained, although stress-related increases of IL-6 temporally predict greater symptom severity in persons inoculated with influenza A. Moreover, experimental vaccinations have been used to examine the disease-specific and integrated *in vivo* action of the immune system in relation to psychological stress.

As reviewed in this volume (Chapter 7), HIV infection also shows a highly variable course. Depression, bereavement, and maladaptive coping responses to stress (including the stress of HIV infection itself) have all been shown to predict the rate of immune system decay in HIV patients. Immune system decline and HIV replication are particularly rapid in patients living under chronic stress (e.g. gay men who conceal their homosexuality) and in patients with high levels of sympathetic nervous system activity (e.g. socially inhibited introverts).[130,131] Tissue culture studies have shown that sympathetic nervous system neurotransmitters and glucocorticoids can accelerate HIV replication by rendering T lymphocytes more vulnerable to infection and suppressing production of the antiviral cytokines that help cells limit viral replication.[132] Current research is focusing on pharmacological strategies to block the effects of stress neuroendocrine hormones on chronic viral infections such as HIV.

10.5.3 Rheumatoid arthritis: neuroimmune mechanisms

In a negative feedback loop, pro-inflammatory cytokines stimulate the HPA axis resulting in the secretion of glucocorticoids, which in turn suppress the immune response. However, it is thought that in autoimmune disorders such as rheumatoid arthritis (RA) the counter-regulatory glucocorticoid response is not fully achieved. In animals that are susceptible to arthritis, there is a central hypothalamic defect in the biosynthesis of CRH, blunted induction of ACTH and adrenal steroids, and decreased adrenal steroid receptor activation in immune target tissues which together contribute to a weak HPA response (i.e. inability to suppress the progression of an autoimmune response).[133] RA patients also show a relative hypofunctioning of the HPA axis despite the degree of inflammation.[134]

In a meta-analysis of RA studies, Dickens *et al.*[135] found that depression was more common in patients with RA than in healthy controls. Stress and depression can lead to HPA axis activation and increases of pro-inflammatory cytokines, and recent data suggest that stressful events, particularly interpersonal ones, provoke symptoms of disease such as greater pain and functional limitations in RA patients.[136] For example, negative self-beliefs (e.g. helplessness) predicted greater flare activity in a group of patients undergoing a 3-month clinical drug trial. Moreover, the presence of depression in RA patients undergoing stress is associated with exaggerated increases of IL-6, a biomarker predictive of disease progression.[66] Conversely, administration of a psychological intervention that decreases emotional distress produced improvements in clinician-rated disease activity in RA patients, although immunological mediators were not measured.[137]

10.6 Summary

Psychoneuroimmunological research has shown that depression is related to many aspects of immune function, including enumerative changes, functional changes, and changes in the expression of cytokines. The relationship between depression and immune changes is complex, and contradictory findings have been reported partially due to differences in study populations and methodologies. Nevertheless, meta-analyses have shown that a host of specific immunological changes reliably occur in depressed persons. Recent evidence suggests that the immune system may impact on behaviour and that abnormal cytokine expression may contribute to depressive symptoms in certain at-risk populations (e.g. older adults). The mechanisms that lead to increased morbidity and mortality in depression are not fully understood, but initial findings implicate psychoneuroimmunological mechanisms. The future of psychoneuroimmunology in the study of depression will probably be led by studies that are sensitive to the broad nuances of psychological and behavioural determinants and how these factors alter immunity and predict individual differences in progression and severity of specific disease outcomes. Understanding these relationships is critical to the development of behavioural and/or psychopharmacological interventions that have the potential to alter neuroimmune mechanisms and clinical outcomes.

Acknowledgements

The research described in this chapter was supported by National Institutes of Health grants AA10215, AA13239, DA16541, MH55253, AG18367, T32-MH19925, and MOIRR00865; and the Cousins Center for Psychoneuroimmunology at the UCLA Neuropsychiatric Institute.

References

1 **Zorrilla EP, Luborsky L, McKay JR, et al.** (2001). The relationship of depression and stressors to immunological assays: a meta-analytic review. *Brain Behav Immun* **15**: 199–226.

2 **American Psychiatric Association** (2000). *Diagnostic and Statistical Manual of Mental Disorders* (4th edn revised) Washington, DC: American Psychiatric Association.

3 **Rapaport MH, Judd LL, Schettler PJ, et al.** (2002). A descriptive analysis of minor depression. *Am J Psychiatry* **159**: 637–43.

4 **Kessler RC, McGonagle KA, Zhao SY, et al.** (1994). Lifetime and 12-month prevalence of DSM-III-R psychiatric disorders in the United States: results from the National Comorbidity Study. *Arch Gen Psychiatry* **51**: 8–19.

5 **Barrett JE, Barrett JA, Oxman TE, Gerber PD** (1988). The prevalence of psychiatric disorders in a primary care practice. *Arch Gen Psychiatry* **45**: 1100–6.

6 **Barry KL, Fleming MF, Manwell LB, Copeland LA, Appel S** (1998). Prevalence of and factors associated with current and lifetime depression in older adult primary care patients. *Fam Med* **30**: 366–71.

7 **Magni G, Schifano F, de Leo D** (1986). Assessment of depression in an elderly medical population. *J Affect Disord* **11**: 121–4.

8 **Feldman E, Mayou R, Hawton K, Ardern M, Smith EB** (1987). Psychiatric disorder in medical inpatients. *Q J Med* **63**: 405–12.

9 **Berger AK, Small BJ, Forsell Y, Winblad B, Backman L** (1998). Preclinical symptoms of major depression in very old age: a prospective longitudinal study. *Am J Psychiatry* **155**: 1039–43.

10 **Lyness JM, Caine ED, Conwell Y, King DA, Cox C** (1993). Depressive symptoms, medical illness, and functional status in depressed psychiatric inpatients. *Am J Psychiatry* **150**: 910–15.

11 **Hays RD, Wells KB, Sherbourne CD, Rogers W, Spritzer K** (1995). Functioning and well-being outcomes of patients with depression compared with chronic general medical illnesses. *Arch Gen Psychiatry* **52**: 11–19.

12 **Bruce ML, Leaf PJ, Rozal GP, Florio L, Hoff RA** (1994). Psychiatric status and 9-year mortality data in the New Haven Epidemiologic Catchment Area Study. *Am J Psychiatry* **151**: 716–21.

13 **Herrmann C, Brand-Driehorst S, Kaminsky B, Leibing E, Staats H, Rüger U** (1998). Diagnostic groups and depressed mood as predictors of 22-month mortality in medical inpatients. *Psychosom Med* **60**: 570–7.

14 **Rovner BW** (1993). Depression and increased risk of mortality in the nursing home patient. *Am J Med* **94**: 19S–22S.

15 **Frasure-Smith N, Lespérance F, Talajic M** (1993). Depression following myocardial infarction: impact on 6-month survival. *JAMA* **270**: 1819–25.

16 **Frasure-Smith N, Lespérance F, Talajic M** (1995). The impact of negative emotions on prognosis following myocardial infarction. Is it more than depression? *Health Psychol* **14**: 388–98.

17 **Benca RM, Obermeyer WH, Thisted RA, Gillin JC** (1992). Sleep and psychiatric disorders: a meta analysis. *Arch Gen Psychiatry* **49**: 651–68.

18 **Dew MA, Hoch CC, Buysse DJ, et al.** (2003). Healthy older adults' sleep predicts all-cause mortality at 4 to 19 years of follow-up. *Psychosom Med* **65**: 63–73.

19 **Owens MJ, Nemeroff CB** (1991). Physiology and pharmacology of corticotropin-releasing factor. *Pharmacol Rev* **91**: 425–73.

20 **Friedman EM, Irwin M** (1995). A role for CRH and the sympathetic nervous system in stress-induced immunosuppression. *Ann NY Acad Sci* **771**: 396–418.

21 Friedman EM, Irwin M (1997). Modulation of immune cell function by the autonomic nervous system. *Pharmacol Ther* **74**: 27–38.

22 Irwin M, Brown M, Patterson T, Hauger R, Mascovich A, Grant I (1991). Neuropeptide Y and natural killer cell activity: findings in depression and Alzheimer caregiver stress. *FASEB J* **5**: 3100–7.

23 Madden KS, Sanders VM, Felten DL (1995). Catecholamine influences and sympathetic neural modulation of immune responsiveness. *Annu Rev Pharmacol Toxicol* **35**: 417–48.

24 Sanders VM, Straub RH (2002). Norepinephrine, the beta-adrenergic receptor, and immunity. *Brain Behav Immun* **16**: 290–332.

25 Moynihan JA, Stevens SY (2001). Mechanisms of stress-induced modulation of immunity in animals. In Cohen N (ed.) *Psychoneuroimmunology*. San Diego, CA: Academic Press, 227–50.

26 Dhabhar FS, Miller AH, McEwen BS, Spencer RL (1996). Stress-induced changes in blood leukocyte distribution. Role of adrenal steroid hormones. *J Immunol* **157**: 1638–44.

27 Irwin M, Caldwell C, Smith TL, Brown S, Schuckit MA, Gillin JC (1990). Major depressive disorder, alcoholism, and reduced natural killer cell cytotoxicity: role of severity of depressive symptoms and alcohol consumption. *Arch Gen Psychiatry* **47**: 713–19.

28 Irwin M, Smith TL, Gillin JC (1987). Low natural killer cytotoxicity in major depression. *Life Sci* **41**: 2127–33.

29 Maes M, Lambrechts J, Bosmans E, *et al.* (1992). Evidence for a systemic immune activation during depression: results of leukocyte enumeration by flow cytometry in conjunction with monoclonal antibody staining. *Psychol Med* **22**: 45–53.

30 Kronfol Z, Turner R, Nasrallah H, Winokur G (1984). Leukocyte regulation in depression and schizophrenia. *Psychiatry Res* **13**: 13–18.

31 Irwin M, Patterson TL, Smith TL, *et al.* (1990). Reduction of immune function in life stress and depression. *Biol Psychiatry* **27**: 22–30.

32 Herbert TB, Cohen S (1993). Depression and immunity—a meta-analytic review. *Psychol Bull* **113**: 472–86.

33 Evans DL, Folds JD, Petitto JM, *et al.* (1992). Circulating natural killer cell phenotypes in men and women with major depression. *Arch Gen Psychiatry* **49**: 388–95.

34 Schleifer SJ, Keller SE, Bond RN, Cohen J, Stein M (1989). Major depressive disorder and immunity: Role of age, sex, severity, and hospitalization. *Arch Gen Psychiatry* **46**: 81–7.

35 Kronfol Z, House JD (1985). Depression, hypothalamic-pituitary adrenocortical activity and lymphocyte function. *Psychopharmacol Bull* **21**: 476–8.

36 Kronfol Z, Silva J, Jr, Greden J, Dembinski S, Gardner R, Carroll B (1983). Impaired lymphocyte function in depressive illness. *Life Sci* **33**: 241–7.

37 Albrecht J, Helderman JH, Schlesser MA, Rush AJ (1985). A controlled study of cellular immune function in affective disorders before and during somatic therapy. *Psychiatry Res* **15**: 185–93.

38 Syvalahti E, Eskola J, Ruuskanen O, Laine T (1985). Nonsuppression of cortisol in depression and immune function. *Prog Neuropsychopharmacol Biol Psychiatry* **9**: 413–22.

39 Schleifer SJ, Keller SE, Siris SG, Davis KL, Stein M (1985). Depression and immunity: Lymphocyte function in ambulatory depressed patients, hospitalized schizophrenic patients, and patients hospitalized for herniorrhaphy. *Arch Gen Psychiatry* **42**: 129–33.

40 Kronfol Z, House JD, Silva J, Greden J, Carroll BJ (1986). Depression, urinary free cortisol excretion, and lymphocyte function. *Br J Psychiatry* **148**: 70–3.

41 Calabrese JR, Skwerer RG, Barna B, *et al.* (1986). Depression, immunocompetence, and prostaglandins of the E-series. *Psychiatry Res* **17**: 41–47.

42 Lowy MT, Reder AT, Gormley GJ, Meltzer HY (1988). Comparison of *in vivo* and *in vitro* glucocorticoid sensitivity in depression: relationship to the dexamethasone suppression test. *Biol Psychiatry* **24**: 619–30.

43 Maes M, Bosmans E, Suy E, Minner B, Raus J (1989). Impaired lymphocyte stimulation by mitogens in severely depressed patients. A complex interface with HPA-axis hyperfunction, noradrenergic activity and the aging process. *Br J Psychiatry* **155**: 793–8.

44 Altshuler LL, Plaeger-Marshall S, Richeimer S, Daniels M, Baxter LR, Jr (1989). Lymphocyte function in major depression. *Acta Psychiatr Scand* **80**: 132–6.

45 Darko DF, Gillin JC, Risch SC, et al. (1989). Mitogen-stimulated lymphocyte proliferation and pituitary hormones in major depression. *Biol Psychiatry* **26**: 145–55.

46 Kronfol Z, Nair M, Goodson J, Goel K, Haskett R, Schwartz S (1989). Natural killer cell activity in depressive illness: preliminary report. *Biol Psychiatry* **26**: 753–6.

47 Cosyns P, Maes M, Vandewoude M, Stevens WJ, DeClerck LS, Schotte C (1989). Impaired mitogen-induced lymphocyte responses and the hypothalamic-pituitary-adrenal axis in depressive disorders. *J Affect Disord* **16**: 41–8.

48 Bartoloni C, Guidi L, Antico L, et al. (1990). Psychological status of institutionalized aged: Influences on immune parameters and endocrinologic correlates. *Int J Neurosci* **51**: 279–81.

49 McAdams C, Leonard BE (1993). Neutrophil and monocyte phagocytosis in depressed patients. Prog Neuropsychopharmacol *Biol Psychiatry* **17**: 971–84.

50 Birmaher B, Rabin BS, Garcia MR, et al. (1994). Cellular immunity in depressed, conduct disorder, and normal adolescents: role of adverse life events. *J Am Acad Child Adolesc Psychiatry* **33**: 671–8.

51 Stein M, Miller AH, Trestman RL (1991). Depression, the immune system, and health and illness. *Arch Gen Psychiatry* **48**: 171–7.

52 Irwin M (2000). Depression and immunity. In Ader R, Felten D, Cohen N (eds) *Psychoneuroimmunology* (3rd edn) San Diego, CA: Academic Press, 383–98.

53 Irwin M (2002). Psychoneuroimmunology of depression: clinical implications (Presidential Address). *Brain Behav Immun* **16**: 1–16.

54 Mohl PC, Huang L, Bowden C, Fischbach M, Vogtsberer K, Talal N (1987). Natural killer cell activity in major depression. *Am J Psychiatry* **144**: 1619.

55 Kronfol Z (2003). Cytokine regulation in major depression. In: Kronfol, Z (ed). *Cytokines and mental health* Boston, MA: Kluwer Academic, 259–80.

56 Seidel A, Arolt V, Hunstiger M, Rink L, Behnisch A, Kirchner H (1995). Cytokine production and serum proteins in depression. *Scand J Immunol* **41**: 534–8.

57 Irwin M, Costlow C, Williams H, Artin KH, Chan CY, Stinson DL (1998). Cellular immunity to varicella-zoster virus in patients with major depression. *J Infect Dis* **178**: 5104–8.

58 Dhabhar FS (2000). Acute stress enhances while chronic stress suppresses skin immunity. The role of stress hormones and leukocyte trafficking. *Ann NY Acad Sci* **917**: 876–93.

59 Hickie I, Hickie C, Lloyd A, Silove D, Wakefield D (1993). Impaired *in vivo* immune responses in patients with melancholia. *Br J Psychiatry* **162**: 651–7.

60 Shinkawa M, Nakayama K, Hirai H, Monma M, Sasaki H (2002). Depression and immunoreactivity in disabled older patients. *J Am Geriatr Soc* **50**: 198–9.

61 Maes M, Smith R, Scharpe S (1995). The monocyte-T-lymphocyte hypothesis of major depression. *Psychoneuroendocrinology* **20**: 111–16.

62 Maes M, Scharpe S, Van Grootel L, et al. (1992). Higher alpha 1-antritrypsin, haptoglobin, ceruloplasmin and lower retinol binding protein plasma levels during depression: further evidence for the existence of an inflammatory response during that illness. *J Affect Disord* **24**: 183–92.

63 Musselman DL, Miller AH, Porter MR, *et al.* (2001). Higher than normal plasma interleukin-6 concentrations in cancer patients with depression: preliminary findings. *Am J Psychiatry* **158**: 1252–7.

64 Maes M, Meltzer HY, Bosmans E, *et al.* (1995). Increased plasma concentrations of interleukin-6, soluble interleukin-6, soluble interleukin-2 and transferrin receptor in major depression. *J Affect Disord* **34**: 301–9.

65 Lespérance F, Frasure-Smith N, Theroux P, Irwin M. (2004) Association between major depression, and levels of soluble intercellular adhesion molecule, interleukin-6 and C-reactive protein in patients with recent acute coronary syndromes. *Am J Psychiatry* **161**: 271–7.

66 Zautra AJ, Yocum D, Villanueva I, *et al.* (2004) Immune activation and depression in women with rheumatoid arthritis. *J Rheumatol* **31**, 457–63.

67 Miller AH (2003). Cytokines and sickness behavior: implications for cancer care and control. *Brain Behav Immun* **17** (Suppl 1): S132–4.

68 Irwin M, Miller C (2000). Decreased natural killer cell responses and altered interleukin-6 and interleukin-10 production in alcoholism: an interaction between alcohol dependence and African-American ethnicity. *Alcohol Clin Exp Res* **24**: 560–9.

69 Irwin M, Mascovich A, Gillin JC, Willoughby R, Pike JL, Smith TL (1994). Partial sleep deprivation reduces natural killer cell activity in humans. *Psychosom Med* **56**: 493–8.

70 Irwin M, McClintick J, Costlow C, Fortner M, White J, Gillin JC (1996). Partial night sleep deprivation reduces natural killer and cellular immune responses in humans. *FASEB J* **10**: 643–53.

71 Irwin M, Smith TL, Gillin JC (1992). Electroencephalographic sleep and natural killer activity in depressed patients and control subjects. *Psychosom Med* **54**: 10–21.

72 Cover H, Irwin M (1994). Immunity and depression: insomnia, retardation and reduction of natural killer cell activity. *J Behav Med* **17**: 217–23.

73 Castanon N, Leonard BE, Neveu PJ, Yirmiya R (2002). Effects of antidepressants on cytokine production and actions. *Brain Behav Immun* **6**: 569–74.

74 Goujon E, Parnet P, Aubert A, Goodall G, Dantzer R (1995). Corticosterone regulates behavioral effects of lipopolysaccharide and interleukin-1β in mice. *Am J Physiol* **269**: R154–9

75 Barden N (1999). Regulation of corticosteroid recetpor gene expression in depression and antidepressant action. *J Psychiatry Neurosci* **24**: 25–39.

76 Yirmiya R, Weidenfeld J, Pollak Y, *et al.* (1999). Cytokines, 'depression due to a general medical condition', and antidepressant drugs. *Adv Exp Med Biol* **461**: 283–316.

77 Yaron I, Shirazi L, Judovich R, *et al.* (1999). Fluoxetine and amitriptyline inhibit nitric oxide, prostaglandin E2, and hyaluronic acid production in human synovial cells and synovial tissue cultures. *Arthritis Rheum* **42**: 2561–8.

78 Hindmarch F (2001). Expanding the horizons of depression: beyond the monoamine hypothesis. *Hum Psychopharmacol* **16**: 203–18.

79 Irwin M, Lacher U, Caldwell C (1992). Depression and reduced natural killer cytotoxicity: a longitudinal study of depressed patients and control subjects. *Psychol Med* **22**: 1045–50.

80 Schleifer SJ, Keller SE, Bartlett JA (1999). Depression and immunity: clinical factors and therapeutic course. *Psychiatry Res* **85**: 63–9.

81 Frank MG, Hendricks SE, Johnson DR, Wieseler JL, Burke WJ (1999). Antidepressants augment natural killer cell activity: *in vivo* and *in vitro*. *Neuropsychobiology* **39**: 18–24.

82 Kim Y, Suh IB, Kim H, *et al.* (2002). The plasma levels of interleukin-12 in schizophrenia, major depression, and bipolar mania: effects of psychotropic drugs. *Mol Psychiatry* **7**: 1107–14.

83 Kenis G, Maes M (2002). Effects of antidepressants on the production of cytokines. *Int J Neuropsychopharmacol* **5**: 401–12.

84 Pike JL, Smith TL, Hauger R, *et al.* (1997). Chronic life stress alters sympathetic neuroendocrine and immune responsivity to an acute psychological stressor in humans. *Psychosom Med* **59**: 447–57.

85 Campagnolo DI, Keller SE, DeLisa JA, Glick TJ, Sipski ML, Schleifer SJ (1994). Alteration of immune system function in tetraplegics: a pilot study. *Am J Phys Med Rehabil* **73**: 387–40.

86 Campagnolo JR, Bartlett JA, Keller SE, Sanchez R, Oza R (1997). Impaired phagocytosis of *Staphylococcus aureus* in complete tetaplegics. *Am J Phys Med Rehabil* **76**: 276–80.

87 Irwin M, Daniels M, Risch SC, Bloom E, Weiner H (1988). Plasma cortisol and natural killer cell activity during bereavement. *Biol Psychiatry* **24**: 173–8.

88 Besedovsky HO, del Rey A (1996). Immune-neuro-endocrine interactions: facts and hypotheses. *Endocr Rev* **17**: 64–102.

89 McEwen BS, Biron CA, Brunson KW, *et al.* (1997). The role of adrenocorticoids as modulators of immune function in health and disease: neural, endocrine and immune interactions. *Brain Res Brain Res Rev* **23**: 79–133.

90 Schobitz B, Reul JM, Holsboer F (1994). The role of the hypothalamic–pituitary–adrenocortical system during inflammatory conditions. *Crit Rev Immunol* **8**: 263–91.

91 Turnbull AV, Rivier CL (1999). Regulation of the hypothalamic–pituitary–adrenal axis by cytokines: actions and mechanisms of action. *Physiol Rev* **79**: 1–71.

92 Maes M, Bosmans E, Meltzer HY, Scharpe S, Suy E (1993). Interleukin-1β: a putative mediator of HPA axis hyperactivity in major depression? *Am J Psychiatry* **150**: 1189–93.

93 Cohen S, Miller G (2000). Stress, immunity and susceptibility to upper respiratory infection. In Ader R, Felten D, Cohen N (eds) *Psychoneuroimmunology* (3rd edn). San Diego, CA: Academic Press, 499–509.

94 Sopori ML, Kozak W (1998). Immunomodulatory effects of cigarette smoke. *J Neuroimmunol* **83**: 148–56.

95 Rosecrans JA, Karin LD (1998). Effects of nicotine on the hypothalamic-pituitary-axis (HPA) and immune function: Introduction to the Sixth Nicotine Round Table Satellite, American Society of Addiction Medicine Nicotine Dependence Meeting. *Psychoneuroendocrinology* **23**: 95–102.

96 McAllister-Sistilli CG, Caggiula AR, Knopf S, Rose CA, Miller AL, Donney EC (1998). The effects of nicotine on the immune system. *Psychoneuroendocrinology* **23**: 175–87.

97 Andreoli AV, Keller SE, Rabaeus M, Marin P, Bartlett JA, Taban C (1993). Depression and immunity: age, severity, and clinical course. *Brain Behav Immun* **7**: 279–92.

98 Jung W, Irwin M (1999). Reduction of natural killer cytotoxic activity in major depression: interaction between depression and cigarette smoking. *Psychosom Med* **61**: 263–70.

99 Mendall MA, Patel P, Asante M, *et al.* (1997). Relationship of serum cytokine concentrations to cardiovascular risk factors and coronary heart disease. *Heart* **78**: 237–77.

100 Linkins RW, Comstock GW (1990). Depressed mood and development of cancer. *Am J Epidemiol* **132**: 962–72.

101 Schuckit MA (1986). Genetic and clinical implications of alcoholism and affective disorder. *Am J Psychiatry* **143**: 140–7.

102 Irwin M (2003). Cytokines, immunity, and disordered sleep. In Kronfol Z (ed) *Cytokines and Mental Health*. Boston, MA: Kluwer Academic, 403–21.

103 Hall M, Baum A, Buysse DJ, Prigerson HG, Kupfer DJ, Reynolds CF, III (1998). Sleep as a mediator of the stress–immune relationship. *Psychosom Med* **60**: 48–51.

104 Irwin M, Clark C, Kennedy B, Christian Gillin J, Ziegler M (2003). Nocturnal catecholamines and immune function in insomniacs, depressed patients, and control subjects. *Brain Behav Immun* **17**, 365–72.

105 Savard J, Laroche L, Simard S, Ivers H, Morin CM (2003). Chronic insomnia and immune functioning. *Psychosom Med* **65**: 211–21.

106 Irwin M, Gillin JC, Dang J, Weissman J, Phillips E, Ehlers CL (2002). Sleep deprivation as a probe of homeostatic sleep regulation in primary alcoholics. *Biol Psychiatry* **51**: 632–41.

107 Irwin M, Miller C, Gillin JC, Demodena A, Ehlers CL (2000). Polysomnographic and spectral sleep EEG in primary alcoholics: an interaction between alcohol dependence and African–American ethnicity. *Alcohol Clin Exp Res* **24**: 1376–84.

108 Redwine L, Dang J, Hall M, Irwin M (2003). Disordered sleep, nocturnal cytokines, and immunity in alcoholics. *Psychosom Med* **65**: 75–85.

109 Besedovsky H, Sorkin E, Felix D, Hass H (1977). Hypothalamic changes during the immune response. *Eur J Immunol* **7**: 323–5.

110 Watkins LR, Maier SF (1999). Implications of immune-to-brain communication for sickness and pain. *Proc Natl Acad Sci USA* **96**: 7710–13.

111 Berkenbosch F, VanOers J, DelRey A, Tilders F, Besedovsky H (1987). Corticotropin-releasing factor-producing neurons in the rat activated by interleukin-1. *Science* **238**: 524–6.

112 Dantzer R (2001). Cytokine-induced sickness behavior. Where do we stand? *Brain Behav Immun* **15**: 7–24.

113 Watkins LR, Maier SF (2000). The pain of being sick: implications of immune-to-brain communication for understanding pain. *Annu Rev Psychol* **51**: 29–57.

114 Opp MR, Toth LA (2003). Neural–immune interactions in the regulation of sleep. *Front Biosci* **8**: D768–79.

115 Irwin M, Rinetti G, Redwine L, Motivala S, Dang J, Ehlers C (2004). Nocturnal proinflammatory cytokine-associated sleep disturbances in abstinent African American alcoholics. *Brain Behav Immun* **18(4)**: 349–60.

116 Bower JE, Ganz PA, Aziz N, Fahey JL (2002). Fatigue and proinflammatory cytokine activity in breast cancer survivors. *Psychosom Med* **64**: 604–11.

117 Gupta S, Aggarwal S, See D, Starr A (1997). Cytokine production by adherent and non-adherent mononuclear cells in chronic fatigue syndrome. *J Psychiatr Res* **31**: 149–56.

118 Cannon JG, Angel JB, Abad LW, *et al.* (1997). Interleukin-1 beta, interleukin-1 receptor antagonist, and soluble interleukin-1 receptor type II secretion in chronic fatigue syndrome. *J Clin Immunol* **17**: 253–61.

119 Capuron L, Gumnick JF, Musselman DL, *et al.* (2002). Neurobehavioral effects of interferon-alpha in cancer patients: phenomenology and paroxetine responsiveness of symptom dimensions. *Neuropsychopharmacology* **26**: 643–52.

120 Musselman DL, Lawson DH, Gumnick JF, *et al.* (2001). Paroxetine for the prevention of depression induced by high-dose interferon alfa. *N Engl J Med* **344**: 961–6.

121 Capuron L, Ravaud A (1999). Prediction of the depressive effects of interferon alfa therapy by the patient's initial affective state. *N Engl J Med* **340**: 1370.

122 Reichenberg A, Yirmiya R, Schuld A, *et al.* (2001). Cytokine-associated emotional and cognitive disturbances in humans. *Arch Gen Psychiatry* **58**: 445–52.

123 Kubera MA, Symbirtsev A, Basta-Kaim A, Borycz J, Roman A, Papp M, Claesson M (1996). Effect of chronic treatment with imipramine on interleukin 1 and interleukin 2 production by splenocytes obtained from rats subjected to a chronic mild stress model of depression. *Pol J Pharmacol* **48(5)**: 503–6.

124 Sluzewska A, Rybakowski JK, Laciak M, Mackiewicz A, Sobieska M, Wiktorowicz K (1995). Interleukin-6 serum levels in depressed patients before and after treatment with fluoxetine. *Ann NY Acad Sci* **762**: 474–6.

125 Landmann R, Schaub B, Link S, Wacker HR (1997). Unaltered monocyte function in patients with major depression before and after three months of antidepressive therapy. *Biol Psychiatry* **41**: 675–81.

126 Black PH, Garbutt LD (2002). Stress, inflammation and cardiovascular disease. *J Psychosom Res* **52**: 1–23.

127 Redwine L, Snow S, Mills P, Irwin M (2003). Acute psychological stress: effects on chemotaxis and cellular adhesion molecule expression. *Psychosom Med* **65**: 598–603.

128 Goebel MU, Mills PJ, Irwin MR, Ziegler MG (2000). Interleukin-6 and tumor necrosis factor-alpha production after acute psychological stress, exercise, and infused isoproterenol: differential effects and pathways. *Psychosom Med* **62**: 591–8.

129 Sheridan JF, Dobbs C, Brown D, Zwilling B (1994). Psychoneuroimmunology: stress effects on pathogenesis and immunity during infection. *Clin Microbiol Rev* **7**, 200–12.

130 Cole SW, Naliboff BD, Kemeny ME, Griswold MP, Fahey JL, Zack JA (2001). Impaired response to HAART in HIV-infected individuals with high autonomic nervous system activity. *Proc Natl Acad Sci USA*, **98**: 12695–700.

131 Cole SW, Kemeny ME, Taylor SE (1997). Social identity and physical health: accelerated HIV progression in rejection-sensitive gay men. J Pers Soc Psychol **72**(2): 320–35.

132 Cole SW, Korin YD, Fahey JL, Zack JA (1998). Norepinephrine accelerates HIV replication via protein kinase A-dependent effects on cytokine production. *J Immunol* **161**(2): 610–6.

133 Sternberg EM, Chrousos GP, Wilder RL, Gold PW (1992). The stress response and the regulation of inflammatory disease. *Ann Int Med* **117**: 854–866.

134 Crofford LJ, Kalogeras KT, Mastorakos G, *et al.* (1997). Circadian relationships between interleukin (IL)-6 and hypothalamic–pituitary–adrenal axis hormones: Failure of IL-6 to cause sustained hypercortisolism in patients with early untreated rheumatoid arthritis. *J Clin Endocrinol Metab* **82**: 1279–83.

135 Dickens C, McGowan L, Clark-Carter D, Creed F (2002). Depression in rheumatoid arthritis: A systematic review of the literature with meta-analysis. *Psychosom Med* **64**: 52–60.

136 Zautra AJ, Smith BW (2001). Depression and reactivity to stress in older women with rheumatoid arthritis and osteoarthritis. *Psychosom Med* **63**: 687–96.

137 Smyth JM, Stone AA, Hurewitz A, Kaell A (1999). Effects of writing about stressful experiences on symptom reduction in patients with asthma or rheumatoid arthritis: a randomized trial [see comments]. *JAMA* **281**(14): 1304–9.

Chapter 11

Wound healing and psychoneuroimmunology

Eric V. Yang and Ronald Glaser

11.1 Introduction

Injuries are common occurrences in everyday life. In order to survive, humans have maintained the ability to regenerate tissues in order to heal injuries. Epithelial tissues, such as the skin and the epithelial lining of the digestive tract and the respiratory system, regenerate most easily, while other tissues, such as liver, bone, and skeletal muscle, can undergo repair to varying degrees. Since the skin is our shield from the environment and a means of interacting with it, it is constantly subjected to various insults and injuries.

Wounds are categorized as either acute or chronic. Acute wounds are those that heal in a timely fashion, while chronic wounds are, according to the Wound Healing Society, those 'that have failed to proceed through an orderly and timely process to produce an anatomic and functional integrity or proceed through the repair process without establishing a sustained and functional result'.[1] Common injuries to the skin include cuts, abrasions, and burns. Poor treatment of a wound can result in delayed healing and/or an unsightly scar.

Several factors, including psychological stress, have been shown to affect the process of wound healing. In this chapter we discuss the process of wound healing in response to injury to the skin, i.e. cutaneous wound healing, focusing on the impact of psychological stress on this process. We direct the reader to recent excellent publications for a more detailed discussion of the many processes involved in wound healing.[2–5]

11.2 The biological/clinical context

11.2.1 The cutaneous wound-healing process

The adult human skin consists of two tissue layers: the epidermis, composed of the keratinized stratified epithelial cells, and the underlying collagen-rich dermis. Additionally, it contains epithelially derived appendages, i.e. hair and sweat glands, that project into the dermis. Injury to the skin triggers a precise set of developmental processes programmed to regain its physical and functional integrity.[5–7] Cutaneous wound healing comprises distinct but temporally overlapping processes including clot formation, inflammation, cellular migration and proliferation, wound contraction, and remodelling (Fig. 11.1). The relative importance of these stages, the speed at which

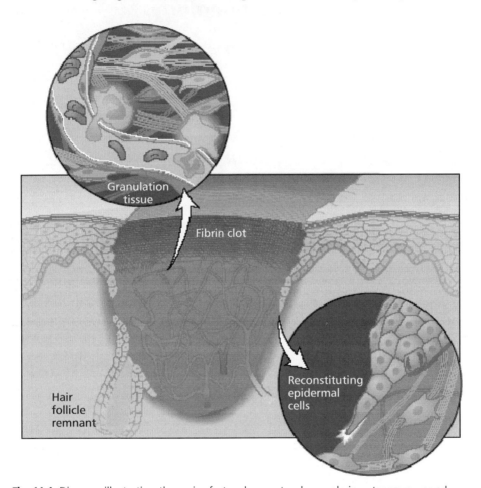

Fig. 11.1 Diagram illustrating the major factors known to play a role in cutaneous wound healing. During clot formation, plasma factors and platelets released from damaged blood vessels form a fibrin clot to temporarily cover the injured area. Within hours after wounding, epithelial cells and remnants of epithelial appendages (e.g. hair follicles) migrate from the wound edge. During the inflammatory phase, inflammatory cells (depicted as blue cells) respond to chemoattractants, escape from the blood vessels through the modulation of integrin expression and secretion of MMPs, and invade the wound site. The presence of cytokines and growth factors secreted by inflammatory cells in the wound further attracts fibroblasts and endothelial cells. The proliferation of these cells and subsequent angiogenesis in the wound result in the formation of the granulation tissue. Remodelling of the wound results in scar formation. (Reproduced with permission from P. Martin (1997) *Science* **276**: 738–46.)

healing occurs, and the extent of scar formation depend on the degree of tissue loss and the depth of the wound. For example, in partial-thickness wounds remnants of cutaneous appendages are left behind and therefore heal rapidly with minimal or no scarring. However, deeper wounds, which are characterized by the loss of more epidermal and dermal components, have a progressively slower rate of wound healing and increased scar formation. For instance, healing of full-thickness wounds, in which the entire dermis is lost, depends to a greater extent on the proliferative phase and wound contraction and results in significant scarring. Studies of human and animal models have identified many of the key cellular players and regulatory growth factors, including extracellular matrix (ECM) related signals, cytokines, and growth factors, involved in cutaneous wound healing.[8,9] In this chapter, we give an overview of the major aspects of acute wound healing of injured skin.

11.2.1.1 Clot formation

Following injury, blood coagulation at the wound site is the first and perhaps the most important process in cutaneous wound healing. Its purpose is to prevent further blood loss and to protect the wound from contamination by the environment, and therefore it is critical for the survival of the injured individual. The release of platelets from damaged vessels exposes them to the connective tissue and factors released by damaged cells. These platelets aggregate in the early extracellular matrix of the wound, called the provisional matrix, which is composed mainly of fibrin, fibronectin, vitronectin, thrombospondin, and type I and IV collagen. Contact of platelets with collagen and with each other, which is mediated by fibrinogen and von Willebrand factor, triggers their aggregation and stimulates the release of molecules stored in granules. These factors, which include platelet-derived growth factor (PDGF), transforming growth factor α (TGF-α), TGF-β, fibroblast growth factor 2 (FGF-2), platelet-activating factor (PAF), monocyte chemotactic protein 1 (MCP-1), interleukin 8 (IL-8), growth-regulated oncogene α (GRO-α), and serotonin, are important for initiating healing.[10–13] For example, both PDGF and TGF-β are multifunctional and play roles in the recruitment of cells to the wound site and the subsequent modulation of cell activity. PDGF is chemotactic for neutrophils and monocytes and thus helps to initiate the inflammatory phase. In addition, PDGF and TGF-β induce the migration of fibroblasts from the dermis at the wound margin to the site of injury.

11.2.1.2 The inflammatory phase

One of the major functions of the wound inflammatory response is to bring inflammatory cells to the wound site. This is achieved by a combination of factors including increased vascular permeability proximal to the injury and chemotaxis. The inflammatory phase can be divided into early inflammation, which is dominated by neutrophils, and late inflammation, which is characterized by an abundance of macrophages and lymphocytes.

As previously mentioned, a number of chemoattractants from platelets and injured tissue, including fragments of the extracellular matrix, PDGF, tumour necrosis factor α (TNF-α), IL-1, complement factors, and platelet factor IV, are present at the site of injury. Release of these molecules and changes in the expression patterns of cell adhesion molecules subsequently promote the invasion of the site of injury by neutrophils, monocytes, and lymphocytes.[8,14–17] These factors initially induce a rapid migration of neutrophils to the wound site within hours of wounding and become the predominant immune cell type within the first 24–48 h after injury. During their migration, the neutrophils are activated and secrete matrix metalloproteinases (MMPs). MMPs belong to a family of over 20 structurally related endopeptidases that together can degrade components of the extracellular matrix, including those of the provisional matrix and the basement membrane. The secretion of the MMPs elastase and collagenase allows neutrophils to pass through the basement membrane surrounding the blood vessels and escape to the extravascular space. In normal healing, the function of neutrophils is limited to the removal of bacteria contaminating the wound. Therefore, in the absence of infection, the neutrophils undergo programmed cell death (apoptosis), are phagocytosed by macrophages, and have no role in subsequent phases of wound healing.

As neutrophils migrate to the wound, monocytes and lymphocytes are attracted to the injured area by chemotactic factors such as PDGF and subsequently become abundant during the late inflammation phase. While neutrophils have been shown not to be essential to wound healing in the absence of an infection, the presence of macrophages and lymphocytes is critical for this process. In response to the cytokines and growth factors released by neutrophils, such as IL-8, monocytes subsequently accumulate at the site of injury within 48–96 h after wounding. Responding to the wound environment, the infiltrating monocytes are activated and differentiate into macrophages. These phagocytic cells further facilitate the removal of bacteria, neutrophils that have gone through apoptosis, and fragments of damaged tissue, a process referred to as debridement. Apart from their role in debridement of the wound, macrophages are also the major source of cytokines that are important for the healing process, which suggests that they play an integral role in the regulation of wound healing.[18,19] This idea is supported by the results of experiments by Liebovich and Ross[20] showing that depletion of macrophages from wounds in guinea pigs by using hydrocortisone or antimacrophage serum severely delayed debridement and fibroblast proliferation, and thus significantly inhibited wound healing. Furthermore, Danon et al.[21] observed that defective healing in aged mice can be restored by transfer of macrophages from young mice.

The other major component of late inflammation is the lymphocyte. The importance of T lymphocytes in wound healing has been suggested by experiments showing that systemic depletion of T lymphocytes with an anti-CD3 monoclonal antibody can impair wound healing in mice.[22,23] T lymphocytes, particularly CD4+ T lymphocytes, are sources of cytokines that are important for wound healing including IL-1, IL-2, TNF-α, epidermal growth factor (EGF), and TGF-β.[13] It is of interest that surgical wounds in humans contain a higher level of CD4+ T helper cells a week after surgery, while CD8+ T cytotoxic/suppressor cells are observed later prior to wound closure,[14] suggesting that CD4+ T cells may have a stimulatory effect on wound healing while CD8+ T cells may have a downregulatory influence. Although 10–15% of lymphocytes in human wound tissue are B cells, a function for this immune cell in wound healing has yet to be described. However, Cowin et al.[24] hypothesized that B-cell-derived IL-6 may be important for the maintenance of the fibroblast proliferation and matrix deposition.

11.2.1.3 Re-epithelialization and proliferation phase

The inflammatory phase is followed by, but overlaps with, the re-epithelialization stage of wound healing. Within hours of injury, epithelial cells begin to migrate from the epidermal wound edge and from any residual epithelial appendages such as hair follicles and sweat glands (Fig. 11.1). The migrating epithelial cells move into the wound site by extending temporary cytoplasmic protrusions called lammelopodia. Re-epithelialization has been observed to occur in several ways. In one mechanism, there is an apparent interchange of positions among cells at the wound edge, with the epithelial cells 'leapfrogging' over one another. In another model, epithelial cells migrate across a wound in a chain, with each cell maintaining its position. Migrating epithelial cells undergo phenotypic changes brought about by modifications in the cytoskeleton, as well as modulation of cell–cell and cell–matrix contacts. Several factors in the wound have been shown to be stimulatory for epithelial cell migration during re-epithelialization. These include changes in calcium concentration, exposure to fragments of ECM components, loss of cell–cell interactions, and the presence of growth factors and cytokines including EGF, TGF-β, and FGF-7.

As epithelial cells continue to migrate into the wound within 1 or 2 days after injury, EGF, TGF-α, and FGF stimulate those at the wound margin to proliferate. Proteases (such as MMPs) may also be important factors for epithelial proliferation by cleaving growth factors sequestered in the ECM and releasing them into the wound environment. As migrating epithelial cells move over and through the provisional matrix, they make contact with ECM molecules through integrin receptors and begin to secrete MMPs and proteases belonging to the urokinase plasminogen activator (uPA)–plasmin system that remodel the ECM. After the wound is fully covered by the epithelium, migration ceases and basal epithelial cells proliferate to produce a stratified keratinized epithelium.

Chemotactic and mitogenic factors produced during the inflammatory phase also attract fibroblasts and endothelial cells to the wound site and then stimulate them to proliferate, resulting in what is called the granulation tissue. This fragile tissue is composed of a matrix of fibrin, fibronectin, glycosaminoglycans, proliferating fibroblasts and endothelial cells, infiltrating macrophages and lymphocytes, and a high density of blood vessels, giving it a granular red appearance.

The formation of new blood vessels (angiogenesis) is necessary to provide a blood supply to the healing wound in order to deliver the necessary energy-providing factors to highly metabolic cells. Under the influence of mitotic factors such as FGF and VEGF, endothelial cells in the walls of vessels at the wound margin proliferate and form capillary buds. The endothelial cells are activated and secrete serine proteases and MMPs that allow them to digest the wound matrix and migrate into the granulation tissue in response to chemotactic stimuli such as PDGF and FGF-2.

11.2.1.4 Wound contraction

In addition to the chemotactic factors described above, other factors involved in the induction of fibroblast migration are MMPs and their endogenous inhibitors known as tissue inhibitors of metalloproteinases (TIMPs) and proteases of the uPA–plasmin pathway. Mitogenic factors such as FGF, PDGF, and insulin-like growth factor 1 (IGF-1) stimulate fibroblasts to proliferate as they invade the wound. Within days, these cells replace macrophages as the most abundant cell type in the wound. They then undergo phenotypic change to form specialized fibroblasts known as myofibroblasts[25] which align into arrays parallel to the wound surface. Myofibroblasts have cytoskeleton-dependent contractile features that facilitate wound closure by exerting tension on the granulation tissue. After wound closure, myofibroblasts undergo apoptosis and are removed by phagocytic cells, and the wound tension decreases.[26]

11.2.1.5 Remodelling

Remodelling of the wound matrix is the last step of wound healing. Remodelling (both synthesis and degradation) of collagen fibres in the provisional matrix allows the wound to gain strength by reorienting the fibres and hence forming scar tissue. The resulting scar is less cellular than normal skin and does not achieve the same tensile strength as uninjured skin.

Collagen degradation also requires members of the MMP family previously discussed. MMPs are produced by a number of cell types including macrophages, fibroblasts, and epithelial cells. Cytokines, growth factors, hormones, and contact with ECM components can regulate the expression of MMPs at several levels. For example, pro-inflammatory cytokines such as TNF-α and IL-1 appear to be major inductive factors, while TGF-β inhibits collagenase (MMP-1) production and induces synthesis of TIMPs.

Remodelling can occur for several months or years after injury as the healed wound becomes covered with mature tissue. The relative weakness of the scar compared with normal skin results from the difference in the collagen fibre bundle orientation and abnormal molecular cross-linking, i.e. the collagen fibres in normal skin are arranged relatively randomly whereas more of the fibres run in parallel in scar tissue. Apart from the usually undesirable appearance of scar tissue, it tends to contract abnormally so that normal function (e.g. arm and leg movements) can be lost if there are large areas of scarring such as those that occur after burn wounds. In addition, as skin appendages are not replaced in human cutaneous wound healing, large areas of scarring can also significantly affect the respiratory function of the skin and can often lead to mortality.

11.2.2 Factors affecting wound healing

Several factors which can affect the rate of wound healing have been described. They can result in failure of the wound to heal in a timely manner and thus lead to delayed or chronic wound healing.[2,27] These factors can be categorized as clinician-induced, local, and systemic.

Clinician-induced factors are those that clinicians introduce either locally on the wound or systemically to treat a related or unrelated medical condition. They include wound dressings, medications, and other treatments.[28–32]

Local factors are those that affect wound healing at the actual site of injury and include the presence of foreign materials and bacterial infection.[33–36] The effect of bacteria on the wound depends on the balance between the quantity of bacteria and the individual's immune status. The inability of the host's immune system to control bacterial growth in the wound results in infection. Over-abundance of bacteria in the wound can compete with the patient's cells for nutrients and oxygen, and their metabolic byproducts can be toxic to cells participating in wound-healing processes.

Finally, systemic factors are those that affect the individual as a whole and have indirect effects on the wound. These include nutrition, advancing age, and psychological stress. Since the wound-healing process requires the expenditure of a large amount of energy, an adequate intake of nutrients is necessary for its proper progression. Therefore malnutrition may cause delays in this process or even result in chronic wounds.[37–39] The ageing process is another factor that has been shown to have negative effects on wound healing.[40–45] This may be due to the well-known decrements in immune function[46] and increased MMP expression[40,47] associated with the ageing process. Finally, there is a growing literature that shows that psychological stress can affect the wound-healing process. This association is the focus of this chapter.

Although these factors are traditionally classified into separate groups, Ennis and Meneses[2] have proposed an 'overlap model' in which several factors in one, two, or all three categories are present and interact with each other to influence the progression of wound healing.

11.3 Theoretical basis for the role of psychoneuroimmunology

As the inflammatory phase of wound healing has been shown to be a significant stage in cutaneous wound healing, we will begin by briefly reviewing the effects of psychological stress on immune function and health.[48,49]

11.3.1 Roles of the hypothalamic–pituitary–adrenal and sympathetic–adrenal–medullary axes

The effect of stress on the immune response appears to be mediated by bidirectional interactions between the central nervous, endocrine, and immune systems.[48,50–52] Stress-induced activation of the hypothalamic–pituitary–adrenal (HPA) axis influences the immune system by the release of neuroendocrine hormones from the pituitary gland. Responses to signals from the HPA axis are mediated by receptors for neuro-endocrine hormones and neuropeptides on lymphoid and myeloid cells, allowing them either to activate or to downregulate their activities. In addition, receptors for the catecholamines epinephrine and norepinephrine are present on the surfaces of these cells, enabling them to respond to signals from the sympathetic–adrenal–medullary (SAM) axis. Immune cells can be stimulated to release cytokines such as IL-1, which in turn stimulate the increased production of corticotrophin-releasing hormone (CRH) by the hypothalamus. CRH induces the secretion of adrenocorticotropic hormone (ACTH) and cortisol by the pituitary gland and the adrenal cortex, respectively.[53] These 'stress' hormones can subsequently dysregulate immune responses and have potentially detrimental effects on an individual's well-being, including delaying wound healing.

In addition to cytokine production, lymphocytes are capable of producing hormones such as ACTH, growth hormone, and prolactin.[54–57] It has also been shown that various aspects of the immune response, such as proliferation of B and T cells, cytokine production, antibody production, chemotaxis of monocytes and neutrophils, and natural killer (NK) cell cytotoxicity, can be affected by glucocorticoids as well as by peptides such as ACTH, endorphins, substance P, and somatostatin.[58]

Furthermore, primary and secondary lymphoid organs, including bone marrow, thymus, spleen, and lymph nodes, are innervated by noradrenergic sympathetic and peptidergic nerve fibres of the autonomic nervous system.[59,60] Norepinephrine, substance P, and other neurotransmitters are released at neuroeffector junctions and can affect immune cells in the immediate proximity (e.g. within the microenvironment of a lymph node) or at a distance, thereby regulating their function. Together, these indicate that stressors can activate the central nervous system and the HPA and SAM axes to release several 'stress' hormones that can mediate changes in the function and trafficking of immune cells.

11.3.2 Evidence of stress-related cytokine dysregulation

As mentioned above, lymphocytes, monocytes–macrophages, and granulocytes have been shown to express receptors for many neurotransmitters.[59] Thus it has been shown that catecholamines can indirectly cause changes in immune activities such as lymphocyte trafficking and proliferation, antibody production, and cell lysis through the regulation of cyclic adenosine $3',5'$-monophosphate (cAMP) levels.[61] In addition, it has been shown that the treatment of isolated peripheral blood leucocytes (PBLs) with catecholamines *in vitro* results in the suppression of IL-12 synthesis and an increase in IL-10 production.[62] Furthermore, our group has shown that norepinephrine and cortisol have no significant effect on IL-10 production in PBLs stimulated with *Candida*, a potent stimulator of Th1 cytokines, but reduced the production of interferon-γ (IFN-γ), thereby markedly decreasing the Th1 (IFN-γ)/Th2 (IL-10) ratio of cytokine production in these human PBLs.[63]

Studies utilizing an academic stress paradigm showing that psychological stress can result in the dysregulation of the balance of Th1 and Th2 cytokine synthesis is supported by *in vitro* studies. For instance, observations by Marshall *et al.*[64] suggest that psychological stress experienced by medical students taking examinations can produce a shift in the Th1–Th2 cytokine balance towards a Th2 response. Work in our laboratory suggest that chronic stress may also induce such a shift in Th1–Th2 cytokine patterns in older individuals.[65] Thus there is a tendency to shift the pattern of cytokine synthesis produced by Th1 cells, which are involved in cell-mediated immune function, to Th2 cells, which are important for antibody production.

This stress-induced tendency for a Th1–Th2 shift has also been supported by studies using animal models. For example, restraint-stressed mice showed evidence of a shift in the Th1–Th2 balance towards Th2 dominance. A significant decrease NK cell activity, decreased IFN-γ production by splenocytes stimulated with Concanavalin A (Con A), and a simultaneous rise in serum corticosterone levels were observed after 24 h of restraint. However, restraint stress did not affect the ability of Con A-stimulated splenocytes to produce IL-4.[66] We believe that a stress-associated shift in Th1 and Th2 cytokine production may be a simplistic interpretation of what may be a much more complicated interaction. Data from our laboratory and others have shown that stress-induced dysregulation of the immune response can affect both antibody and T-cell responses at the same time.[67–69] Further studies are required to help elucidate the mechanisms involved in stress-induced dysregulation of the immune response.

11.4 Empirical evidence for the effects of stress on wound healing

The studies described in section 11.2.1 have shown that cytokines and immune cells play important roles in cutaneous wound healing. Several studies have explored the role of stress-associated immune changes on the wound-healing process in humans and in animal models.

11.4.1 Human studies

11.4.1.1 Descriptive studies

The effects of psychological stress on wound healing is an area of interest in the field of psychoneuroimmunology.[70] Several studies have shown the direct impact of psychological stress on the physical and functional integrity of the skin.[71–73] Garg et al.[72] described the relationship between psychological stress and epidermal permeability barrier function in 27 medical, dental, and pharmacy students. They assessed psychological state using Perceived Stress and Profile of Mood States scores. Cellophane tape stripping was used to disrupt the barrier function of the forearm skin. Since a primary function of the skin is to prevent the evaporation of water from the body, barrier function was assessed by measuring water evaporation from the stripped area, a measure known as transepidermal water loss (TEWL). As the epidermis recovers its barrier function, evaporation decreases. TEWL measurements were obtained simultaneously with behavioural measurements during final examinations (high stress) and immediately after two vacation periods (low stress). A negative association between recovery of barrier function and perceived psychological stress during the examination period was observed. In addition, this study showed that the greatest decline in barrier function recovery was observed in individuals who experienced the largest increases in perceived psychological stress between the low- and high-stress periods.

Another interesting study showed that psychological stress associated with impending divorce can have a negative effect on recovery of skin barrier function.[71] Twenty-eight healthy women, aged between 21 and 45, who were going through the process of marital separation were tested for skin barrier recovery after tape stripping as described in the previous study. They were compared with a control group composed of age-matched and self-described 'happy' subjects. TEWL was measured from the cheek area of the face before and after tape stripping. Barrier recovery was determined by the level of TEWL measured 3 h and 24 h after barrier disruption. The results showed that psychological stress associated with marital dissolution was related to slower rates of skin barrier recovery. Taken together, these observations suggest that re-establishment of the structural and functional integrity of injured skin is affected by psychological stress.

11.4.1.2 Mechanistic studies

As already described, injury to the skin triggers a precise sequence of developmental events (cutaneous wound healing) in which the inflammatory response plays a major role. Since psychological stress has been shown to have the ability to cause dysregulation of cytokine production and in the immune response (see section 11.3.2), several studies have tested the hypothesis that stress-induced cytokine dysregulation is part of the mechanism related to delays in the early phases of wound healing.

Altemus et al.[73] showed that stress-related disruption of skin barrier function is associated with cytokine and immune dysregulation. This study investigated the effect of three different stressors (psychological interview stress, sleep deprivation, and exercise) on the recovery of skin barrier function after tape stripping. The effects of stress on plasma levels of cytokines and hormones (cortisol, norepinephrine, IL-1β,

IL-10, and TNF-α), NK cell activity, and absolute numbers of the PBLs were also assessed. It was found that the 25 women who participated in the interview stress paradigm exhibited a delay in the recovery of skin barrier function. This was associated with increased levels of plasma cortisol, norepinephrine, IL-1β, IL-10, and TNF-α, and an increase in NK cell number and activity. The increase in NK cell activity was presumably related to trafficking of cells to the peripheral blood. In addition, sleep deprivation decreased skin barrier function recovery and increased plasma IL-1β, TNF-α, and NK cell activity in 11 female participants. Finally, the 10 female subjects who participated in exercise stress activity did not show any change in skin barrier function recovery, but exhibited an increase in NK cell activity and circulating numbers of both cytolytic T lymphocytes and helper T cells in the peripheral blood.[73] These observations support the hypothesis that stress-related disruption of skin barrier function is mediated by modulation of immune function and endocrine, cytokine, and growth factor levels.

Several studies from our laboratory have supported the hypothesis that dysregulation of cytokine production and immune function mediate stress-associated delays in wound healing. In order to assess the impact of stress-associated changes in the inflammatory response, we recruited 13 women who cared for dementia patients and 13 well-matched control subjects.[74] Subjects were wounded by creating a 3.5-mm diameter full-thickness punch biopsy in the forearm. Thus all subjects started out with the same size wound at the same anatomical site. The process of wound healing was monitored every 2–3 days by comparing the wound size with a standard dot. Completion of wound healing took 24% longer in caregivers compared with non-caregivers. In addition, LPS-stimulated IL-1β gene expression by isolated PBLs was significantly lower in PBLs obtained from caregivers than in PBLs obtained from control subjects.

In a follow-up study, we utilized the blister wound model described by Kuhns et al.[17] which allowed us to study the effect of stress on cytokine production directly at a wound site on the arm (Fig. 11.2). Suction blister wounds were created on the forearms of 36 women (mean age, 57 years). Women reporting higher perceived stress exhibited significantly lower protein levels of IL-1α and IL-8 at these wound sites. In addition, subjects with lower levels of both cytokines in chamber fluid bathing the wound site after 24 h reported more stress and negative affect, and they had higher levels of salivary cortisol than those who had high cytokine levels. These data suggest that a possible mechanism by which psychological stress affects the local wound environment is through the control of pro-inflammatory cytokine production.[75]

Work by Marucha et al.[76] shows that the stress-associated delays in wound healing seen in dermal wounds are also observed in mucosal wounds. In this study, two 3.5-mm punch biopsy wounds were placed on the hard palates of 11 dental students, with the first wound created during summer vacation (non-stress period) and the second created on the contralateral side 3 days before their first major examination

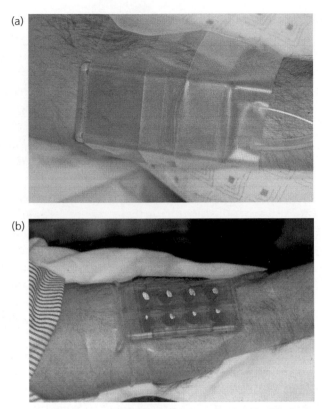

Fig. 11.2 (a) Photograph of the plastic template used to prepare the blister wounds. The template was taped to the surface of the forearm and a vacuum applied until blisters formed approximately 1–1.5 h later. This gentle suction separated the junction of the epidermis and dermis, creating eight sterile 8-mm blisters. (b) Photograph of a plastic plate containing eight chambers. Each chamber was able to hold approximately 1 ml of chamber fluid. Using a syringe, the template wells were filled with 0.8–1.0 ml of 70% autologous serum in Hanks' balanced salt solution. The top was sealed with sterile tape. Blister chamber fluid was removed with a syringe for analysis at various time-points after blister induction.[17,75,81]

(stress period). The progress of wound healing was monitored with photographs taken daily after wounding. This study showed that the wounds took an average of 40% longer to heal completely during examinations. In addition, IL-1β gene expression was 68% lower in PBLs obtained during examinations, suggesting that IL-1β, which is known to be an important pro-inflammatory cytokine for wound healing, is a candidate molecule for the mediator of stress-related effects on mucosal wound healing.

In a subsequent study, we explored the effects of the stress-related activation of HPA and SAM axes, and the resulting cytokine dysregulation, on MMP expression. As previously described, MMPs have been shown to be important factors in cutaneous wound-healing processes.[77] Using the blister chamber wound model described earlier on UVB-exposed forearm skin of healthy individuals, we investigated whether stress- or mood-associated neuroendocrine alteration is sufficient to modulate MMP expression at the site of injury. UV irradiation of skin has been shown to upregulate MMP expression.[78–80] A positive association between plasma norepinephrine and MMP-2 protein levels and a negative correlation between plasma cortisol and MMP-2 levels were found. The data suggest that activation of the HPA and SAM axes, even in individuals within the normal range of depressive symptoms, could mediate MMP levels and wound healing in blister wounds.[81]

Additionally, we explored the possibility that relaxation could buffer the impact of stress on wound healing. Blister fluid was collected from the forearms of 47 participants (25 participants engaged in relaxation training and 22 well-matched controls) 22 h after suction blister formation and assayed for IL-1β, IL-8, TNF-α, and MMP-2 and MMP-9 protein levels. We observed that control participants who reported increased stress at the start of the study had higher MMP-2 and MMP-9 levels in blister fluid. In contrast, there was no association between stress and MMP levels for participants who engaged in relaxation techniques, suggesting an apparent buffering of stress-related effects on MMP levels. All participants demonstrated a significant positive association between MMPs and IL-1β, IL-8, and TNF-α in the blister fluid 22 h after blistering. However, conducting analyses separately for controls and relaxation participants indicated that these associations existed only for relaxation subjects (E. V. Yang et al., unpublished data). The absence of an association between MMPs and cytokines for individuals who did not receive a relaxation intervention indirectly suggests that stress-associated cytokine dysregulation may be impacting the course of wound healing. Elevated MMP-2 and MMP-9 levels associated with higher perceived stress imply that the inflammatory stage of wounds in these subjects was longer than normal and further substantiates our previous hypothesis that delay in cutaneous wound healing is a result of a delay in the early phases of the wound-healing process.[76,82] Failure to resolve the inflammatory response initiated by injury in a timely fashion results in poor wound healing because of the wound's inability to re-establish the ECM, support cell proliferation, and remodel.[83] This study suggests that relaxation techniques may modify the effects of psychological stress on wound-healing processes through modulation of cytokine and MMP expression. It further adds to the data suggesting that relaxation/stress-intervention methods may modify the detrimental effects of psychological stress on physiological processes.

While the human studies described above were performed in a laboratory setting, a recent study by Broadbent et al.[84] examined the effect of psychological stress on wound healing in a clinical setting. This study examined the effect of pre-operative stress and worry (assessed 1 week prior to surgery) on wound healing following surgery for inguinal hernia in 36 patients. Wound fluid was collected over the first 20-h post-operative period to measure levels of IL-1, IL-6, and MMP-9. The analyses also included information on patient self-report of recovery and data on LPS-stimulated cytokine response of PBLs. The results showed that greater pre-operative perceived stress was negatively correlated with levels of IL-1 in the wound fluid, and greater worry about the operation was associated with lower MMP-9 levels in the wound fluid. Patients who expressed more worry experienced a more painful, poorer, and slower recovery following surgery. This study suggests that pychological stress associated with surgery impaired the inflammatory response and degradation of the ECM in the wound, leading to more painful, poorer, and slower surgical recovery.

The apparent inconsistency between our results and those of Broadbent and colleagues with regard to the relationship between psychological stress and MMP-9 expression is due to the difference in the experimental designs of the two studies, i.e. the timing of stress assessment prior to measurement of MMP expression, the type of wound, and the type of stressor studied. This difference demonstrates that the mechanism involved in stress-related effects on wound healing is complex and is modulated by a variety of factors, making comparisons of studies using different methodologies difficult. However, these studies support the critical roles of the immune response and ECM remodelling in the timely progression of wound healing discussed in section 11.2.1.

11.4.2 **Animal models**

Animal models of wound healing have supported results in humans and have provided some insight into the mechanism of stress-associated effects on cutaneous wound healing. Padgett et al.[85] subjected 6–8-week-old female hairless SKH-1 mice to restraint stress (RST) 3 days before the creation of a dorsal 3.5-mm sterile punch wound and for 5 days thereafter. Photography and image analysis were used to compare the rate of wound healing between the RST group and control mice that were wounded but not restrained. Wounds on control mice were observed to heal an average 3.10 days faster than mice subjected to RST. In addition, wounds of RST mice exhibited less inflammation at 1, 3, and 5 days after wounding. Serum corticosterone levels in the RST mice were higher (162.5 ng/ml) than in control mice (35.7 ng/ml). Treatment of RST mice with the glucocorticoid receptor antagonist RU40555 restored wound healing to rates comparable to those in control mice. Further analysis using the reverse transcriptase polymerase chain reaction (RT-PCR) showed that RST mice had significantly lower IL-1β and KGF-1 mRNA levels than controls 1 day after wounding, and significantly higher IL-1α and IL-1β mRNA levels than controls 5 days after wounding.[86] These studies support the hypothesis that stress-associated delays in cutaneous wound healing are mediated by activation of the HPA axis and dysregulation of cytokine and growth factor expression.

11.5 **Directions for future research**

In this review we have presented data from human and animal models that explore the interactions among the central nervous, endocrine, and immune systems and the effects of different stressors on cellular immunity. These studies demonstrate that psychological stressors have the ability to modulate the cellular immune response and produce changes that are large enough to have biological consequences on wound healing. While the effects of psychological stress on the immune aspects of cutaneous wound healing have been described, the stress-associated effects on the expression of other major players implicated in wound healing have not yet been fully elucidated.

As our group and others have now begun to ask questions regarding the effects of stress-related cytokine/immune dysregulation on other factors involved in cutaneous wound healing (e.g. growth factors, MMPs, and members of the uPA–plasmin system), the regulatory factors involved in the expression of these molecules need to be explored. Additionally, the role of transcription factors (such as those belonging to the members of the AP-1 family) in the regulation of gene expression of these factors needs to be investigated. In addition to using PCR and *in situ* hybridization to examine stress-associated effects on known players in wound healing, novel techniques such as microarray analysis of gene expression can lead to the discovery of other factors whose expression is affected by psychological stress. Studies designed to elucidate further the mechanism of stress-related delays in wound healing would be of interest from both the basic scientific and clinical points of view.

Furthermore, the observations discussed in this chapter involve the study of the early stages of wound healing. Therefore there is a need to extend these studies to the intermediate and late phases of wound healing. For example, *in situ* hybridization and immunohistochemistry can be utilized to study wound healing in the RST mouse model and to describe the temporal and spatial regulation of factors involved in intermediate and late stages of wound healing such as the proliferation and remodelling stages.

As scars are cosmetically unpleasant and can also lead to debilitating effects on an individual such as a burns patient, the examination of stress-related effects on scar formation is another area worthy of research. Studies of stress-related changes in collagen formation and orientation, as well as expression of proteases, will have an impact on the control of scar formation after stressful surgery and recovery from serious burns. A recent study has shown that RST mice exhibited an increase in the gene expression of the plasminogen activator inhibitor 1 (PAI-1), another key player in the uPA–plasmin enzyme system, in hepatocytes, renal tubular epithelial cells, adrenomedullar chromaffin cells, neural cells in the para-aortic sympathetic ganglion, vascular smooth muscle cells, and adipocytes.[87] A similar stress-related regulation of PAI-1 gene expression may also be observed during cutaneous wound healing.

The studies of stress-associated immunoregulation reviewed here are of great interest to both basic scientists and clinicians. Whereas these results implicate stress in the dysregulation of the cellular immune response in healthy individuals, the implications of these observations for individuals whose cellular immune response is in some way compromised, such as organ transplant patients, individuals affected by AIDS, and the elderly, is of greater importance. Greater understanding of the signalling mechanisms that result in the dysregulation of the cellular immune response will better enable the medical community to tackle the problems that stressed and/or ageing patients encounter during recovery from surgery or other injuries.[88] For example, it has been reported that the trauma due to injury itself (e.g. surgery) is associated with the suppression of immune function.[89–91] This decreased immune function may be manifested in delayed recovery from surgery. In addition, other negative behaviours that are associated with stress, such as smoking, alcohol, and nutrition status, have been shown to have unfavourable effects on the wound-healing process.[38,92,93] Understanding the mechanisms underlying these relationships will allow the development of stress intervention modalities, both behavioural (e.g. relaxation) and pharmacological (e.g. MMP inhibitors), that may help to reduce the impact of stress on wound healing.

References

1 Lazarus GS, Cooper DM, Knighton DR, *et al* (1994). Definitions and guidelines for assessment of wounds and evaluation of healing. *Arch Dermatol* **130**: 489–93.

2 Ennis WJ, Meneses P (2002). Factors impeding wound healing. In Kloth L, McCulloch JM (eds) *Wound Healing: Alternatives in Management* (3rd edn). Philadelphia, PA: F. A. Davis, 68–96.

3 Monaco JL, Lawrence WT (2003). Acute wound healing: an overview. *Clin Plast Surg* **30**: 1–12.

4 Yamaguchi Y, Yoshikawa K (2001). Cutaneous wound healing: an update. *J Dermatol* **28**: 521–34.

5 Falanga V (ed) (2001). *Cutaneous Wound Healing*. London: Martin Dunitz.

6 Singer AJ, Clark RA (1999). Cutaneous wound healing. *N Engl J Med* **341**: 738–46.

7 Martin P (1997). Wound healing—aiming for perfect skin regeneration. *Science* **276**: 75–81.

8 Agaiby AD, Dyson M (1999). Immuno-inflammatory cell dynamics during cutaneous wound healing. *J Anat* **195**: 531–42.

9 Scheid A, Meuli M, Gassmann M, Wenger RH (2000). Genetically modified mouse models in studies on cutaneous wound healing. *Exp Physiol* **85**: 687–704.

10 Martin P, Hopkinson-Woolley J, McCluskey J (1992). Growth factors and cutaneous wound repair. *Prog Growth Factor Res* **4**: 25–44.

11 Kiritsy CP, Lynch AB, Lynch SE (1993). Role of growth factors in cutaneous wound healing: a review. *Crit Rev Oral Biol Med* **4**: 729–60.

12 Steed DL (1997). The role of growth factors in wound healing. *Surg Clin North Am* **77**: 575–86.

13 Gillitzer R, Goebeler M (2001). Chemokines in cutaneous wound healing. *J Leukoc Biol* **69**: 513–21.

14 Boyce DE, Jones WD, Ruge F, Harding KG, Moore K (2000). The role of lymphocytes in human dermal wound healing. *Br J Dermatol* **143**: 59–65.

15 Hart J (2002). Inflammation. 1: Its role in the healing of acute wounds. *J Wound Care* **11**: 205–9.

16 Hart J (2002). Inflammation. 2: Its role in the healing of chronic wounds. *J Wound Care* **11**: 245–9.

17 Kuhns D, DeCarlo E, Hawk D, Gallin J (1992). Dynamics of the cellular and humoral components of the inflammatory response elicited in skin blisters in humans. *J Clin Invest* **89**: 1734–40.

18 Riches DWH (1996). Macrophage involvement in wound repair, remodeling and fibrosis. In Clark RAF (ed) *The Molecular and Cellular Biology of Wound Repair* (2nd edn). New York: Plenum Press, 95–141.

19 Rappolee DA, Mark D, Banda MJ, Werb Z (1988). Wound macrophages express TGF-alpha and other growth factors *in vivo*: analysis by mRNA phenotyping. *Science* **241**: 708–12.

20 Leibovich SJ, Ross R (1975). The role of the macrophage in wound repair. A study with hydrocortisone and antimacrophage serum. *Am J Pathol* **78**: 71–100.

21 Danon D, Kowatch MA, Roth GS (1989). Promotion of wound repair in old mice by local injection of macrophages. *Proc Natl Acad Sci USA* **86**: 2018–20.

22 Barbul A (1990). Immune aspects of wound repair. *Clin Plast Surg* **17**: 433–42.

23 Peterson JM, Barbul A, Breslin RJ, Wasserkrug HL, Efron G (1987). Significance of T-lymphocytes in wound healing. *Surgery* **102**: 300–5.

24 Cowin AJ, Brosnan MP, Holmes TM, Ferguson MW (1998). Endogenous inflammatory response to dermal wound healing in the fetal and adult mouse. *Dev Dyn* **212**: 385–93.

25 Darby I, Skalli O, Gabbiani G (1990). Alpha-smooth muscle actin is transiently expressed by myofibroblasts during experimental wound healing. *Lab Invest* **63**: 21–9.

26 Desmouliere A, Redard M, Darby I, Gabbiani G (1995). Apoptosis mediates the decrease in cellularity during the transition between granulation tissue and scar. *Am J Pathol* **146**: 56–66.

27 Burns JL, Mancoll JS, Phillips LG (2003). Impairments to wound healing. *Clin Plast Surg* **30**: 47–56.

28 Zamboni WA, Browder LK, Martinez J (2003). Hyperbaric oxygen and wound healing. *Clin Plast Surg* **30**: 67–75.

29 Vazquez JR, Short B, Findlow AH, Nixon BP, Boulton AJM, Armstrong DG (2003). Outcomes of hyaluronan therapy in diabetic foot wounds. *Diabetes Res Clin Pract* **59**: 123–7.

30 Brower MC, Johnson ME (2003). Adverse effects of local anesthetic infiltration on wound healing. *Reg Anesth Pain Med* **28**: 233–40.

31 Thomas A, Harding KG, Moore K (2000). Alginates from wound dressings activate human macrophages to secrete tumour necrosis factor-alpha. *Biomaterials* **21**: 1797–1802.

32 Harding KG, Jones V, Price P (2000). Topical treatment: which dressing to choose. *Diabetes Metab Res Rev* **16** (Suppl 1): S47–50.

33 Bowler PG (2002). Wound pathophysiology, infection and therapeutic options. *Ann Med* **34**: 419–27.

34 Scanlon E, Stubbs N (2002). To use or not to use? The debate on the use of antiseptics in wound care. *Br J Community Nurs Woundcare* September: 8,10,12.

35 Hunt TK, Hopf HW (1997). Wound healing and wound infection. What surgeons and anesthesiologists can do. *Surg Clin North Am* **77**: 587–606.

36 Wysocki AB (2002). Evaluating and managing open skin wounds: colonization versus infection. *AACN Clin Issues* **13**: 382–97.

37 Patten JA (1995). Nutrition and wound healing. *Compendium* **16**: 200–14.

38 Thomas DR (1996). Nutritional factors affecting wound healing. *Ostomy Wound Manage* **42**: 40–51.

39 Todorovic V (2002). Food and wounds: nutritional factors in wound formation and healing. *Br J Community Nurs Woundcare* September: 43–4,46,48.

40 Ashcroft G, Horan M, Herrick S, Tarnuzzer R, Schultz G, Ferguson M (1997). Age-related differences in the temporal and spatial regulation of matrix metalloproteinases (MMPs) in normal skin and acute cutaneous wounds of healthy humans. *Cell Tissue Res* **290**: 581–91.

41 Khorramizadeh M, Tredget E, Telasky C, Shen Q, Ghahary A (1999). Aging differentially modulates the expression of collagen and collagenase in dermal fibroblasts. *Mol Cell Biochem* **194**: 99–108.

42 **Ashcroft GS, Horan MA, Ferguson MW** (1995). The effects of ageing on cutaneous wound healing in mammals. *J Anat* **187**: 1–26.

43 **Ashcroft GS, Horan MA, Ferguson MW** (1997). The effects of ageing on wound healing: immunolocalisation of growth factors and their receptors in a murine incisional model. *J Anat* **190**: 351–65.

44 **Ashcroft GS, Horan MA, Ferguson MW** (1998). Aging alters the inflammatory and endothelial cell adhesion molecule profiles during human cutaneous wound healing. *Lab Invest* **78**: 47–58.

45 **Swift ME, Burns AL, Gray KL, DiPietro LA** (2001). Age-related alterations in the inflammatory response to dermal injury. *J Invest Dermatol* **117**: 1027–35.

46 **Horan MA, Ashcroft GS** (1997). Ageing, defence mechanisms and the immune system. *Age Ageing* **26**(Suppl 4): 15–19.

47 **Kylmaniemio M, Autio P, Oikarinen A** (1995). Influence of aging, localization, glucocorticoids and isotretinoin on matrix metalloproteases 2 (MMP-2) and 9 (MMP-9) in suction blister fluids. *Arch Dermatol Res* **287**: 434–8.

48 **Rabin BS** (1999). *Stress, Immune Function, and Health: The Connection*. New York: Wiley–Liss.

49 **Ader R, Felten DL, Cohen N (eds)** (2001). *Psychoneuroimmunology* (3rd edn). San Diego, CA: Academic Press.

50 **Besedovsky HO, del Rey A** (1991). Physiological implications of the immune-neuro-endocrine network. In Ader R, Felten DL, Cohen N (eds) *Psychoneuroimmunology* (2nd edn). San Diego, CA: Academic Press, 589–608.

51 **Besedovsky HO, del Rey A** (1996). Immune-neuro-endocrine interactions: facts and hypotheses. *Endocr Rev* **17**: 64–102.

52 **Besedovsky HO, del Rey A** (2002). Introduction: immune-neuroendocrine network. *Front Horm Res* **29**: 1–14.

53 **Chrousos GP, Gold PW** (1992). The concepts of stress and stress system disorders. Overview of physical and behavioral homeostasis. *JAMA* **267**: 1244–52.

54 **Malarkey WB, Zvara BJ** (1989). Interleukin-1-β and other cytokines stimulate ACTH release from cultured pituitary cells of patients with Cushing's disease. *J Clin Endocrin Metab* **69**: 196–9.

55 **Sabharwal P, Glaser R, LaFuse W, et al** (1992). Prolactin synthesized and secreted by human peripheral blood mononuclear cells: An autocrine growth factor for lymphoproliferation. *Proc Natl Acad Sci USA* **89**: 7713–16.

56 **Smith EM, Blalock JE** (1981). Human lymphocyte production of corticotropin and endorphin-like substances: association with leukocyte interferon. *Proc Natl Acad Sci USA* **78**: 7530–4.

57 **Varma S, Sabharwal P, Sheridan JF, Malarkey WB** (1993). Growth hormone secretion by human peripheral blood mononuclear cells detected by an enzyme-linked immunoplaque assay. *J Clin Endocrinol Metab* **76**: 49–53.

58 **Blalock JE** (1989). A molecular basis for bidirectional communication between the immune and neuro-endocrine systems. *Physiol Rev* **69**: 1–32.

59 **Felten DL** (1991). Neurotransmitter signalling of cells of the immune system: important progress, major gaps. *Brain Behav Immun* **5**: 2–8.

60 **Schorr E, Arnason B** (1999). Interactions between the sympathetic nervous system and the immune system. *Brain Behav Immun* **13**: 271–8.

61 **Madden K, Livnat S** (1991). *Catecholamine Action and Immunologic Reactivity* (2nd edn). New York: Academic Press.

62 Elenkov IJ, Papanicolau DA, Wilder RL, Chrousos GP (1996). Modulatory effects of glucocorticoids and catecholamines on human interleukin-12 and interleukin-10 production: clinical implications. *Proc Assoc Am Physicians* **108**: 374–81.

63 Malarkey WB, Wang J, Cheney C, Glaser R, Nagaraja H (2002). Human lymphocyte growth hormone stimulates interferon gamma production and is inhibited by cortisol and norepinephrine. *J Neuroimmunol* **123**: 180–7.

64 Marshall GJ, Agarwal S, Lloyd C, Cohen L, Henninger E, Morris G (1998). Cytokine dysregulation associated with exam stress in healthy medical students. *Brain Behav Immun* **12**: 297–307.

65 Glaser R, MacCallum RC, Laskowski BS, Malarkey WB, Sheridan JF, Kiecolt-Glaser JK (2001). Evidence for a shift in the Th-1 to Th-2 cytokine response associated with chronic stress and aging. *J Gerontol A Biol Sci Med Sci* **56**: M477–82.

66 Iwakabe K, Shimada M, Ohta A, *et al* (1998). The restraint stress drives a shift in Th1/Th2 balance toward Th2-dominant immunity in mice. *Immunol Lett* **62**: 39–43.

67 Glaser R, Kiecolt-Glaser JK, Malarkey WB, Sheridan JF (1998). The influence of psychological stress on the immune response to vaccines. *Ann NY Acad Sci* **840**: 649–55.

68 Vedhara K, Cox NK, Wilcock GK, *et al* (1999). Chronic stress in elderly carers of dementia patients and antibody response to influenza vaccination. *Lancet* **353**: 627–31.

69 Jabaaij L, Grosheide P, Heijtink R, Duivenvoorden H, Ballieux R, Vingerhoets A (1993). Influence of perceived psychological stress and distress on antibody response to low dose rDNA hepatitis B vaccine. *J Psychosom Res* **37**: 361–9.

70 Marucha PT, Sheridan JF, Padgett D (2001). Stress and wound healing. In Ader R, Felten DL, Cohen N (eds) *Psychoneuroimmunology* (3rd edn). San Diego, CA: Academic Press, 613–26.

71 Muizzuddin N, Matsui MS, Marenus KD, Maes DH (2003). Impact of stress of marital dissolution on skin barrier recovery: tape stripping and measurement of trans-epidermal water loss (TEWL). *Skin Res Technol* **9**: 34–8.

72 Garg A, Chren MM, Sands LP, *et al* (2001). Psychological stress perturbs epidermal permeability barrier homeostasis: implications for the pathogenesis of stress-associated skin disorders. *Arch Dermatol* **137**: 53–9.

73 Altemus M, Rao B, Dhabhar FS, Ding W, Granstein RD (2001). Stress-induced changes in skin barrier function in healthy women. *J Invest Dermatol* **117**: 309–17.

74 Kiecolt-Glaser JK, Marucha PT, Malarkey WB, Mercado AM, Glaser R (1995). Slowing of wound healing by psychological stress. *Lancet* **346**: 1194–6.

75 Glaser R, Kiecolt-Glaser J, Marucha P, MacCallum R, Laskowski B, Malarkey W (1999). Stress-related changes in proinflammatory cytokine production in wounds. *Arch Gen Psychiatry* **56**: 450–6.

76 Marucha P, Kiccolt-Glaser J, Favagehi M (1998). Mucosal wound healing is impaired by examination stress. *Psychosom Med* **60**: 362–5.

77 Steffensen B, Hakkinen L, Larjava H (2001). Proteolytic events of wound-healing—coordinated interactions among matrix metalloproteinases (MMPs), integrins, and extracellular matrix molecules. *Crit Rev Oral Biol Med* **12**: 373–98.

78 Fisher G, Choi H, Bata-Csorgo Z, *et al* (2001). Ultraviolet irradiation increases matrix metalloproteinase-8 protein in human skin *in vivo*. *J Invest Dermatol* **117**: 219–26.

79 Fisher G, Datta S, Talwar H, *et al* (1996). Molecular basis of sun-induced premature skin ageing and retinoid antagonism. *Nature* **379**: 335–9.

80 Fisher G, Wang Z, Datta S, Varani J, Kang S, Voorhees J (1997). Pathophysiology of premature skin aging induced by ultraviolet light. *N Engl J Med* **337**: 1419–28.

81 Yang EV, Bane CM, MacCallum RC, Kiecolt-Glaser JK, Malarkey WB, Glaser R (2002). Stress-related modulation of matrix metalloproteinase expression. *J Neuroimmunol* **133**: 144–50.

82 Kiecolt-Glaser JK, Marucha PT, Malarkey WB, Mercado AM, Glaser R (1995). Slowing of wound healing by psychological stress. *Lancet* **346**: 1194–6.

83 Ayala A, Chung C-S, Grutkoski PS, Song GY (2003). Mechanisms of immune resolution. *Crit Care Med* **31**(Suppl): S558–71.

84 Broadbent E, Petrie KJ, Alley PG, Booth RJ (2003). Psychological stress impairs early wound repair following surgery. *Psychosom Med* **65**: 865–9.

85 Padgett DA, Marucha PT, Sheridan JF (1998). Restraint stress slows cutaneous wound healing in mice. *Brain Behav Immun* **12**: 64–73.

86 Mercado AM, Padgett DA, Sheridan JF, Marucha PT (2002). Altered kinetics of IL-1 alpha, IL-1 beta, and KGF-1 gene expression in early wounds of restrained mice. *Brain Behav Immun* **16**: 150–62.

87 Yamamoto K, Takeshita K, Shimokawa T, *et al* (2002). Plasminogen activator inhibitor-1 is a major stress-regulated gene: implications for stress-induced thrombosis in aged individuals. *Proc Natl Acad Sci USA* **99**: 890–5.

88 Padgett DA, Glaser R (2003). How stress influences the immune response. *Trends Immunol* **24**: 444–8.

89 Slade MS, Simmons RL, Yunis E, Greenberg LJ (1975). Immunodepression after major surgery in normal patients. *Surgery* **78**: 363–72.

90 Balfour HHJ, Slade MS, Kalis JM, Howard RJ, Simmons RL, Najarian JS (1977). Viral infections in renal transplant donors and their recipients: a prospective study. *Surgery* **81**: 487–92.

91 Schäffer M, Barbul A (1998). Lymphocyte function in wound healing and following injury. *Br J Surg* **85**: 444–60.

92 Silverstein P (1992). Smoking and wound healing. *Am J Med* **93**: 22S–4S.

93 Benveniste K, Thut P (1981). The effect of chronic alcoholism on wound healing. *Proc Soc Exp Biol Med* **166**: 568–75.

Chapter 12

Behavioural interventions and psychoneuroimmunology

Michael H. Antoni

12.1 Introduction

Many different types of behavioural interventions are used in research and clinical applications within the field of health psychology. Many of these have been shown to produce improvements in mood, quality of life, health behaviours, and endocrine and immune system functioning. Some of these effects may be more or less relevant to patients with specific diseases or health conditions. This chapter will focus on summarizing what we know about the effects of some of the more commonly employed behavioural interventions on these variables, with special attention to those interventions that have been tested in psychoneuroimmunology (PNI) paradigms.

This chapter is organized into sections describing different behavioural interventions and the theoretical basis for their mechanisms of action, sections laying out the theoretical basis of how these behavioural interventions impact on the immune system and possible immune-related health outcomes, sections summarizing the empirical evidence for the effects of these interventions on psychosocial, endocrine, and immunological functioning including studies of different PNI paradigms that have been applied to various populations. In the final section we focus on directions for future research with new populations and emerging health questions. The overall goal will be to show how behavioural interventions may be used both to illuminate basic PNI mechanisms and to produce clinically relevant health outcomes.

The most commonly used behavioural interventions in PNI research include relaxation and imagery techniques, cognitive–behavioural stress management, and exercise training, but there is a body of work examining the effects of other techniques such as massage, biofeedback, hypnosis, and expressive writing, and other forms of psychotherapeutic approach such as supportive–expressive therapy. We begin with a description of these techniques and refer to them collectively as behavioural interventions.

12.2 The clinical context

12.2.1 Relaxation and imagery techniques

Relaxation techniques teach participants ways to reduce anxiety, tension, and other forms of stress response. These skills may also help participants to achieve a sense of mastery over some of the many stressful circumstances in their lives. Moreover, by 'taking the edge off' acute emotional or somatic stress responses, participants can make better use of some of the cognitive, behavioural, and interpersonal skills that are often embedded in multimodal stress management programmes.[1] The primary relaxation strategies taught in most stress management programmes are progressive muscle relaxation (PMR) and some form of mental imagery. Some of these exercises teach participants systematically to reduce tension throughout all their major muscle groups, while others teach the participants ways to use mental imagery to bring about a total state of relaxation.

We know that stress responses are often characterized by sympathetic nervous system (SNS) activation, with concomitant activity in the sympathetic–adrenal–medullary (SAM) and hypothalamic–pituitary–adrenal (HPA) systems. Affective processes such as anxiety often accompany these responses and may manifest themselves in physical symptoms or tension. PMR was originally developed by Jacobson in 1938 and later adapted by Bernstein and Borkovec[2] as a means of counteracting muscle tension and other symptoms of anxiety. Jacobson proposed that the relaxed physical state brought about by PMR would counter physical symptoms of anxiety.

Empirical evidence for the influence of relaxation training on SNS-related indices includes reported decreases in the blood pressure of hypertensives (relative to controls) using relaxation training with biofeedback.[3,4] McGrady et al.[3] also found significant decreases in urinary and plasma cortisol levels among hypertensives after relaxation training. PMR training combined with biofeedback also significantly improved glucose tolerance in a group of non-insulin-dependent diabetics relative to a no-treatment control group.[5] Since neither insulin secretion nor action changed as a result of treatment, it is plausible that hepatic glucose uptake was increased, suggesting that relaxation training effects may have been mediated by decreased SNS activity.

Direct evidence for the effects of relaxation on specific SNS-related indices includes PMR-related reductions in galvanic skin responses[6] and decreases in heart rate, respiration, and electromyographic (EMG) activity.[7] In a review of the physiological effects of PMR, Borkovec and Sides[8] concluded that this method is most effective in bringing about changes in the autonomic nervous system when the programme involves several sessions and is controlled by the subject, and when physiological 'overactivity' is a pathognomic aspect of the presenting problem. This technique is particularly relevant for PNI research as the effects of stressors on the immune system are believed to be mediated in part by elevations or dysregulation of neuroendocrine systems that are affected by anxiety and tension.[9]

12.2.2 Massage

Massage therapy provides a useful paradigm for studying relaxation because it does not require effort on the part of the participant and is easy to monitor objectively (i.e. one knows how much massage a participant is receiving).[10] One group examined the effects of daily massage on HIV-infected men.[11] This massage intervention represented what one might receive in daily massage therapy and thus may overestimate the impact of massage as it is typically practised and received by the general population. The intervention included a full body massage with the application of several types of strokes (effleurage, petrissage, stroking, stretching, etc.) provided in 45-min sessions, 5 days per week over a 4-week period. Significant interactions (increase during the massage period; no change or decrease during the control period) were found for natural killer (NK) cell number, NK cell count, soluble CD8, and the cytotoxic subset of CD8 cells. However, no changes in disease progression markers (CD4, CD4/CD8 ratio, β_2-microglobulin, neopterin) were observed during the massage period. The massages were also associated with reports of significant decreases in anxiety and significant increases in relaxation, and these changes were significantly correlated with increases in NK cell number. Finally, there was a significant reduction in 24-h urinary free cortisol, and a trend towards a decrease in urinary epinephrine and norepinephrine. Thus there appeared to be a significant impact on psychological, neuroendocrine, and some immune measures relevant to cytotoxic capacity. However, it is important to note that this was not a randomized design, and massage did not impact on disease progression markers for HIV. This study needs to be replicated with a larger group and a randomized design.

12.2.3 Biofeedback, imagery, and hypnosis

There have been a few studies in which relaxation was combined with other techniques such as biofeedback and hypnosis to examine mood and immune effects in various populations. Here we focus on studies with HIV+ individuals and those with cancer. Taylor[12] examined the effect of an intervention combining PMR, biofeedback, meditation, and hypnosis on mood, self-esteem, and CD4 cell counts in HIV+ men. Intervention group participants completed 20 1-h sessions over a 10-week period. Each session involved 15 min discussing home practice and general training issues, 15 min of PMR, 20 min of EMG biofeedback training, 10 min of meditation, and 10 min of hypnosis, where the subject visualized himself becoming increasingly relaxed. Subjects in the intervention group showed decreases in the State Trait Anxiety and POMS scales and increases in self-esteem over the course of treatment. CD4 counts increased for the intervention group and decreased for the control group, but no differences in the change scores between the groups were observed from post-treatment to 1-month follow-up. The changes in CD4 cell count should be interpreted with caution as no information is provided on antiretroviral drug therapy, and the data were taken from subject medical records rather than being coordinated with the collection of psychosocial data. In a related study, Auerbach et al.[13] randomly assigned HIV+ men to an intervention consisting of 8 weeks of training in thermal biofeedback, guided imagery, and hypnosis, or to a wait-list control group. The intervention was associated with reduced self-reported symptoms of HIV (fever, fatigue, pain, headache, nausea, and insomnia) and increased vigour and hardiness relative to controls. However, there was no change in anxiety, depression, or CD4+ cell number.

Gruber et al.[14] designed a 9-week programme that included relaxation and biofeedback for women with early-stage breast cancer. They found that breast cancer patients completing this stress reduction intervention showed decreases in distress and increases in lymphocyte proliferative responses and NK cell count, although there were no effects on survival. Other groups have explored the effects of hypnosis in persons dealing with cancer. Studies which more directly tested the effects of hypnosis on individuals dealing with cancer have reported some changes in immune system parameters. Other studies, to be summarized in a later section, have focused on the effects of relaxation training in combination with other stress management techniques designed to change the ways in which stressors are appraised and resources are obtained for managing those stressors.

12.2.4 Physical exercise

Exercise training is one of the most commonly employed behavioural interventions in health psychology;[15] it is sometimes referred to as a stress management technique, and has been associated with decreased levels of mood and distress (depression and anxiety) as well as alterations in immune system parameters in a variety of populations.

Most studies evaluating the effects of exercise on immune parameters have been conducted with HIV-infected persons. In one study asymptomatic gay men who did not know their HIV status were randomly assigned to a 10-week group exercise intervention or a measurement-only control group.[16] The exercise intervention consisted of a stationary bicycle ergometry interval aerobic exercise for 45 min, 3 days per week, with a maximum intensity of 80% of predicted maximum heart rate. Men were enrolled in the intervention for 5 weeks before blood was drawn for the HIV test, received notification of their status within 72 h, and then continued for another 5 weeks in whichever group to which they had initially been assigned. Psychosocial measures and blood samples were taken 72 h before and 1 week after notification of HIV antibody status. HIV+ exercisers showed no significant change in anxiety or depression scores pre- and post-notification, whereas those in the control group had significant increases in both anxiety and depression.[16] HIV+ exercisers also maintained their CD4 cell number, NK cell number, and NK cell count, while those in the control group had a significant decrease in NK cell count and a non-significant decrease in CD4 cell count.

After completion of the 10-week exercise training programme, Both HIV+ and HIV− exercisers showed significant decreases in antibody titres to Epstein–Barr virus (EBV) and HIV− exercisers had significant decreases in human herpes virus type 6 (HHV-6), suggesting better immunological control of these latent viruses, whereas the HIV+ controls showed no change.[17] Another interesting immune result of the 10-week exercise programme[18] was that seronegative exercisers had a significant increase in CD4 cell counts, whereas HIV+ exercisers had a non-significant increase. Finally, an analysis of follow-up data 2 years after notification found that those who attended more exercise sessions were less likely to have progressed to AIDS,[19] even after controlling for CD4 count at study entry.

A few other studies have examined the effects of exercise training on HIV+ individuals. Schlenzig et al.[20] randomly assigned 28 people to either two 1-h sessions per week for 8 weeks or a no-treatment control condition. The intervention included supervised sports activities designed to develop cardiovascular endurance. After the intervention the participants showed reductions in anxiety and depression, and these mood changes were correlated with increases in CD4 cell counts. Other studies of exercise in HIV-infected persons have tested programmes differing in length and type of training activities. Rigsby et al.[21] randomly assigned HIV+ persons to either a 12-week exercise group or a counselling control group. The exercise group increased in flexibility, strength, and cardiorespiratory fitness. Both the exercise and counselling groups showed significant decreases in Beck depression scores and a non-significant trend towards increased CD4 cell counts. Florijn et al.[22] tested the effects of a sports training programme among HIV+ persons. Those randomized to the exercise intervention received endurance training, gymnastics, games, and relaxation in 90-min weekly sessions. The exercise group showed decreases in depression, fatigue, and anger, and an increase in vigour and quality of life. They also showed a preservation of CD4 and CD8 counts, while the control group showed reductions in these immune parameters. The effects of these programmes on immune status are not totally clear and are likely to depend to a large degree on participants' ability to maintain excellent compliance.[23] The largest sustained immune effects of exercise may only be achieved by those individuals who are able to train at the level necessary to modulate stress hormone levels (e.g. cortisol) on a more continuous basis. This may be the case in populations beyond HIV+ men.

12.2.5 Cognitive–behavioural stress management techniques

Cognitive-based stress management (CBSM) techniques have been applied in a number of health psychology arenas including health promotion and disease prevention, disease detection, and modulating the effects of medical treatments. CBSM interventions have been tailored for persons with chronic illnesses such as asthma,[24] rheumatoid arthritis,[25] and peptic ulcer.[26] Additionally, cognitive techniques have been used to reduce the side effects of medical treatments including postoperative pain after Caesarean section,[27] pain associated with cancer,[28] control of acute and chronic pain,[29] and, more recently, the effects of surgery and adjuvant therapies such as radiation and chemotherapy in persons with breast cancer[30] and prostate cancer.[31]

Two basic assumptions underlie the use of CBSM techniques. First, individuals are seen as active processors of stimuli from their environments. The amount of threat, arousal, or 'stress' individuals experience when encountering a stressor or challenge is determined by both their appraisal of the stimulus and their perception of available resources.[32] Importantly, thoughts, feelings, behaviours, and the social elements often interact.[33] Thus cognitions can affect emotions, tension levels, and behaviours. Similarly, feelings can facilitate or inhibit cognitions that can affect the behavioural responses as a function of the social context.[32] A second assumption underlying CBSM is that individuals can be taught new patterns of thinking, feeling, and behaving to help them achieve a sense of mastery and self-efficacy over challenges, and subsequently achieve better control over emotional states and maladaptive behaviours.[32] According to this perspective, an individual's appraisals, beliefs, attitudes, cognitive coping strategies, and expectancies are important mediators in many realms of health, disease, and responses to treatment.[32]

Several techniques have been developed to address the cognitive and behavioural aspects of how people respond to stressors and challenges in their lives. These include techniques designed to modify one's appraisals of stressors (cognitive restructuring), techniques focused on teaching new cognitive coping strategies concerning how coping energies are allocated (coping effectiveness training), and techniques that teach more efficient interpersonal skills (anger management and assertiveness training).

Cognitive–behavioural interventions are believed to work, especially in stressed individuals, by modifying stressor appraisals and furnishing the person with an available coping response,[32] changing maladaptive cognitive distortions (e.g. mind-reading, black-and-white thinking[34]), decreasing hopeless thoughts,[35] and increasing perceptions of self-efficacy, personal control, and mastery.[36] Some interventions studied to date have used one or more of these techniques in combination and are often referred to collectively as cognitive–behavioural stress management (CBSM) or cognitive–behavioural therapy (CBT). Most PNI studies examining the effects of these interventions have used group formats. Thus social support was 'built into' these interventions as a component beyond the specific cognitive or interpersonal techniques being taught.

12.2.5.1 Cognitive restructuring

At the centre of most of the CBSM interventions reviewed above is a technique called cognitive restructuring. Here, through in-session activities and homework assignments, participants become aware of, learn to challenge, and ultimately refute and replace self-defeating cognitive appraisals of stressors that are related to their difficulties in achieving psychological adjustment.[37]

Increasing their awareness of stressor appraisals is thought to diminish the likelihood of extreme reactions (e.g. catastrophizing) and may prevent participants from giving up prematurely and/or allocating energy to unproductive responses to the situation. It is plausible that a more efficient initial appraisal of stressful circumstances may also affect the magnitude and duration of neuroendocrine responses to challenge, with possible effects on immunological parameters and health outcomes in vulnerable populations (e.g. persons diagnosed with HIV infection, or patients undergoing treatment for cancer). Alternatively, more efficient processing of illness-related stressors may also facilitate the adoption and maintenance of health-promoting behaviours such as adequate diet, exercise and medication management.[30,38]

12.2.5.2 Coping skills training

Another set of cognitive–behavioural techniques focuses more directly on teaching people cognitive and behavioural coping responses to challenges. One can think of these techniques as being the next logical step after one has clarified the appraisal of the stressful situation as accurate (i.e. via cognitive restructuring). Typically, participants are introduced to the notion of coping responses to stressors after they have spent several weeks learning cognitive restructuring. Some programmes simply teach people to avoid using obviously destructive coping responses (e.g. denial, violence, substance use), while others are more sophisticated in attempting to improve the 'efficiency' of the coping response. There have been numerous studies supporting the idea that individual differences in coping actions and resources play a substantial role in amplifying, diminishing, or otherwise 'moderating' a wide range of environmental burdens.[39,40]

'Matching' coping strategies to stressor characteristics is the main feature of an intervention called coping effectiveness training.[41] Participants are taught to choose problem-focused coping strategies (e.g. active coping, planning) for dealing with the controllable aspects of stressful situations and emotion-focused strategies (e.g. venting, relaxation, seeking emotional support) in order to deal with the uncontrollable or unchangeable aspects of stressful situations.

12.2.5.3 Anger management

Owing to the chronic burdens and limitations of having a medical disease as well as the inappropriate reactions of friends and family members once they learn the diagnosis, an individual may experience a variety of difficult emotions including anger, fear, sadness, and anxiety. For instance, some women report feeling very angry and frustrated at having breast cancer after they had spent years maintaining a healthy lifestyle.[30] Other women report being infuriated by the lack of understanding on the part of their husbands or family members who attempt to minimize the sense of loss and fear that emerges after learning the diagnosis. Some HIV-infected individuals may be extremely resentful of the implication by others that they 'deserved' to contract HIV because of their 'lifestyle'.[42]

The set of cognitive–behavioural techniques referred to as anger management teaches people to be aware of the situations in their lives capable of eliciting anger responses, the ways in which they express anger, and strategies for changing their responses so that they are most productive in ensuring that their needs are met. By providing an opportunity for expressing frustrations, anger and other negative emotions these techniques may in turn facilitate the development of cognitive insight and resolution of the distress state more quickly.[43] A by-product of better anger management may be improved social support as members of one's network may be more willing to provide support if one is vocal about one's needs and not explosive in communications of these needs. Expressing negative emotions in a supportive environment may influence some aspects of immune system functioning in ways that may be similar to expressive writing.[44–47]

12.2.5.4 Assertiveness training

Assertiveness training teaches individuals some basic 'styles' of communication (passive, passive–aggressive, aggressive, and assertive) and the advantages and disadvantages of each. They are then given exercises to examine the style that is closest to their own and asked to monitor how the use of this approach is related to their mood as well as the likelihood of them ensuring that their needs are met. The rationale for assertiveness training is similar to that for anger management. If one cannot communicate emotional reactions and behavioural intentions clearly, interpersonal conflict is likely to occur and persist, and may be accompanied by stress symptoms and physiological changes characterizing protracted 'stress responses' (elevated SNS activation), which in turn may affect aspects of immune system functioning.

12.2.5.5 Social support building

Research has provided evidence that social support can moderate the effects of stress on health,[48] neuroendocrine parameters,[49,50] and immune system functioning.[51,52] Unemployed men receiving high levels of emotional support from their wives and families have been shown to suffer less physiological strain[50] and display lower catecholamine levels[49] than their low-support counterparts. In addition, low social support states (e.g. loneliness) have been associated with elevated urinary cortisol levels, lower NK cell count, poorer control of latent herpes virus infections, and diminished T-lymphocyte responsivity.[53–56] Work with patients with breast cancer has shown that seeking social support as a major coping strategy and receiving high levels of support from a spouse predicts a higher NK cell count.[57] Among women with ovarian cancer, better social support was associated with lower levels of the angiogenesis-promoting cytokine vascular endothelial growth factor (VEGF), which may have implications for metastasis and tumour growth rates.[58] Recent findings indicate that improvements in social support during CBSM explain some of its beneficial effects on mood[59] and components of the immune system in HIV-infected individuals.[52]

Earlier work suggested that the more active components of social support (e.g. engaging and interacting with supportive others), as opposed to passive components (e.g. distraction from troubles), have the strongest stress-buffering effects.[60] Social support building is provided subtly in several aspects of stress management interventions. For group-based programmes the presence of other persons sharing the same diagnosis or similar challenges may increase perceptions of communality and decrease a sense of social isolation. Use of role-playing exercises involving group members further facilitates cohesiveness. Many stress management techniques are also helpful in raising participants' awareness of resources and limitations within their social networks as well as strategies for improving specific sources of support. Some of these programmes deal more explicitly with teaching new techniques for building social support networks,[30] presenting different 'shades' of social support (including sources of support more useful for informational than emotional purposes) that some of us are often unaware of as resources in our environment. Efficient support seeking may involve best matching the types of support chosen (e.g. emotional) with the particular aspects of the stressful situation (e.g. uncontrollable aspects).[51]

12.2.5.6 Use of CBSM techniques

The CBSM techniques discussed so far are likely to be most powerful if taught as an integrated set of strategies that can be employed in a variety of situations. By using flow diagrams, interventionists can help participants to see how to sequence the use of these new tools as they encounter and work through different situations.

12.2.6 Supportive–expressive therapy

Another type of psychosocial intervention, often classified as existential/experiential group therapy or supportive expressive therapy (SET),[61] has been designed to address the adjustment issues faced by individuals dealing with later-stage cancers and other life-threatening diseases[62] or disease-related losses such as bereavement.[63] This intervention approach is designed to help individuals express and work through anxieties (e.g. death anxieties[64]), ventilate negative feelings, provide emotional support, and encourage individuals to pursue positive goals and activities. Some have suggested that these interventions offer the opportunity for group participants to share their strategies for dealing with disease-related stressors, the chance for them to help one another, a sense of universality, and a buffer to the sense of isolation that many of them face.[65] Thus the existential/experiential interventions, in theory, appear to address the issues of social isolation, emotional suppression, loss of self-esteem, and hopelessness that may accompany a chronic or life-threatening illness. It remains to be tested whether patients with early-stage disease (stage 1 or 2 breast cancer or early symptomatic HIV infection) might benefit more from cognitive–behavioural interventions that allow them to move on with their lives, whereas those with advanced disease (metastatic cancer or AIDS) might benefit more from SET group support programmes that focus on pain management, existential challenges, and end-of-life issues.[66] Despite the appeal of SET interventions for people with such conditions and a single study showing effects on survival time in women with metastatic breast cancer,[67] little is known about their effects on neuroendocrine or immune system parameters that might contribute to health outcomes.

12.3 Theoretical basis for the role of psychoneuroimmunology in behavioural intervention research

Several recent surveys polling the opinions of physicians about the effectiveness of alternative medical interventions such as exercise, biofeedback, acupuncture, massage, and hypnosis have suggested that the majority of practitioners view these techniques as at least moderately effective and as 'legitimate medical practices'.[68] While solid empirical tests of the efficacy of many of these practices are still lacking, the extensive body of PNI research documenting interactions of behavioural, neural, endocrine, and immune systems across a wide variety of species and situations is often used to justify their existence (see Chapters 1 and 2).

Implicit in much human PNI research is the notion that psychosocial factors relate to immune system changes by way of stress- or mood-induced changes in hormonal regulatory systems, resulting in neuroendocrine elevations and imbalances.[11] However, it is important to note that several neuroendocrine system responses are known to be altered as a function of an individual's appraisal of (i.e. controllable versus uncontrollable) and coping response to (i.e. active versus passive) stressful stimuli. Immunological decrements and elevations in adrenocortical hormones have also been observed in those reporting significant degrees of loneliness,[69] suggesting that the degree of disruption in personal ties and social support may contribute significantly to the degree of immune system decrements observed during stressful periods. Given that perceived loss of control, and social losses such as divorce and bereavement, have been related to alterations in some of these immunomodulatory hormones,[70] it can be reasoned that many PNI relationships might be mediated, in part, by neurohormonal changes that are linked to an individual's appraisals of, coping responses to, and resources available for dealing with environmental stimuli (reviewed by Schneiderman et al.[71]). In people undergoing stressful circumstances, perceptions of a loss of personal control, helplessness/hopelessness, and low self-efficacy have all been associated with immunological decrements.[72] Passive coping strategies[73] and insufficient emotional expression about traumatic or highly stressful events[47,74,75] have been associated with decreased lymphoproliferative responses (LPRs) to mitogens and elevated antibody titres to EBV and HIV disease status. Finally, interpersonal processes such as social support,[76] marital distress,[77] and hostile interactions between marital partners[78] have also been related to decrements in several cellular immune function measures.

It is generally agreed that efforts to characterize the mechanisms underlying stressor–immune interactions in humans must take into account these appraisal, coping, and interpersonal processes since they can moderate the nature, degree, and duration of neuroendocrine responses. Recent theoretical models proposing stress-associated neuroanatomical changes involving structures critical for HPA[79] and SAM[80] hormonal regulation and efficient neuroimmune interactions have laid the groundwork for a new breed of investigations designed to identify the mechanisms underlying the negative health consequences of chronic and repeated stressor exposure. Terms such as 'allostatic load' have been promulgated to reflect the sum total of successful and unsuccessful attempts to manage a lifetime of stressors and challenges.[79] Presumably the most effective psychosocial interventions for helping stressed and distressed individuals handle the challenges in their lives while optimizing physical health will need to consider the role of psychosocial (e.g. appraisals, coping, social support), neuroendocrine [HPA, hypothalamic–pituitary–gonadal (HPG), and SAM hormonal regulation], and immunological (cell trafficking, functionality, and regulation) mechanisms that explain the negative physical sequelae that often appear during and after stressful experiences. It is reasonable that those interventions that are of greatest value are the ones that are found to be effective in individuals whose immune systems are compromised due to a medical disease or condition, a medical treatment, or other conditions (e.g. ageing, malnutrition, sleep deprivation) known to be associated with immunological deficits. The following section focuses on some of the empirical evidence that has been gathered on the effects of behavioural interventions in some of these populations, with a major focus on individuals dealing with viral or neoplastic disease.

12.4 Empirical evidence

The first systematic studies of the effects of behavioural intervention on immune parameters in healthy young and older subjects were performed in the 1980s. Relaxation and guided imagery have been shown to modulate lymphocyte proliferative response to challenge and NK cell count in healthy subjects.[81–83] Kiecolt-Glaser et al.[81] found a 30% increase in NK cell count in healthy adults living in a retirement home following a month of muscle relaxation training. These authors also found an association between practising relaxation and increases in CD4 cell counts in healthy medical students.[82] This work and related studies of relaxation, guided imagery, physical exercise, and hypnosis in other healthy and medical populations provided some of the impetus for full-scale PNI studies of behavioural interventions in medical populations for whom immune system modulation might have clinical benefits. In the last decade the bulk of this applied work has focused on people with cancers and HIV infection.[84] However, most of these studies have been based on small samples of persons at risk for, recently diagnosed with, or currently being treated for these conditions. It is reasonable to consider these studies separately in light of the point in the continuum of medical risk, diagnosis, and treatment, as the timing of such interventions may dictate their form, determine their effectiveness, and identify their place in clinical practice. In the following we discuss some of the work being done in each of these domains as it relates to cancer and HIV infection. Later we will suggest some frontier areas that appear to be ripe for the development of new PNI intervention research.

12.4.1 Recovery from immune compromising medical treatment in cancer

Cancers frequently studied in the psycho-oncology literature which have documented immune system involvement include malignant melanoma,[85] breast cancer,[86] and cervical cancer.[87] Psychosocial factors such as active coping have been shown to predict greater survival time,[88] while repressive coping has been related to poorer survival in melanoma patients.[89] Breast cancer patients have significantly more life stressors prior to the discovery of the primary tumour,[90] and those experiencing elevated life stressors may be at risk for a relapse or shortened survival time after treatment,[91] though other work refutes this.[92] The reactions of breast cancer patients to the stress of diagnosis (e.g. distress, depression, maintaining a 'fighting spirit') may also predict the course of disease.[93] Poor expression of anger,[94] stoicism,[94] repressiveness,[95] and lack of social support[96] have also been related to poorer prognosis in breast cancer patients.

12.4.1.1 Immunological 'complications' of medical treatment for cancer

There are many points within the experience of cancer where PNI research is particularly relevant. One is the time period surrounding initial medical treatment for the tumorous growth. Contemporary medical treatments for a wide range of human cancers often involve curative treatments such as surgery together with adjuvant therapies such as cytotoxic chemotherapy or radiation administered either before (neoadjuvant) or after surgery. Patients undergoing these procedures are under enormous stress. During the treatment phase, people's predominant emotional reactions include feelings of fear and grief. Here, maladaptive responses might include avoidance, postoperative reactive depression, and prolonged postoperative grief reaction.[97]

There is also a body of work indicating that adjuvant therapy for cancers (including chemotherapy, radiation, and endocrine therapy) can have significant immunomodulatory effects including reductions in NK cell count.[98,99] Antineoplastic agents such as Taxol have been shown to impair NK cell activity to K562 in a concentration-dependent fashion, and interfere with the induction of lymphokine-activated killer (LAK) cell activity and lymphocyte proliferation in IL-2 cultures.[100] Together, treatment-associated changes in immune cell numbers associated with cytotoxic responses (NK cells and CD3+ CD8+ cells), lymphocyte proliferation, and NK cell activity may make postsurgery patients more vulnerable to poorer surveillance of cancer-related antigens over the recovery period and possibly to recurrence of disease over the longer term.

Since each of these medical interventions may have downregulatory effects on the immune system, there is the potential for stressors to compound the temporary immunological deficits during and after these phenomena, thus paving the way for negative health effects in cancer patients undergoing treatment. It follows that a stress management intervention at this critical juncture may act to mitigate some of these immunomodulatory changes and may also set the stage for a faster recovery to presurgical or preadjuvant levels of immune system functioning.[30]

Since both stressors and surgery have been associated with decrements in immune functioning,[101] stress-reducing psychosocial interventions administered just before cancer surgery might optimize postsurgical immune status, possibly reducing the risk of opportunistic infection and the growth of cancer cells (e.g. micrometastases) mechanically 'spread' by the surgical procedure. One recent pilot study showed that patients with breast cancer receiving two 90-min sessions of information, problem-solving, relaxation, and psychosocial support showed a tendency towards lower declines in IFN-γ production by peripheral blood mononuclear cells after surgery than those receiving standard care.[102] It is possible that larger effects would have been evident with a longer intervention, although there are clearly practical limitations on what can be done presurgically. Although these results suggest that stress reduction techniques used prior to breast cancer surgery may help buffer the immune system during an otherwise potentially vulnerable period, the health implications of these findings are unclear at present.

Other techniques studied in patients with cancer include contingency management, biofeedback, progressive muscle relaxation, hypnosis, autogenic training, guided imagery, and stress innoculation training.[103] The majority of cognitive–behavioural interventions that have been tested empirically on patients with cancer have included combinations or 'packages' of these techniques, and many seem to include both relaxation and tension reduction (e.g. progressive muscle, autogenics, guided imagery), coping skills training, and problem-solving techniques.[103]

12.4.1.2 Behavioural intervention effects

Relatively few of these interventions have been evaluated for immunological effects in individuals dealing with cancer.[104] A few studies have suggested that psychosocial interventions may be capable of modulating NK cell count,[105] LPR to mitogens,[106,107] lymphocyte numbers,[108] and serum cortisol levels[109] in breast cancer patients at different stages of disease. Only one study to date has demonstrated a relationship between a psychosocial intervention and both immune functioning and disease course in cancer patients.[110] Malignant melanoma patients assigned to a 6-week stress reduction group showed improvements in coping and reductions in distress which were followed by increases in IFN-stimulated NK cell count 6 months later.[111] This team found that malignant melanoma patients assigned to the intervention group showed increases in NK cell count over a 6-month follow-up period and a greater disease-free interval and survival rate at 6-year follow-up than standard-care controls. While baseline NK cell count and intervention-related changes in active coping both predicted disease course, changes in NK cell count did not predict either disease-free interval or survival over time.[88] A widely publicized study also demonstrated that metastatic breast cancer patients assigned to a long-term expressive supportive group therapy group lived twice as long as similar women assigned to standard care.[67] It is possible that the opportunity for emotional expression, processing, and assimilation offered in these groups acted as one mechanism contributing to the greater longevity seen in group members. Alternatively, the built-in social support offered by this type of intervention could also play a central role in their effects on health. Importantly, both emotional disclosure[112] and social support[76] have been associated with aspects of immune system functioning in other populations.

We have heeded this advice by using randomized experimental designs to test the effects of a standardized intervention (group-based CBSM), restricting our intervention studies to patients with specific cancer types and stages (early- to mid-stage breast cancer in the period during or shortly after adjuvant treatment); detailing the types of medical treatment that patients received (e.g. surgery only, surgery plus radiation, surgery plus chemotherapy, etc), and controlling for clinicopathological prognostic risk factors in each of these studies. Specifically, we have monitored a specific set of immune measures during the 10-week CBSM intervention period among women diagnosed with stage 1–3 breast cancer at a point 4–8 weeks after surgery but before the onset of chemotherapy or radiation therapy. We conduct our post-intervention blood draws 3 months after the conclusion of our intervention at a point when, in most cases, adjuvant therapy has been completed. Our work has shown that women assigned to CBSM shortly after surgery for stage 1 and 2 breast cancer show decreases in cortisol[113] and testosterone after the completion of the 10-week group,[114] and increases in lymphocyte proliferative responses to anti-CD3 challenge after the completion of adjuvant therapy.[107] Interestingly, each of these physiological changes was greatest in women who showed the greatest psychological improvement (increase in benefit finding) during the intervention.

12.4.2 Preventing cancer recurrence and metastasis

The relevance of these short-term changes in the immune system for longer-term quality of life and health outcomes in these cancer patients is unclear at this time and remains a mystery in the literature, as no study to date has shown that participation in a psychosocial intervention has effects on long-term (5-year follow-up) quality of life and health outcomes that operate through immunological changes occurring during or shortly after these interventions. The only study that has demonstrated both immunological (NK cell activity) and survival effects for a similar form of psychosocial intervention in patients with early-stage malignant melanoma[115,116] was unable to demonstrate that physical health effects at 6- or 10-year follow-up were mediated by initial immunological changes. In order to address this question, one needs reasonably sized samples of similarly treated patients for whom adequate controls are in place for medical treatments, clinicopathological prognostic risk factors, behavioural risk factors for recurrence, and relevant immune indices. We continue to follow women at regular time intervals to assess the short- and longer-term effects of the intervention on immune variables that may be predictive of retarded disease progression/relapse.

Some broad methodological issues that remain for studies evaluating the efficacy of psychosocial interventions for improving psychosocial adjustment, quality of life, and physical health in patients with cancer and other health conditions include the following:

(1) the need for a standardized, valid, and reliable set of assessment instruments to monitor changes and predictors of change in psychosocial, endocrine, and immunological parameters over time;

(2) the need to utilize information on genetic factors (e.g. family cancer history), disease type/stage, treatment type and duration, demographic and sociocultural (e.g. ethnicity) factors, spiritual beliefs, and personality and contextual characteristics that could moderate intervention effects on adjustment.

Importantly, because of the large role played by genetic factors, unmeasured biological events, and environmental events on disease outcomes, PNI disease research is likely to require large-scale clinical trials in order to arrive at definitive answers.[117]

12.4.3 Reconstituting immune function in conjunction with successful antiviral treatment for HIV infection

Given existing evidence that experimentally induced and naturally occurring stressors, perceived loss of control, social isolation, and depression are related to decrements in the numbers and functions of immune cells known to be altered by HIV infection, it can be reasoned that these psychosocial and behavioural factors might influence immunological status and, possibly, disease course in HIV+ individuals.[118] Similarly, stress management interventions that target these factors might provide both psychological and physical benefits for infected people, especially for those in the early stages of this chronic disease before the virus has established a stranglehold on the immune system and other physiological regulatory processes.[119] Because T-helper (CD4) cells are depleted in the advanced stages of HIV infection,[120] increases in qualitative aspects of HIV itself (e.g. mutation and replication rate)[121] and of lymphocytes (e.g. proliferation and cytotoxicity) might be important in predicting those HIV-infected individuals who do and do not develop opportunistic infections quickly. Innate immune functions such as NK cell activity may compensate in conferring protection against extant viral infections. Since herpes viruses such as EBV or HSV are often poorly controlled in the context of HIV-induced defects in CD4-cell-directed cytotoxic function[122] it is plausible that NK cell activity, which may be partially preserved in HIV infection, could help to survey and control these and other infections in the HIV-infected host. Conversely, stress-induced impairments in NK cell activity may permit herpes virus reactivation and other pathogenic challenges to go unchecked in HIV-infected individuals[123] with the subsequent effects of increased HIV replication.[124]

Stressful events interpreted by HIV-infected individuals as beyond their control may lead to social isolation, loneliness, anxiety, and depressed affect, which may accompany alterations in some neurohormones (e.g. peripheral catecholamine and cortisol elevations) due to SNS activation and dysregulation of the HPA axis. These neuroendocrine changes may also be accompanied by changes in the immune system (redistribution of lymphocytes and decrements in functions concerning LPR and NK cell activity) via interactions between neural and neuroendocrine signals at the immune cell membrane, intracellular cyclic nucleotide activation, and altered production of cytokines such as IL-1, IL-2, and IFN-γ. Since these structural and functional aspects of the immune system are known to decline progressively across the course of HIV infection,[121] it can be further hypothesized that superimposing stressor-induced changes in the functioning of the immune system may increase the rate at which infected people develop clinical symptoms caused by opportunistic infections and neoplasias.

Psychosocial factors that have been related to the rate of decline of CD4 cells over time in HIV-infected gay men include stressful life events,[125] depressive symptoms,[126] fatalistic appraisals,[127] denial coping,[128] distraction coping,[129] and social support,[130] although other studies have failed to find any associations between CD4 cell count declines and these psychosocial variables.[131] Generally the most consistent evidence for associations between these variables comes from studies restricted to more homogeneous samples (e.g. gay men at the earlier stages of disease) followed over periods greater than 12 months.

There is growing evidence that stress-reducing interventions such as CBSM may be capable of lowering antibody titres to herpes viruses such as EBV,[17] HHV-6,[17] and genital herpes (HSV-2)[132] in conjunction with anxiety and dysphoria reductions in HIV-infected men. HIV+ men assigned to CBSM also show decreases in 24-hour urinary cortisol in association with decreases in depression levels.[133] In another study HIV+ men showed decreases in 24-h urinary norepinephrine in association with reductions in anxiety levels.[134] Longer-term follow-up of these men revealed that those in a CBSM intervention revealed greater numbers of CD8+ cytotoxic suppressor cells[134] and CD4+ CD45 RA+ CD29+ transitional naive T cells[135] 6–12 months after the intervention. These studies also showed that men with the greatest decreases in norepinepherine during the 10-week CBSM intervention showed the greatest CD8+ cell counts at follow-up,[134] while those showing the greatest reductions in cortisol showed the greatest transitional naive T-cell counts at follow-up.[136] As mentioned previously, other workers have observed that HIV-infected men receiving another form of stress reduction, massage therapy, showed increases in CD8 cytotoxic cells, NK cell number, and NK cell activity in parallel with decreased anxiety and 24-h urinary cortisol output.[13] Two studies following participants over the post-intervention period revealed that greater distress reductions appeared to predict slower rates of immunological decline up to 2 years later.[19,136] These studies indicate the potential efficacy of stress management interventions for increasing psychological adjustment, improving neuroendocrine regulation, and normalizing immune functioning and health status in HIV+ people in the early and middle stages of the disease.

Individuals participating in the majority of HIV studies were all gay or bisexual men, congruent with the predominant AIDS incidence patterns occurring in the 1980s. It should be noted that women now make up over 15% of all AIDS cases and current incidence patterns for HIV infection suggest that this proportion will increase.[137] The shifting demographic patterns of the HIV–AIDS epidemic make it imperative to develop techniques to help other HIV-infected populations, such as Black inner-city women, to manage their disease. Preliminary data indicate that CBSM techniques may impact on both the psychological and immune functioning of HIV+ Black women. Among HIV+ women, a 10-week CBSM intervention buffered increases in depressed mood and declines in CD4+ CD3+ cell counts over a 10-week period compared with the control group.[138] Another trial is evaluating the effects of a similar intervention in women who have already developed AIDS. To date this intervention has been shown to improve quality of life in this population; immune results are still pending.[61]

The arrival of protease inhibitors and triple combination therapies in the treatment arena has brought about important improvements in the health care of AIDS patients.[139] The resulting treatment philosophy for HIV/AIDS now more than ever views HIV infection as a chronic disease in which patient management is critical. The key here is consistent adherence to a demanding medication schedule in the context of an already stressful daily existence. Failure to adhere rigidly to specific guidelines can not only compromise the effects of the particular protease inhibitor being used, but can also reduce the efficacy of other related compounds to which cross-resistance has developed.

Psychosocial interventions that provide information, skills, and support to patients can facilitate adherence to difficult medication protocols. Since interventions such as CBSM can decrease anxiety and tension levels as well as denial and depressed affect, they may in turn facilitate adherence to medical treatment regimens. The improvements in immune function that have been associated with these psychosocial interventions raises the interesting question of whether CBSM can help reconstitute the compromised immune system once pharmacological agents such as protease inhibitors have contained the virus.[139] These latter questions constitute the focus of the ongoing work using stress management interventions to address medical treatment issues in the growing populations of HIV-infected persons who are attempting to manage their disease.

12.5 Directions for future research

Beyond these diseases and syndromes just noted it is also plausible that PNI mechanisms may play an important role in determining health outcomes for patients who are more vulnerable to disease after undergoing treatments such as surgery, chemotherapy, radiation therapy, and tissue transplantation. Optimal health and recovery following these procedures probably requires a rate and degree of immune system recovery or reconstitution that will outpace infection by opportunistic pathogens. It should be kept in mind that while some of the PNI studies conducted to date show evidence that stressors may contribute to disease processes by way of related immune system changes, it is also possible that these associations are mediated by stress-induced changes in diet, sleep, physical exercise, medication adherence, and substance use, all of which have been independently associated with physical health changes as well as with many components of the immune system.[123,140] Therefore it is critical to control for a wide range of health behavioural factors that could explain apparent associations between stressors, emotional reactions and physiological changes when investigating PNI research questions.

12.5.1 Prevention of cancer in high-risk hosts: carcinogenic viral infections

The role of the immune system in the initiation, promotion, and recurrence of different types of carcinomas in humans is an area of continuing debate.[141] While extensive reviews of PNI research within the context of some specific cancers are available,[140,142] a consensus on the role of the immune system in the course of human cancers is still lacking. There is some evidence that psychosocial variables and related immune system indices are associated with a greater likelihood of developing precancerous changes in certain populations, although the best PNI evidence in this regard comes from persons with cancers that have a viral etiology. This is believed to be because these cancers have greater immunogenicity (due to the presence of viral antigens), a logical assumption for the role of immune surveillance in disease development. One population that has received some attention in the PNI literature is women at risk for cervical neoplasia associated with human papilloma virus (HPV).[142] One paradigm for studying PNI influences on the development of this disease is to study persons who are immuno-compromised due to infection with HIV and who have been exposed to a cervical-cancer-associated virus such as HPV-16 or HPV-18. Among women at increased risk for cervical carcinoma due to co-infection with HIV and human HPV-16/18, a promoter of cervical cancer, greater pessimism was associated with lower NK cell cytotoxicity.[143] In a separate study, more negative life events prospectively predicted greater declines in NK cell number,[144] greater risk of an HSV-2 outbreak,[145] and a greater likelihood of developing or persisting squamous intraepithelial lesions (SILs) over a 1-year follow-up in HIV+ HPV+ women.[146]

Among HIV+ women who are co-infected with carcinogenic viruses such as HPV, stress management interventions may retard SIL promotion and other opportunistic pathogens over time, possibly through buffering decrements in immune system components (e.g. CD8 cells and NK cell activity) that are critical for controlling HPV infection and other viruses such as HSV-2. Our group is examining the psychological, immune and health effects of a 10-week CBSM intervention in HIV+ HPV+ women who have not yet developed AIDS. A major goal of this study is to test whether CBSM can reduce the likelihood that these women will develop the first stages of cervical neo-plasia (SIL). Other viral-associated cancers may present equally plausible models for testing the effects of stress management and other behavioural interventions on health outcomes by way of immune system alterations. Some of these include HPV-associated anal carcinoma in men, HPV-associated head and neck cancers in men and women, HHV-8-associated Kaposi's sarcoma, and EBV-associated Burkitt's lymphoma and nasopharyngeal carcinoma. It is plausible that one place to begin this line of work would be in persons who are most vulnerable to these neoplastic processes owing to a background of immunosuppression secondary to HIV infection.

12.5.2 Decreasing susceptibility to other diseases in treated cancer patients

One intriguing target for future intervention research in psycho-oncology involves the proposed link between stress and susceptibility to infectious disease.[147] It has been sug-gested that since stress is associated with increased susceptibility to upper respiratory infections[148] and bacterial infections,[149] patients treated for cancer, especially those who are emotionally distressed and receiving chemotherapy or other immunosuppress-ive adjuvant therapies, may be vulnerable to stress-associated opportunistic infec-tions,[147] a major health problem in patients with cancer.[149]

12.5.3 Decreasing the likelihood of relapse of cancer after treatment

Another issue of interest to PNI researchers concerns the role of psychosocial factors, behavioural interventions, and immune system functioning in preventing the return of cancer once a patient has been medically treated. Newly treated patients with cancer are vulnerable to distress and loss of positive experiences,[104] and this may reduce cellu-lar immune functions[150,151] that survey the development of metastases.[141,152] Thus psychosocial interventions may provide both mental and physical health benefits, with the latter potentially mediated by intervention-associated changes in specific endocrine and/or immune functions.[141,84] Psychosocial interventions may also facilitate positive adaptations (enhanced relationships, positive emotional growth) that have direct effects on immune system functions such as NK cell count.[53] The cytolytic activity of NK cells and cytotoxic T cells is believed to play an important role in the host response against spontaneous tumours, especially in dealing with shed tumour cells and thus possibly preventing metastases.[153]

Poorer social support[96] and greater distress levels[152] have also been related to decre-ments in NK cell activity among patients with early-stage breast cancer. In one of these studies, early-stage breast cancer patients with greater distress after surgery had lower NK cell activity by 15 months after surgery, predicting a shorter time to recurrence over the 5- to 8-year follow-up.[96] In a related study with early-stage breast cancer patients, greater NK cell activity was associated with patients' perceptions of emotional support from their spouse, greater perceived support from their physician, and seeking social support as a coping strategy.[53] Thus distress, coping strategies, and inadequate social support experienced by cancer patients during the period following surgery could contribute to persisting decrements in immune function, possibly increasing the risk of regional and distant metastases over longer periods.

Several studies have evaluated cognitive–behavioural strategies with patients with cancer, including the use of progressive muscle relaxation with colon carcinoma and melanoma patients, progressive muscle relaxation, imagery, and biofeedback with patients with metastatic cancers of mixed primary sites, group-based multimodal CBSM for women with early- to mid-stage breast cancer, and structured problem-oriented cognitive therapy (based on Beck's cognitive therapy for anxiety and depression) with patients with mixed cancer types. The latter programme focuses on reducing anxiety and depressive symptoms and provides coping skills to help patients develop a 'fighting spirit'.

12.5.4 Key methodological issues

12.5.4.1 Measurement issues

There are now numerous immunological measures (and multiple assay systems for each of these) available for describing changes in quantitative aspects (e.g. enumerating lymphocyte subpopulations, cells with activation markers, intracellular concentrations of pro-cytotoxic substances such as perforin and granzymes) and qualitative aspects (e.g. proliferation, cytotoxicity, antibody production, cytokine production) of the immune system. Recent positive trends in the measurement technologies available for PNI research in cancer include the use of antigen-specific functional assays (e.g. antigen-specific cytotoxicity tests that use breast-cancer-associated cell lines), and the use of stimulated or 'enhanced' function tests (e.g. mitogen-induced cytokine production by lymphocytes, cytokine-enhanced NK cell cytotoxicity using recombinant IL-2 or IFN-γ). Many of these have been widely used in animal studies but are yet to be fully exploited in studies of human cancers. It is unlikely that a single immune measure will be found that is an indicator of long-term health in patients with specific cancers; thus researchers track patterns of changes in several indicators.

In choosing an immunological battery to study, for instance, breast cancer patients in a stress management intervention trial, one may focus on specific immunological measures that have previously been shown to relate to psychosocial variables expected to change during the intervention. Impairments in NK cell activity and LPR to mitogens have been related to depressive symptoms[154] and uncontrollable life events such as bereavement.[155] Since stress management interventions have been shown to reduce depression,[43,133] it is plausible to hypothesize that cancer patients participating in stress management may reveal increases in NK cell activity and lymphoproliferative responses. Therefore at this point in time a comprehensive assessment of immune system status in patients with breast cancer going through a stress management intervention might include the following: lymphocyte cell counts and subpopulations of cells with specific functions; immune system functions such as NK cell activity and LAK activity against breast cancer antigens such as MCF7, and lymphocyte proliferative responses to anti-CD3 stimulation; immune system soluble mediators such as the Th1 cytokines IL-2, IL-12, and IFN-γ, and Th2 cytokines, such as IL-4 and IL-10.

12.5.4.2 Theoretical issues

As Andersen *et al.*[140] note, research at the interface of behavioural oncology and immunology has methodological challenges. They recommend that studies use an experimental design, focus on a specific cancer type and stage [favouring certain types (breast, ovary/cervix, prostate) and early rather than later stages], and use participants who are homogeneous on well-established clinicopathological prognostic factors (e.g. nodal status, hormone receptor status, and menopausal status in the case of breast cancer).[140] A major issue concerns the timing of the stress management intervention and immune assessments. The potentially huge effects of surgery and related anaesthesia, as well as adjuvant therapies such as chemotherapy and radiation, on immune system status must be taken into account in any PNI studies conducted with cancer patients.[101] On the one hand, trying to evaluate the effects of a behavioural intervention on immune parameters during such medical interventions may make it very difficult to demonstrate the effects of stress management. On the other hand, if the study is well controlled, it may be possible to evaluate whether stress management helps to mitigate the stress-induced immunosuppression in cancer patients receiving immunosuppressive treatments like chemotherapy, thereby facilitating immune 'recovery' after the completion of their course of adjuvant therapy.

12.5.4.3 Examining mechanisms of disease

A major issue that plagues health psychology research in HIV/AIDS and cancer is the near absence of any studies relating psychosocial factors and interventions to changes in subclinical markers of disease progression before the point at which disease-related symptoms, relapse, metastasis, or death occurs. This greatly precludes our ability to understand the mechanisms by which psychosocial factors may influence health outcomes in these patients. A few studies have related psychosocial interventions to increases in survival time and disease-free intervals, but these offered very little in the way of mind–body mechanisms to explain their findings. It is important in 'survival' studies to monitor disease activity markers that are relevant to the progression of HIV infection and growth of cancers in general, and others that are specific to the opportunistic pathogen or cancer being studied.

There is currently a great deal of interest in monitoring changes in HIV viral load after the implementation of behavioural interventions, although it is important to note that any intervention-related changes must be carefully interpreted in light of both health behaviour mechanisms (e.g. medication adherence, substance use, sexual activity) and affective–PNI mechanisms. Other subclinical disease markers that may emerge as useful in behavioural intervention studies with HIV-infected persons include measures of apoptosis and concentrations of opportunistic pathogens in the circulation and in target tissue (e.g. HPV viral load in cervical smears).

In terms of behavioural intervention studies with cancer patients, both general and more specific subclinical markers of disease activity are now available for monitoring changes over time. Some of these measure substances associated with the promotion of angiogenesis, a process underlying the assembly of the blood supply for tumours (e.g. VEGF), while others can measure tumour antigens such as CA15–3 for breast cancer and prostate specific antigen (PSA) for prostate cancer patients.

VEGF is a promoter of tumour angiogenesis, the process by which tumour cells recruit capillaries for their blood supply.[156] Angiogenesis has an important role in the progression of solid tumours.[157] The serum levels of VEGF are reported to be significantly higher in cancer patients than in healthy subjects.[158] Elevated levels of VEGF may be produced by defects in p53,[159] but this work is equivocal.[160] Of greater interest to health psychology researchers is recent evidence that VEGF levels appear to be related to psychosocial factors such as social support,[58] and that these associations may be mediated by HPA (cortisol) and SNS (norepinephrine) hormones.[161] Specifically, ovarian cancer patients with better social support showed lower levels of VEGF.[58] Follow-up *in vitro* studies showed that norepinepherine stimulated production of VEGF from an ovarian cancer cell line and these effects were compounded in the presence of cortisol,[161] providing a possible mechanism whereby stress might promote carcinogenesis in patients with ovarian cancer. Similar studies have yet to be performed in patients with breast and prostate cancers, and in those cancers for which angiogenesis may also play a key role (e.g. melanoma[162]). Future research should monitor levels of relevant disease progress in markers in breast and prostate survivors over the long term after behavioural intervention and correlate their levels with measures of quality of life, endocrine function, and physical health.

In addition to monitoring levels of VEGF as a subclinical disease marker, one can monitor more organ-specific disease markers. PSA is thought to be highly specific for prostate tissue and may be increased in prostate cancer, benign prostatic hyperplasia (BPH), and prostatitis. It is secreted into the prostatic ducts and serves to liquefy semen at ejaculation.[163] CA 15-3 is a circulating adenocarcinoma-associated antigen belonging to a family of high-molecular-weight glycoproteins normally present in human milk fat globule membranes. It is a marker that is considered useful in monitoring the clinical course of breast cancer patients. Whereas elevated levels are only present in a small percentage of patients with localized disease, two-thirds of cases with metastatic disease will have significantly elevated levels.[164] It may be useful to examine longer-term effects of behavioural interventions on PSA levels in men previously treated for prostate cancer and to correlate PSA levels at follow-up with psychosocial factors, HPG hormones (e.g. testosterone), immune measures such as NK cell activity, and physical status indicators. Similar designs can be developed for women with breast cancer or individuals previously treated for a cancer for which such subclinical disease markers are available.

In sum, while there are a growing number of studies demonstrating PNI associations in patients with different types of cancer, the health relevance of these associations remains largely unknown at present. There is some suggestion across these studies that psychosocial factors are more likely to be associated with disease course in younger women and those at earlier stages of disease,[165] although at least one study[67] challenges this generalization. Nevertheless, it is critical that future PNI research with cancer patients controls for factors such as age, stage of disease, and ongoing adjuvant therapies such as chemotherapy, radiation, hormonal therapy, and immunotherapy, since each of these can have a significant effect on immunological measures such as NK cell count[98] and LPR to mitogens.[100] Although the role of the immune system in acting as a surveillance system for human cancers is still controversial, tumour-specific immune responses related to prognosis have been documented for certain cancers such as cervical carcinoma and malignant melanoma, and efforts are underway to develop immunotherapies for some of these.[166] Other immunological avenues that may be relevant for cancer control which are now under close scrutiny include those immune system components controlling apoptosis[167] and angiogenesis.[168] Future PNI research with cancer patients may be able to capitalize on some of these developments to establish a firmer link between psychosocial factors and health outcomes in these vulnerable populations.

12.5.5 Understanding the role of sickness behaviour in cancer patients undergoing treatment

A growing body of research suggests that certain treatments for medical conditions such as cancer (e.g. chemotherapy) may induce cytokine dysregulation associated with a constellation of symptoms collectively referred to as 'sickness behaviour'. These symptoms, including fatigue, cognitive difficulties (e.g. memory problems), sleep problems, pain, and general malaise, can have huge effects on the quality of life of cancer patients.[169] To date there have been no systematic studies of behavioural interventions designed to modify sickness behaviour *per se*. However, there is work indicating that behavioural interventions may be effective in modulating fatigue levels,[103] improving sleep quality,[170] improving mild cognitive symptoms, and many more studies showing that these interventions can affect pain perceptions.[171] It is plausible that PNI mechanisms underlying sickness behaviour may be helpful in identifying the underlying mechanisms of action for these interventions in order to make them more targeted, and possibly tailored for specific conditions.

Many of the quality-of-life target areas in cancer identified in prior reviews involve anxiety symptoms and depressed mood.[172] Another area is persistent fatigue, clearly one of the most common experiences of patients treated for cancer.[173,174] Cancer-related fatigue has many sources.[175] One is the medical/physical conditions associated with disease, surgery and adjuvant treatment, and concurrent systemic disorders.[173] Cancer-related fatigue may also stem from sleep disorders, lack of exercise, chronic pain, and use of centrally acting drugs.[176] Fatigue may also co-occur with anxiety or depressive states, and assessments capable of differentiating these factors are important.[173,177] The factors just noted—anxiety, depression, fatigue, and sleep problems—probably exist in many patients with cancer and may be affected by psychosocial intervention. These phenomena may be influenced by focal concerns in the period after surgery, such as fears about recurrence and about potential damage from adjuvant therapy.[178] Cognitive–behavioural techniques and relaxation training interventions aimed at how people deal with these concerns may reduce fatigue and sleep disruption by targeting mood management and tension/anxiety reduction.

Surprisingly, there have been almost no clinical trials testing the efficacy of psycho-social interventions for decreasing or managing fatigue in patients with cancer. Pharmacological therapies may be warranted in advanced cases with debilitating fatigue.[179] An exciting area of PNI concerns the use of antidepressant medications with anti-inflammatory properties to treat sickness behaviour-related symptoms in cancer patients.[169] Blending education, tension/anxiety reduction, sleep monitoring, cognitive restructuring, and pharmacological treatment for sickness behaviour symptoms may be an optimal 'package' for reducing fatigue in patients with cancer in the period following surgery and during adjuvant therapy. These interventions may affect fatigue levels through a combination of stress management, improved sleep quality, and cytokine regulatory changes. It is important to evaluate such an intervention package in controlled research designs since no study to date has tested the concurrent effects of such techniques on mood, fatigue, and sleep quality in patients with cancer during this period. If successful, this type of intervention could offer physical benefits. For instance, since research suggests that the influence of stressors and psychosocial factors on immune system functioning (NK cell activity) may be mediated by alterations in sleep quality,[180–182] it is possible that psychosocial interventions that improve sleep quality may enhance health outcomes in persons with cancer via PNI mechanisms. Alternatively, these interventions may affect fatigue levels and other aspects of the sickness behaviour constellation by modulating the production of pro-inflammatory cytokines such as IL-6 and TNF.

12.6 Conclusions

What we have learned about PNI associations and underlying mechanisms from young and older healthy subjects, as well as human and animal models of infectious, neo-plastic, and immunoregulatory diseases, may allow researchers to address remaining questions and develop effective behavioural interventions for the large populations of vulnerable persons who might benefit from future advances in this field. Future research should focus on specific at-risk and disease groups, modelling the impact of behavioural interventions using randomized designs, testing theory-driven and standardized interventions, and monitoring reliable and clinically relevant measures of immune system functioning, and then relating these changes to alterations in behavioural and psychosocial processes, on the one hand, and subclinical and symptomatic indicators of disease activity on the other. Only empirically supported interventions that pass through this rigorous process should be considered in clinical practice with these populations.

References

1 **Antoni MH** (1997). Cognitive behavioral stress management for gay men learning of their HIV-1 antibody test results. In Spira J (ed.) *Group Therapy for Patients with Chronic Medical Diseases*. New York: Guilford Press, 55–91.

2 **Bernstein B, Borkovec T** (1973). *Progressive Muscle Relaxation Training: A Manual for the Helping Professions*. Champaign, IL: Research Press.

3 **McGrady A, Woerner M, Bernal GAA, Higgins JT** (1987). Effect of biofeedback-assisted relaxation on blood pressure and cortisol levels in normotensives and hypertensives. *J Behav Med* **10**: 301–10.

4 **Patel CH, North WR** (1975). Randomized controlled trial of yoga and biofeedback in the management of hypertension. *Lancet* **ii**: 93–5.

5 **Surwit RS, Feinglos MN** (1983). The effects of relaxation on glucose tolerance in non-insulin-dependent diabetes. *Diabetes Care* **6**: 176–9.

6 **Brandt K** (1973). The effects of relaxation training with analog HR feedback on basal levels of arousal and response to aversive tones in groups selected according to Fear Survey scores. *Psychophysiology* **11**: 242.

7 **Paul G** (1969). Physiological effects of relaxation training and hypnotic suggestion. *J Abnorm Psychol* **74**: 425–537.

8 **Borkovec TD, Sides JK** (1979). Critical procedural variables related to the physiological effects of progressive relaxation: a review. *Behav Res Ther* **17**: 119–25.

9 **Maier SF, Watkins L, Fleshner M** (1994). Psychoneuroimmunology: the interface between behavior, brain, and immunity. *Am Psychol* **49**: 1004–17.

10 **Ironson G, Antoni MH, Lutgendorf S** (2002). Coping: interventions for optimal disease management. In Chesney M, Antoni MH (eds) *Innovative Approaches to Health Psychology: Prevention and Treatment Lessons from AIDS*. Washington, DC: American Psychological Association Press, 167–96.

11 **Ironson G, Field T, Scafidi F,** *et al.* (1996). Massage therapy is associated with enhancement of the immune system's cytotoxic capacity. *Int J Neurosci* **84**: 205–17.

12 **Taylor DN** (1995). Effects of a behavioral stress management program on anxiety, mood, self esteem, and T-cell count in HIV-positive men. *Psychol Rep* **76**: 451–7.

13 **Auerbach JE, Oleson TD, Solomon GF** (1992). A behavioral medicine intervention as an adjunctive treatment for HIV-related illness. *Psychol Health* **6**: 325–34.

14 **Gruber B, Hersh S, Hall N,** *et al.* (1993). Immunologic responses of breast cancer patients to behavioral interventions. *Biofeedback Self Regul* **18**: 1–22.

15 **Morgan W** (1982). Psychological effects of exercise. *Behav Med Update* **4**: 25–30.

16 **LaPerriere A, Antoni MH, Schneiderman N,** *et al.* (1990). Exercise intervention attenuates emotional distress and natural killer cell decrements following notification of positive serologic status for HIV-1. *Biofeedback Self Regul* **15**: 229–42.

17 Esterling B, Antoni MH, Schneiderman N, *et al.* (1992). Psychosocial modulation of antibody to Epstein–Barr viral capsid antigen and human herpes virus-type 6 in HIV-1 infected and at-risk gay men. *Psychosom Med* **54**: 354–71.

18 LaPerriere A, Fletcher MA, Antoni MH, *et al.* (1991). Aerobic exercise training in an AIDS risk group. *Int J Sports Med* **12**: 1–5.

19 Ironson G, Friedman A, Klimas N, Antoni MH, Fletcher MA, Schneiderman N (1994). Distress, denial, and low adherence to behavioral intervention predict faster disease progression in gay men infected with HIV. *Int J Behav Med* **1**: 90–105.

20 Schlenzig C, Jager H, Rieder H, *et al.* (1989). Supervised physical exercise leads to psychological and immunological improvement in pre-AIDS patients. *Proceedings of the 5th International AIDS Conference.*

21 Rigsby L, Dishman R, Jackson A, Maclean G, Raven T (1992). Effects of exercise training on men seropositive for the human immunodeficiency virus-1. *Med Sci Sports Exerc* **24**: 6–12.

22 Florijn Y, Geiger A (1991). Community based physical activity program for HIV-1 infected persons. *Proceedings of the Biological Aspects of HIV Infection Conference.*

23 LaPerriere A, Goldstein A, Klimas N, *et al.* (1997). Non compliant exercise decreases CD4 cells in early symptomatic HIV-1 infection. Paper presented at the Society of Behavioral Medicine, San Francisco, CA.

24 Bartlett E (1983). Educational self-help approaches in childhood asthma. *J Allergy Clin Immunol* **72**: 545–54.

25 Parker J, Frank R, Beck N, *et al.* (1987). Pain management in rheumatoid arthritis: a ognitive–behavioral approach. Unpublished data, Washington University.

26 Brooks GR, Richardson FC (1980). Emotional skills training: a treatment program for duodenal ulcer. *Behav Ther,* **11**: 198–207.

27 Baumstark K, Beck N (1988). A cognitive–behavioral treatment package for management of postoperative Cesarean-section pain. Paper presented at the 9th Annual Scientific Sessions of the Society of Behavioral Medicine, Boston, MA.

28 Fishman B, Loscalzo M (1987). Cognitive–behavioral interventions in management of cancer pain: principles and applications. *Med Clin North Am* **71**: 271–87.

29 Weisenberg M (1987). Psychological intervention for the control of pain. *Behav Res Ther* **25**: 301–12.

30 Antoni MH (2003). *Stress Management Intervention for Women with Breast Cancer.* Washington, DC: American Psychological Association Press.

31 Penedo FJ, Dahn JR, Molton I, *et al.* (2004). Cognitive–behavioral stress management improves quality of life and stress management skill in men treated for localized prostate cancer. *Cancer* **100**: 192–200.

32 Turk D, Holzman A, Kerns R (1986). Chronic pain. In Holroyd K, Creer T (eds) *Self Management of Chronic Disease: Handbook of Clinical Interventions and Research.* Orlando, FL: Academic Press.

33 Beck A, Rush A, Shaw B, Emery G (1979). *Cognitive Therapy of Depression.* New York: Guilford Press.

34 Simons AD, Garfield SL, Murphy GE (1984). The process of change in cognitive therapy and pharmacotherapy for depression. Changes in mood and cognition. *Arch Gen Psychiatry* **41**: 45–51.

35 Rush AJ, Beck AT, Kovacs M, Weissenburger J, Hollon SD (1982). Comparison of the effects of cognitive therapy and pharmacotherapy on hopelessness and self-concept. *Am J Psychiatry* **139**: 862–6.

36 Breitbart W, Payne D (1998). Pain. In Holland J (ed.) *Textbook of Psycho-oncology*. New York: Oxford University Press, 450–67.

37 Beck A, Emery G (1979). *Cognitive Therapy of Anxiety and Phobic Disorders*. Philadelphia, PA: Center for Cognitive Therapy.

38 Antoni MH (2003). Psychoneuroendocrinology and psychoneuroimmunology of cancer: plausible mechanisms worth pursuing? *Brain Behav Immun* 17: S84–91.

39 Lazarus RS, Folkman S (1984). *Stress, Appraisal and Coping*. New York, NY: Springer.

40 Carver CS, Scheier MF, Weintraub JK (1989). Assessing coping strategies: a theoretically-based approach. *J Pers Soc Psychol* 56: 267–283.

41 Folkman S, Chesney M, McKusick L, Ironson G, Johnson D, Coates T (1991). Translating coping theory into intervention. In Eckenrode J (ed.) *The Social Context of Coping*. New York: Plenum Press, 239–59.

42 Antoni MH, Schneiderman N (1998). HIV/AIDS. In Bellack A, Hersen M (eds) *Comprehensive Clinical Psychology*. New York: Elsevier Science, 237–75.

43 Antoni MH, Lehman J, Kilbourn K, *et al.* (2001). Cognitive–behavioral stress management intervention decreases the prevalence of depression and enhances benefit finding among women under treatment for early-stage breast cancer. *Health Psychol* 20: 20–32.

44 Esterling B, Antoni MH, Kumar M, Schneiderman N (1990). Emotional repression, stress disclosure responses, and Epstein-Barr viral capsid antigen titers. *Psychosom Med* 52: 397–410.

45 Esterling B, Antoni MH, Fletcher MA, Marguilles S, Schneiderman N (1994). Emotional disclosure through writing or speaking modulates latent Epstein-Barr virus reactivation. *J Cons Clin Psychol* 62: 130–40.

46 Lutgendorf S, Antoni M, Kumar M, Schneiderman N (1994). Changes in cognitive coping strategies predict EBV-antibody titre change following a stressor disclosure induction. *J Psychosom Res* 38: 63–78.

47 Pennebaker JW, Kiecolt-Glaser JK, Glaser R (1988). Disclosure of traumas and immune function: health implications for psychotherapy. *J Consult Clin Psychol* 56: 239–45.

48 Cohen S, Wills T (1985). Stress, social support, and the buffering hypothesis. *Psychol Bull* 98: 310–57.

49 Cobb S (1974). Physiological changes in men whose jobs are abolished. *J Psychosom Res* 18: 245–58.

50 Gore S (1978). The effect of social support in moderating the health consequences of unemployment. *J Health Soc Behav* 17: 157–65.

51 Zuckerman M, Antoni MH (1995). Social support and its relationship to psychological physical and immune variables in HIV infection. *Clin Psychol Psychother* 2: 210–19.

52 Cruess S, Antoni MH, Cruess D, *et al.* (2000). Reductions in HSV-2 antibody titers after cognitive behavioral stress management and relationships with neuroendocrine function, relaxation skills, and social support in HIV+ gay men. *Psychosom Med* 62: 828–37.

53 Levy S, Herberman R, Whiteside T, *et al.* (1990). Perceived social support and tumor estrogen/progesterone receptor status as predictors of natural killer cell activity in breast cancer patients. *Psychosom Med* 52: 73–85.

54 Dixon D, Kilbourn K, Cruess S, *et al.* (2001). Social support mediates loneliness and human herpesvirus-type 6 (HHV-6) antibody titers. *J Appl Soc Psychol* 31: 1111–32.

55 Kiecolt-Glaser J, Ricker D, George J, *et al.* (1984). Urinary cortisol levels, cellular immunocompetency, and loneliness in psychiatric inpatients. *Psychosom Med* 46: 15–23.

56 Esterling B, Kiecolt-Glaser J, Glaser R (1996). Psychosocial modulation of cytokine-induced natural killer cell activity in older adults. *Psychosom Med* **58**: 264–72.

57 Levy S, Herberman R (1988). Behavior, immunity, and breast cancer: mechanistic analyses of cellular immunocompetence in patient subgroups. Paper presented at The Society of Behavioral Medicine, Boston, MA.

58 Lutgendorf S, Johnsen E, Holmes R, *et al.* (2002). Social relationships and tumor angiogenesis factors in ovarian cancer patients. *Cancer* **95**: 808–15.

59 Lutgendorf S, Antoni M, Ironson G, *et al.* (1997). Cognitive–behavioral stress management decreases dysphoric mood and herpes simplex virus-type 2 antibody titers in symptomatic HIV-seropositive gay men. *J Consult Clin Psychol* **64**: 31–43.

60 Kobasa S, Maddi S, Puccetti M, Zola M (1985). Effectiveness of hardiness, exercise, and social support as resources against illness. *J Psychosom Res* **29**: 525–33.

61 Classen C, Sephton S, Diamond S, Spiegel D (1998). Studies of life-extending psychosocial interventions. In Holland J (ed.) *Textbook of Psycho-oncology*. New York: Oxford University Press, 730–742.

62 Lechner S, Antoni MH, Lydston D, *et al.* (2003). Cognitive–behavioral interventions improve quality of life in women with AIDS. *J Psychosom Res* **54**: 253–61.

63 Goodkin K, Baldewicz T, Asthana D, *et al.* (2001). A bereavement support group intervention affects plasma burden of HIV-1. *J Hum Virol* **4**: 44–54.

64 Spiegel D, Glafkides M (1983). Effects of group confrontation with death and dying. *Int J Group Psychother* **33**: 433–47.

65 Spiegel D, Bloom J, Yalom I (1981). Group support for patients with metastatic cancer: a randomized prospective outcome study. *Arch Gen Psychiatry* **38**: 527–33.

66 Fawzy I, Fawzy N (1998). Psychoeducational interventions. In Holland J (ed) *Textbook of Psycho-oncology*. New York: Oxford University Press, 676–93.

67 Spiegel D, Bloom J, Kraemer HC, Gottheil E (1989). Effect of psychosocial treatment on survival of patients with metastatic breast cancer. *Lancet* **ii**: 888–91.

68 Fontanarosa P, Lundberg G (1997). Complementary, alternative, unconventional, and integrative medicine. *JAMA* **278**: 2111–12.

69 Kiecolt-Glaser J, Ricker D, George J, *et al.* (1984). Urinary cortisol levels, cellular immunocompetency, and loneliness in psychiatric inpatients. *Psychosom Med* **46**: 15–23.

70 Calabrese J, Kling M, Gold P (1987). Alterations in immunocompetence during stress, bereavement, and depression: focus on neuroendocrine regulation. *Am J Psychiatry* **144**: 1123–34.

71 Schneiderman N, Antoni MH, Ironson G, Fletcher MA, Klimas N, LaPerriere A (1994). HIV-1, immunity and behavior. In Glaser R. (ed.) *Handbook of Human Stress and Immunity*. New York: Academic Press, 267–300.

72 Wiedenfeld SA, O'Leary A, Bandura A, Brown S, Levine S, Raska K (1990). Impact of perceived self-efficacy in coping with stressors on components of the immune system. *J Pers Soc Psychol* **59**: 1082–94.

73 Goodkin K, Blaney N, Feaster D, Fletcher MA (1992). Active coping is associated with natural killer cell cytotoxicity in asymptomatic HIV-1 seropositive homosexual men. *J Psychosom Res* **36**: 635–50.

74 Lutgendorf S, Antoni MH, Schneiderman N, Ironson G, Fletcher MA (1994). Psychosocial interventions and quality of life changes across the HIV spectrum. In Baum A, Dimsdale J (eds) *Perspectives in Behavioral Medicine*. Mahwah, NJ: Erlbaum, 205–39.

75 O'Cleirigh C, Ironson G, Antoni MH, *et al.* (2003). Emotional expression and depth processing of trauma and their relation to long-term survival in patients with HIV/AIDS. *J Psychosom Res* **54**: 225–35.

76 Baron R, Cutrona C, Hicklin D, Russel D, Lubaroff D (1990). Social support and immune function among spouses of cancer patients. *J Pers Soc Psychol* **59**: 344–52.

77 Kiecolt-Glaser J, Fisher L, Ogrocki P, Stout J, Speicher C, Glaser R (1987). Marital quality, marital disruption, and immune function. *Psychosom Med* **49**: 13–34.

78 Kiecolt-Glaser J, Malarkey W, Cacioppo J, Glaser R (1994). Stressful personal relationships: endocrine and immune function. In Glaser R, Kiecolt-Glaser J (eds) *Handbook of Human Stress and Immunity*. San Diego, CA: Academic Press, 321–39.

79 McEwen B (1998). Protective and damaging effects of stress mediators. *N Engl J Med* **338**: 171–9.

80 Felten D (1996). Changes in the neural innervation of lymphoid tissues with age. In Hall N, Altman F, Blumenthal S (eds) *Mind–Body Interactions and Disease and Psychoneuroimmunological Aspects of Health And Disease. Proceedings of Conference on Stress, Immunity and Health*. Washington, DC: Heath Dateline Press, 157–64.

81 Kiecolt-Glaser J, Glaser R, Williger D (1985). Psychosocial enhancement of immunocompetence in a geriatric population. *Health Psychol* **4**: 25–41.

82 Kiecolt-Glaser J, Glaser R, Strain E, *et al.* (1986). Modulation of cellular immunity in medical students. *J Behav Med* **9**: 311–20.

83 Zachariae R, Hansen JB, Andersen M (1994). Changes in cellular immune function after immune specific guided imagery and relaxation in high and low hypnotizable healthy subjects. *Psychother Psychosom* **61**: 74–92.

84 Ironson G, Antoni M, Lutgendorf S (1995). Can psychological interventions affect immunity and survival? Present findings and suggested targets with a focus on cancer and human immunodeficiency virus. *Mind/Body Med*, **1**: 85–110.

85 Fonteneau JF, Le Drean E, Le Guiner S, Gervois N, Diez E, Jotereau, F (1997). Heterogeneity of biologic responses of melanoma-specific CTL. *J Immunol* **15**: 2831–9.

86 Baxevanis C, Reclos G, Gritzapis A, Dedousis G, Missitzis I, Papamichail M (1993). Elevated prostaglandin E2 production by monocytes is responsible for the depressed levels of natural killer and lymphokine-activated killer cell function in patients with breast cancer. *Cancer* **72**: 491–501.

87 Clerici M, Shearer G, Clerici E (1998). Cytokine dysregulation in invasive cervical carcinoma and other human neoplasias: time to consider the Th1/Th2 paradigm. *J Natl Cancer Inst* **90**: 261–3.

88 Fawzy F, Fawzy N, Hyun C, *et al.* (1993). Malignant melanoma. Effects of an early structured psychiatric intervention, coping, and affective state on recurrence and survival 6 years later. *Arch Gen Psychiatry* **50**: 681–9.

89 Rogentine G, Van Krammen D, Fox B *et al.* (1979). Psychological factors in the prognosis of malignant melanoma: a prospective study. *Psychosom Med* **4**: 647–55.

90 Geyer S (1991). Life events prior to manifestation of breast cancer: a limited prospective study covering eight years before diagnosis. *J Psychosom Res* **35**: 355–63.

91 Ramirez A, Craig T, Watson J, Fentiman I, North W, Rubens R (1989). Stress and relapse of breast cancer. *BMJ* **298**: 291–3.

92 Greer S, Morris T, Pettingale K, Haybittle J (1990). Psychological response to breast cancer and 15-year outcome. *Lancet* **i**: 49–50.

93 Pettingale KW, Morris T, Greer S, Haybittle JL (1985). Mental attitudes to cancer: an additional prognostic factor. *Lancet* **i**: 750.

94 Greer S (1991). Psychological responses to cancer and survival. *Psychol Med* **21**: 43–9.

95 Jensen M (1987). Psychobiological factors predicting the course of breast cancer. *J Pers* **55**: 317–42.

96 Levy S, Herberman R, Lippman M, D'Angelo T, Lee J (1991). Immunological and psychosocial predictors of disease recurrence in patients with early-stage breast cancer. *Behav Med* **17**: 67–75.

97 Fawzy F, Fawzy N, Hyun C, Wheeler J (1997). Brief, coping-oriented therapy for patients with malignant melanoma. In Spria J (ed.) *Group Therapy for Medically Ill Patients*. New York: Guilford, 133–64.

98 Tichatschek E, Zielinski C, Muller C, *et al.* (1988). Long-term influence of adjuvant therapy on natural killer cell activity in breast cancer. *Immunotherapy* **27**: 278–82.

99 Brenner B, Margolese R (1991). The relationship of chemotherapeutic and endocrine intervention on natural killer cell activity in human breast cancer. *Cancer* **68**: 482–8.

100 Chuang L, Lotzova E, Cook K, *et al.* (1993). Effect of new investigational drug Taxol on oncolytic activity and stimulation of human lymphocytes. *Gynecol Oncol* **49**: 291–8.

101 van der Pompe G, Antoni M, Heijnen C (1998). The effects of surgical stress and psychological stress on the immune function of operative cancer patients. *Psychol Health* **13**: 1015–26.

102 Larson M, Duberstein P, Talbot N, Caldwell C, Moynihan J (2000). A pre-surgical psychosocial intervention for breast cancer patients: psychological distress and the immune response. *J Psychosom Res* **48**: 187–94.

103 Jacobsen P, Hann D (1998). Cognitive–behavioral interventions. In Holland J (ed.) *Textbook of Psycho-oncology*. New York: Oxford University Press, 717–29.

104 van der Pompe G, Antoni MH, Mulder N, *et al.* (1994). Psychoneuroimmunology and the course of breast cancer, an overview: the impact of psychosocial factors on progression of breast cancer through immune and endocrine mechanisms. *Psychooncology* **3**: 271–88.

105 Anderson BL, Farrar WB, Golden-Kreutz DM, *et al.* (2004). Psychological, behavioural and immune changes after a psychological intervention: a clinical trial. *J Clin Oncol* **22**: 3570–80.

106 van der Pompe G, Antoni MH, Visser A, Heijnen C, deVries M (1996). Psychological and immunological effects of psychotherapy for breast cancer patients: a reactivity study. *Psychosom Med* **58**: 97 (abstr).

107 McGregor B, Antoni MH, Boyers A, *et al.* (2004). Effects of cognitive behavioral stress management on immune function and positive contributions in women with early-stage breast cancer. *J Psychosom Res* **54**: 1–8.

108 Schedlowski M, Jungk C, Schimanski G, Tewes U, Schmoll H (1994). Effects of behavioral intervention on plasma cortisol and lymphocytes in breast cancer patients: an exploratory study. *Psychooncology* **3**: 181–7.

109 van der Pompe G, Duivenvoorden H, Antoni MH, Visser A, Heijnen C (1997). Effectiveness of a short-term group psychotherapy program on endocrine and immune function in breast cancer patients: an exploratory study. *J Psychosom Res* **42**: 453–66.

110 Barraclough J, Pinder P, Cruddas M, Osmond C, Taylor I, Perry M. Life events and breast cancer prognosis. *BMJ* **304**:1078–81.

111 Fawzy F, Kemeny M, Fawzy N, *et al.* (1990). A structured psychiatric intervention for cancer patients. II. Changes over time in immunological measures. *Arch Gen Psychiatry* **47**: 729–35.

112 Petrie KJ, Booth RJ, Pennebaker JW, Davidson KP, Thomas MG (1995). Disclosure of trauma and immune response to a hepatitis B vaccination program. *J Consult Clin Psychol* **63**: 787–92.

113 Cruess DG, Antoni MH, McGregor BA, *et al.* (2000). Cognitive–behavioral stress management reduces serum cortisol by enhancing positive contributions among women being treated for early stage breast cancer. *Psychosom Med* **62**: 304–8.

114 Cruess D, Antoni MH, McGregor B, *et al.* (2001). Cognitive behavioral stress management effects on testosterone and positive growth in women with early-stage breast cancer. International *J Behav Med* **8**: 194–207.

115 Fawzy F, Fawzy N (1994). Psycheducational interventions and health outcomes. In Glaser R, Kiecolt-Glaser J (eds) *Handbook of Human Stress and Immunity*. New York: Academic Press, 365–402.

116 Fawzy F, Canada A, Fawzy N (2003). Malignant melanoma: effects of a brief, structured psychiatric intervention on survival and recurrence at 10-year follow-up. *Arch Gen Psychiatry* **60**: 100–3.

117 Schneiderman N, Antoni MH, Saab PG, Ironson G (2002). Health psychology: psychosocial and biobehavioral aspects of chronic disease management. *Annu Rev Psychol* **52**: 555–80.

118 Kemeny ME (1994). Stressful events, psychological responses and progression of HIV infection. In Glaser R, Kiecolt-Glaser J (eds) *Handbook of Human Stress and Immunity*. New York: Academic Press.

119 Antoni MH, Schneiderman N, Fletcher M, Goldstein D, Laperriere A, Ironson G (1990). Psychoneuroimmunology and HIV-1. *J Consult Clin Psychol* **58**: 38–49.

120 Klimas N, Caralis P, LaPerriere A, *et al.* (1991). Immunologic function in a cohort of HIV type-1 seropositive and negative healthy homosexual men. *J Clin Microbiol* **29**: 1413–21.

121 Pantaleo G, Graziosi C, Fauci AS (1993). The immunopathogenesis of human immunodeficiency virus infection. *N Engl J Med* **328**: 327–35.

122 Biron G, Byron K, Sullivan J (1989). Severe herpes virus infections in an adolescent without natural killer cells. *N Engl J Med* **320**: 1731–5.

123 Kiecolt-Glaser JK, Glaser R (1988). Psychological influences on immunity: implications for AIDS. *Am Psychol* **43**: 892–8.

124 Carbonari M, Fiorilli M, Mezzaroma I, Cherichi M, Aiuti F (1989). CD4 as the receptor for retroviruses of the HTLV family: immunopathogenetic implications. *Adv Exp Med Biol* **257**: 3–7.

125 Leserman J, Petitto J, Perkins D, Folds J, Golden R, Evans D (1997). Severe stress, depressive symptoms, and changes in lymphocyte subsets in human immunodeficiency virus-infected men. *Arch Gen Psychiatry* **54**: 279–85.

126 Burack JH, Barrett DC, Stall RD, Chesney MA, Ekstrand ML, Coates TJ (1993). Depressive symptoms and CD4 lymphocyte decline among HIV-infected men. *JAMA* **270**: 2567–73.

127 Reed GM, Kemeny ME, Taylor SE, Wang HJ, Visscher B (1994). Realistic acceptance as a predictor of decreased survival time in gay men with AIDS. *Health Psychol* **13**: 299–307.

128 Leserman J, Petitto JM, Golden RN, Gaynes BN, Gu H, Perkins DO (2000). The impact of stressful life events, depression, social support, coping and cortisol on progression to AIDS. *Am J Psychiatry* **157**: 1221–8.

129 Mulder C, de Vroome E, van Griensven G, Antoni MH, Sandfort T (1999). Distraction as a predictor of the virological course of HIV-1 infection over a 7-year period in gay men. *Health Psychol* **18**: 107–13.

130 Theorell T, Blomkvist V, Jonsson H, Schulman S, Berntorp E, Stigendal L (1995). Social support and the development of immune function in human immunodeficiency virus infection. *Psychosom Med* **57**: 32–6.

131 Rabkin JG, Williams JBW, Remien RH, Goetz RR, Kertzner R, Gorman JM (1991). Depression, lymphocyte subsets, and human immunodeficiency virus symptoms on two occasions in HIV-positive homosexual men. *Arch Gen Psychiatry* **48**: 111–19.

132 Lutgendorf S, Antoni MH, Ironson G, Klimas N, Fletcher MA, Schneiderman N (1997). Cognitive processing style, mood and immune function following HIV seropositivity notification. *Cogn Ther Res* **21**: 157–84.

133 Antoni MH, Wagner S, Cruess D, *et al.* (2000). Cognitive behavioral stress management reduces distress and 24-hour urinary free cortisol among symptomatic HIV-infected gay men. *Ann Behav Med* **22**: 29–37.

134 **Antoni MH, Cruess D, Wagner S, *et al.*** (2000). Cognitive behavioral stress management effects on anxiety, 24-hour urinary catecholamine output, and T-cytotoxic/suppressor cells over time among symptomatic HIV-infected gay men. *J Consult Clin Psychol* **68**: 31–45.

135 **Antoni MH, Cruess D, Klimas N, *et al.*** (2002). Stress management and immune system reconstitution in symptomatic HIV-infected gay men over time: effects on transitional naive T-cells (CD4+ CD45 RA+ CD29+). *Am J Psychiatry* **159**: 143–5.

136 **Mulder N, Antoni MH, Emmelkamp P, *et al.*** (1995). Psychosocial group intervention and the rate of decline of immunologic parameters in asymptomatic HIV-infected homosexual men. *J Psychother Psychosom* **63**: 185–92.

137 **Centers for Disease Control** (1997). *HIV/AIDS Surveillance Report* **9**: 1–39.

138 **West-Edwards C, Pereira D, Greenwood D, *et al.*** (2001). An investigation of the psychological and immune effects of a cognitive behavioral stress management (CBSM) intervention for HIV+ African American women. *Ann Behav Med* **23**: 12 (abstr).

139 **Schneiderman N, Antoni MH, Ironson G** (1997). Cognitive behavioral stress management and secondary prevention in HIV/AIDS. *Psychol AIDS Exch* **22**: 1–8.

140 **Andersen B, Kiecolt-Glaser J, Glaser R** (1994). A biobehavioral model of cancer stress and disease course. *Am Psychol* **49**: 389–404.

141 **Bovjberg D** (1991). Psychoneuroimmunology: implications for oncology? *Cancer* **67**: 828–32.

142 **Goodkin K, Antoni MH, Fox BH, Sevin B** (1993). A partially testable model of psychosocial factors in the etiology of cervical cancer. II. Psychoneuroimmunological aspects, critique and prospective integration. *Psychooncology* **2**: 99–121.

143 **Byrnes D, Antoni MH, Goodkin K, *et al.*** (1998). Stressful events, pessimism, natural killer cell cytotoxicity, and cytotoxic/suppressor T-cells in HIV+ Black women at risk for cervical cancer. *Psychosom Med* **60**: 714–22.

144 **Pereira D, Antoni MH, Danielson A, *et al.*** (2000). Declines in natural killer cell percentages mediate the effects of high life stress on the incidence of cervical dysplasia in HIV+ black women at risk for cervical cancer. *Psychosom Med* **62**: 105.

145 **Pereira D, Antoni MH, Simon T, *et al.*** (2003). Stress as a predictor of symptomatic genital herpes virus recurrence in women with human immunodeficiency virus. *J Psychosom Res* **54**: 237–44.

146 **Pereira D, Antoni MH, Simon T, *et al.*** (2003). Stress and squamous intraepithelial lesions in women with human papillomavirus and human immunodeficiency virus. *Psychosom Med* **65**: 427–34.

147 **Bovbjerg D, Valdimarsdottir H** (1996). Stress, immune modulation, and infectious disease during chemotherapy for breast cancer. *Ann Behav Med* **18**: S63.

148 **Cohen S, Tyrrell DA, Smith AP** (1991). Psychological stress in humans and susceptibility to the common cold. *N Engl J Med* **325**: 606–12.

149 **White M** (1993). Prevention of infection in patients with neo-plastic disease: use of a historical model for developmental strategies. *Clin Infect Dis* **17**: S355–8.

150 **Herbert T, Cohen S** (1993). Stress and immunity in humans: a meta-analytic review. *Psychosom Med* **55**: 364–79.

151 **Herbert T, Cohen S** (1993). Depression and immunity: a meta-analytic review. *Psychol Bull* **113**: 472–86.

152 **Andersen B, Farrar W, Golden-Kreutz D, *et al.*** (1998). Stress and immune responses after surgical treatment for regional breast cancer. *J Natl Cancer Inst* **90**: 30–6.

153 **Melief C, Kast W** (1991). Cytotoxic T lymphocyte therapy of cancer and tumor escape mechanisms. *Cancer Biol* **2**: 347–53.

154 Irwin M, Patterson T, Smith TL, *et al.* (1990). Reduction of immune function in life stress and depression. *Biol Psychiatry* **27**: 22–30.

155 Irwin M, Caldwell C, Smith T, Brown S, Schuckit M, Gillin C (1990). Major depressive disorder, alcoholism, and reduced natural killer cell cytotoxicity. *Arch Gen Psychiatry* **47**: 713–19.

156 Bergers G, Benjamin L (2003). Tumorigenesis and the angiogenic switch. *Nat Rev Cancer* **3**: 401–10.

157 Beck L, Jr, D'Amore PA (1997). Angiogenesis and markers *FASEB J* **5**: 365–73.

158 Dosquet C, Coudert MC, Lepage E, Cabane J, Richard F (1997). Are angiogenic factors, cytokines, and soluble adhesion molecules prognostic factors in patients with renal cell carcinoma? *Clin Cancer Res* **3**: 2451–8.

159 Kwak C, Jin RJ, Lee C, Park MS, Lee SE (2002). Thrombosondin-1, vascular endothelial growth factor expression and their relationship with p53 status in prostate cancer and benign prostatic hyperplasia. *BJU Int* **89**: 303–9.

160 Agani F, Kirsch DG, Friedman SL, Kastan MB, Semenza GL (1997). p53 does not repress hypoxia-induced transcription of the vascular endothelial growth factor gene. *Cancer Res* **57**: 4474–7.

161 Lutgendorf S, Cole S, Costanzo E, *et al.* (2003). Stress related mediators stimulate vascular endothelial growth factor secretion by two ovarian cancer cell lines. *Clin Cancer Res* **9**: 4514–21.

162 Hendrix M, Seftor E, Hess A, Seftor R (2003). Vasculogenic mimicry and tumour-cell plasticity: lessons from melanoma. *Nat Rev Cancer* **3**: 411–21.

163 Oesterling E, Oesterling JE (1991). Prostate specific antigen: a critical assessment of the most useful tumor marker for adenocarcinoma of the prostate. *J Urol* **143**: 907–23.

164 Bliss P, Fisken J, Roulsten J, Leonard RC (1993). An assessment of the clinical usefulness of two serum markers, CA15 3 and HMFG 2 in localized and metastatic breast cancer. *Dis Markers* **11**: 45–8.

165 Schultz R, Bookwala J, Knapp JE, Scheier MF, Williamson GM (1996). Pessimism, age, and cancer mortality. *Psychol Aging* **11**: 304–9.

166 Osanto S, Brouwenstyn N, Vessen N, Figdor C, Melief C, Schrier P (1993). Clinical protocol. Immunization with interleukin-2-transfected melanoma cells. A phase I–II study of patients with metastatic melanoma. *Hum Gene Ther* **4**: 323–30.

167 Hahne M, Rimoldi D, Schroter M, *et al.* (1996). Melanoma cell expression of fas (Apo-1/CD95) ligand: implications for tumor immune escape. *Science* **274**: 1363–6.

168 Kurtzman S, Miller L, Anderson K, Wang P, Kreutzer D (1997). Cytokine regulation of angiogenesis in human breast cancer. *Proceedings of the Department of Defense Breast Cancer Research Program Meeting 'Era of Hope'*. Washington, DC: Department of Defense, 341–2.

169 Kelley K, Bluthe R, Dantzer R, *et al.* (2003). Cytokine-induced sickness behavior. *Brain Behav Immun* **17**: S112–18.

170 Cruess D (2002). Improving sleep quality in patients with chronic illness. In Chesney M, Antoni M (eds) *Innovative Approaches to Health Psychology: Prevention and Treatment Lessons from AIDS*. Washington, DC: American Psychological Association Press, 235–52.

171 Breitbart W, Payne D (1998). Pain. In Holland J (ed.) *Textbook of Psycho-oncology*. New York: Oxford University Press, 450–67.

172 Payne D, Hoffman R, Theodoulou M, Dosik M, Massie M (1999). Screening for anxiety and depression in women with breast cancer. *Psychosomatics* **40**: 64–9.

173 Portenoy R, Miaskowski C (1998). Assessment and management of cancer-related fatigue. In Berger A (ed) *Principles and Practice of Supportive Oncology*. New York: Lippincott—Raven, 109–80.

174 Vogelzang N, Breitbart W, Cella D, *et al.* (1997). Patient, caregiver, and oncologist perceptions of cancer-related fatigue: results of a tripart assessment survey. The Fatigue Coalition. *Semin Hematol* **34**: 4–12.

175 Piper B, Lindsey A, Dodd M (1991). Fatigue mechanisms in cancer patients: developing nursing theory. *Oncol Nurs Forum* **14**: 17–23.

176 Engstrom C, Strohl R, Rose L, Lewandowski L, Stefanek M (1999). Sleep alterations in cancer patients. *Cancer Nurs* **22**: 143–8.

177 Portenoy R, Itri L (1999). Cancer-related fatigue: guidelines for evaluation and management. *Oncologist* **4**: 1–10.

178 Spencer S, Lehman J, Wynings C, *et al.* (1999). Concerns of a multi-ethnic sample of early stage breast cancer patients and relations to psychosocial well being. *Health Psychol* **18**: 159–69.

179 Breitbart W, Mermelstein H (1992). An alternative psychostimulant for management of depressive disorders in cancer patients. *Psychosomatics* **33**: 352–6.

180 Ironson G, Wynings C, Schneiderman N, *et al.* (1997). Post traumatic stress symptoms, intrusive thoughts, loss and immune function after Hurricane Andrew. *Psychosom Med* **59**: 128–41.

181 Hall M, Baum A, Buysse D, *et al.* (1998). Sleep as a mediator of the stress-immune relationship. *Psychosom Med* **60**: 48–51.

182 Irwin M, Smith T, Gillin J (1992). Electroencephalographic sleep and natural killer activity in depressed patients and control subjects. *Psychosom Med* **54**: 10–21.

Chapter 13

Emotional disclosure and psychoneuroimmunology

Roger Booth

13.1 The clinical context

As humans, we are entwined in social networks. Events happen to us throughout our lives, and we generate stories about those events through our relationships and conversations with families, friends, workmates, society, and culture. These stories help us to make sense of our lives and to describe and define who we are. Sharing our stories with others somehow binds us into the social fabric, but sometimes there are stories which are difficult to tell others and even ourselves. Sometimes when events are upsetting or traumatic, they threaten our capacity to make sense of our lives in acceptable ways and so we find it difficult to accept or acknowledge them. Do such stories also have the power to affect our health adversely and, if so, can we reverse those adverse effects in any way? These questions are central to research that delves into the psychological, physiological, and health effects of emotional disclosure.

13.1.1 What this chapter is about

This chapter will review the effects of studies employing this approach and will also include some studies that have explored the effects of emotional expression in other ways. It is not intended to be an exhaustive review or critique of published emotional disclosure studies, but rather an overview of the field highlighting particular areas of clinical interest and relevance to psychoneuroimmunology.

The chapter begins with description of emotional disclosure as an experimental tool and summarizes some of the early work using it. A theoretical basis for a role of psychoneuroimmunology in mediating the health effects of emotional disclosure is then presented that attempts to integrate psychological and physiological processes within a model of self-generation in which emotions play a central role in expressing who we are. The health effects of emotional disclosure are then explored in healthy volunteers and in primary care (section 13.3) and various illness groups (section 13.4). Section 13.5 asks how emotional disclosures leads to health benefits by exploring behavioural, psychological, and immune mechanisms, and the chapter ends with a discussion of the challenges still remaining in this area and possible directions for future research (section 13.6).

13.1.2 **What is emotional disclosure/expression**

Emotional disclosure is a term most commonly used to describe 'Pennebaker-type' interventions in which volunteers are encouraged to write about traumatic or upsetting events in their lives and to explore their deepest thoughts and feelings about these events in their writing. In the mid-1980s, Pennebaker and colleagues began a series of laboratory-based studies into the health effects of emotionally expressive writing about traumatic or upsetting events. They used a simple randomized control design in which participants were asked to write for 15–20 min every day for 4 days about either traumatic experiences in an emotionally expressive way or mundane events in a descriptive way. All writing was anonymous and confidential. Subjects in the emotional disclosure group were typically given directions of the following type:

> During each of the four writing days, I want you to write about the most traumatic and upsetting experiences of your whole life. You can write on different topics each day or on the same topic for all four days, The important thing is for you to really let go and explore your very deepest thoughts and feelings. Don't worry about sentence structure or grammar or repetition, just continue writing for the full time. All your writing will be completely confidential.

Initial research using this approach employed first-year college students[1] and assessed the effects on physical health following the writing exercise by monitoring student visits to the university health centre over the subsequent 6 months. Those students who had written emotionally about their thoughts and feelings had significantly reduced numbers of doctor visits than did the students who had written descriptively about mundane topics.

13.2 **Theoretical basis for a role for psychoneuroimmunology**

13.2.1 **Interactions in the human world**

In essence, the stories we tell are explanations of the interaction between ourselves and the world in which we live, and they help us to build and maintain an adequate relationship with that world. Consequently, they are important for our human, social, and cultural adaptation. Moreover, as living organisms we must maintain an adequate relationship not only with our sociocultural milieu but also with our biological and physical environments (Fig. 13.1). Our biophysical adaptation is maintained through homeostatic and allostatic physiological processes and through the coordination of our sensory–effector systems (i.e. how we see, hear, touch, taste, and smell the world about us, and how we move within that world). At every moment in our lives, we are disposed to a particular domain of actions that is determined by a combination of the composition of our bodies and the context in which we find ourselves. As our situation (physiological and/or contextual) changes, so the domain of actions available to us changes accordingly. We experience these domains of action as emotions. In other words, emotions are what move us to think, feel, and act in particular ways. When we change from one emotion to another—from joy to fear, for example—the composition

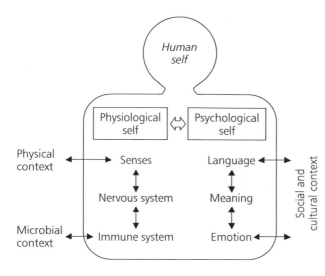

Fig. 13.1 A model of the relationship between the physiological and psychological facets of the human self, and their relationships with each other and with the environments of human life.

of our bodies, our relationship with our context, and the domain of actions available to us all change in a coordinated manner. Similarly, when events change in our lives, our emotions change to reflect that. In one sense, emotions are a little like the gears of a car—changing emotions changes the domain of actions available to us.

Therefore the events of our lives and how we perceive them must always arise for us in a particular emotional context. We label events as upsetting or traumatic because of the emotions they evoke within us, and they affect our physiology in ways that are consistent with that emotional context. Moreover, because we are social beings, we can relive some aspects of events in our lives by talking about them. We might do this in conversation with others, or by ourselves through reflective or ruminative thinking or imagination. Like all other actions in our lives, such conversations bring with them a particular emotional framework. Emotions and physiology, then, mutually influence one another and so we would expect the immune system, as part of our physiology, to be affected by the expression of emotion.

13.2.2 Emotions and the neuroimmune system

Empirical evidence exists to support the contention that the expression of emotions affects the immune system. In particular, emotional expression in a variety of situations has been found to result in short-term changes in immune parameters. For example, in one study volunteers were asked to view emotionally rich videos and to either inhibit or express overt emotions (laughter or weeping). Humorous videos resulted in increased salivary IgA (sIgA) concentrations regardless of whether or not overt laughter was expressed, whereas overt crying was associated with decreased sIgA but inhibition of weeping in the context of the same sad video was not linked to lower sIgA.[2,3] Deliberate expression of particular emotional states also affects immune measures. When method actors were asked to act out various states, affective states such as happiness, anxiety, and depression induced more immune fluctuations than did a neutral state.[4] Compared with the neutral state, all mood states affected several immune parameters. Natural killer (NK) cell percentage and activity and percentage of suppressor/cytotoxic T cells, regardless of the valence or arousal level of the mood induced, and changes in heart rate, physical activity, and cortisol levels contributed to some of these effects.[5] Recalling or reliving emotionally rich experiences also results in immune changes. For example, when healthy volunteers were asked to recall maximally disturbing or maximally pleasurable emotional experiences, they displayed significant cardiovascular activation while recalling the events. Disturbing experiences, in particular, also elicited transient declines in mitogen-induced T-cell proliferation and small changes in NK cell activity.[6] Immunological regulatory factors (cytokines) have also been found to be affected by mood changes. For example, increased secretion of cytokines associated with T-cell proliferation (e.g. IL-2) but not those associated with inflammation (e.g. IL-1 and IL-6) was observed in response to mild induced negative emotional changes, while the reverse (i.e. increased inflammatory cytokines but not T-cell proliferative cytokines) occurred following positive mood changes.[7]

Expressing emotion in interpersonal situations is associated with changes in physical appearance (e.g. facial features and muscle tension) and behaviour (e.g. aggression, hostility, submission). Because these involve our physiology, we would expect there to be concomitant changes in nervous system activity and possibly immune system activity as well. At Ohio State University, a series of experiments were conducted to investigate such changes in situations of interpersonal conflict. Married couples were asked to engage in discussion with one another in the laboratory to solve a problem or to attempt to resolve a conflict. Blood samples and physiological measures were taken before, during, and after the 30-min discussion. Hostile or negative behaviour during conflict was closely linked to changes in serum hormone levels. It was associated with decreased levels of prolactin and increases in epinephrine, norepinephrine, adrenocorticotropic hormone (ACTH), and growth hormone, but not cortisol.[8] Among wives, escalation of negative behaviour during conflict accounted for around 20% of the variance in the rates of change of cortisol, ACTH, and norepinephrine (but not epinephrine), while the endocrine data of husbands did not show significant relationships with negative behaviour.[9]

These neuroendocrine hormonal changes were also mirrored by short-term effects on immune variables. In a study involving 90 newlywed couples, negative behaviour during marital conflict was associated with immunological downregulation. Relative to low-negative subjects, those who exhibited more negative or hostile behaviours during a 30-min discussion of marital problems showed greater decrements in functional immunological assays (NK cell cytotoxicity and T-lymphocyte proliferative response to mitogenic stimulation) and larger increases in the numbers of circulating

T lymphocytes over the subsequent 24 h. Women were more likely than men to show negative immunological changes. Highly hostile behaviours also led to larger increases in blood pressure that remained elevated for longer.[10] In another study, differences in the physiological effects of displaying anger during conflict were evident depending on whether the subjects were categorized as high or low in cynical hostility.[11] Display of anger among men high in cynical hostility was associated with greater elevations in systolic and diastolic blood pressure, and cortisol, and increases in NK cell numbers and NK cell cytotoxicity, whereas in men low in cynical hostility, anger was associated with smaller increases in heart rate and NK cell cytotoxicity.

13.2.3 Can we explain emotional disclosure health effects in terms of psychoneuroimmunology?

Clearly, expression of emotion is associated with short-term changes in physiology, nervous system activity, and some immune measures, but do these short-term effects provide any way of explaining the longer-term health benefits of emotional disclosure or emotionally expressive writing? The short answer is 'no', because these short-term effects are indicative of the expressive behaviours themselves rather than of any perceptual and psychological changes associated with potential health benefits. Although there are short-term physiological and neuroimmune effects of emotional disclosure, the health benefits (see later) are associated with more enduring changes of perception, and therefore it is longer-term or dispositional changes in neuroimmune activity and/or behaviour that are likely to be informative.

How then might we explore the link between emotional disclosure and immune function? What facets of immune system activity within people's lives are likely to be central? One way of answering these questions is to return to the nature of the immune system itself in the context of living organisms (see Fig. 13.1). In order for living organisms to remain adapted to their environments they must be sensitive to changes in those environments. Through our five 'traditional' senses of sight, sound, smell, taste, and touch we can respond to aspects of our environment both automatically and voluntarily. For example, if I see something terrifying I can voluntarily close my eyes to shut out the sight. Alternatively, if my eyes sense an object approaching at speed, they will trigger an automatic blink reaction to protect my eyeballs from damage. In both examples, my body will automatically adapt with changes in endocrine secretions, digestive system activity, musculature, breathing, heart rate, and blood circulation. These changes arise coherently in order that I can continue to generate myself and maintain an adequate relationship with my environment. However, some environmental changes are not readily detected by our traditional five senses. These include many microorganisms that we cannot see, hear, taste or smell, yet if we had no means of sensing them within our bodies, they might readily compromise our biological integrity. Fortunately, within our bodies, the immune system acts as an internal sensory system[12] receptive to changes such as those associated with microorganisms.

Therefore the sensory mechanics of my body allows me to apprehend information about my physical and microbial environments. How I respond to that information is determined by the state of my body at the time and how the information is 'perceived' by me. Something sensed as a threat or potentially dangerous will trigger bodily changes designed to handle that threat. For example, the 'fight-or-flight' response of the sympathetic nervous system mobilizes my body for rapid physical action by promoting vigilance, blood circulation, and energy for muscle activity, while concomitantly inhibiting activities not immediately necessary, such as digestion and immune function. Here, the nervous system and the immune system are acting in a coordinated manner to optimize the use of energy in the body and to maintain adaptation in relation to a transiently threatening life situation. This is one reason why events perceived as acutely 'stressful' lead to short-term immune decrements. Neuroimmune coordination is also evident when internal 'dangers' (e.g. associated with an infection) are sensed by the immune system. In such cases, the immune recognition system triggers changes that promote immune effector function designed to deal with the infectious agent, while at the same time signalling the nervous system to alter the physiological disposition of the body to support the immune effector requirements. These physiological changes have been termed 'sickness' or 'illness' behaviours and include such things as increased body temperature, increased need for sleep, loss of appetite, and decreased physical and social activity.[13]

13.2.4 Generation and maintenance of self

Our immune systems act to maintain the integrity of our bodies by sensing molecular shapes and determining whether particular shapes are appropriate within the context of our bodies. In other words, the immune system is involved in the physical process of 'self–non-self discrimination'; it functions to detect and protect against potentially dangerous material arising within our bodies.[14] In achieving this, it acts as part of an extended network of communications within the body that includes extensive links with the nervous system. Therefore physical 'self' is maintained in relation to an ever-changing environment through the activity of the neuroimmune network in the body. However, as humans we have another 'self', which we might call a psychosocial self. This 'self' distinguishes us from other humans and arises out of the language that we use to describe and make sense of our relationships. It arises as a consequence of a particular human life history in the following way. As children we learn to coordinate with others through a variety of gestures; we learn to 'make sense' of patterns of behaviours and sensations, and to associate them with particular meanings. As we become adept at this, we learn to distinguish objects, and eventually to distinguish one special object that we each call 'myself'. When we become 'self-conscious', we become aware of 'self' as distinct from 'other' and we conceptually associate 'self' with our own bodies. As we learn to live in human society, we learn to ascribe meanings to forms of communication and to make sense of those meanings in terms of our 'selves'.[15] Therefore our psychosocial selves could be considered as descriptive narratives of the life stories of our bodies and the events that happen to them.

Clearly, psychosocial self is not the same as physiological self, but it influences it. Many aspects of our nervous systems and other parts of our body change as a result of the psychological value or meaning we attach to our sensory experiences. Through this physical 'emotional' response, our psychosocial domain provides a semantic layer, conditioning our senses and modulating our biological responses. Further, the physiological processes central to maintaining the integrity of my physical self (i.e. immune and nervous systems) affect how my psychosocial self functions. We have already discussed 'illness' behaviours arising from immune responses to infections. Illness behaviour effects extend also to our moods and emotions—how we feel about ourselves and others, and how we perceive and interpret our world. They are evident not only as a consequence of infections,[13] but also as a result of other illnesses associated with immune activity such as allergies and autoimmune conditions.[16,17]

In summary, as humans, we have two levels of self-construction: a psychosocial level and a physiological level. Yet each of us experiences 'self' as a coherent whole, and so our psychosocial and physiological selves must operate in a coordinated and coherent manner. Further, because in both cases the 'self' arises in concert with that which is 'non-self' (i.e. our psychosocial, cultural, and physical context or environment), the processes of self-generation operate to maintain both the self–non-self distinction and an adequate relationship between self and non-self. This means that there will always be a 'harmony of purpose' between the psychosocial and physiological self-generative processes.[18,19] How we find meaning and purpose in the flow of our lives affects how we interpret our experiences and, accordingly, how we generate our psychosocial selves, and in turn our physiological selves. The meaningful patterns of our existence modulate the psycho-physiological link such that 'like a piece of jazz music, we are constantly improvised to meet the internal and external demands of our daily lives. Each of us has a theme that is our identity and a repertoire of being that we use to adapt biologically and existentially'.[20]

This then provides a broad conceptual framework for understanding the relationship between emotional disclosure and psychoneuroimmunology. Emotional disclosure is effective when it leads to changes in the manner of constituting the psychosocial self. Such changes might arise in a various ways. For example, the meaning of the disclosed events could be reinterpreted during the expressive writing process to be more coherent with the individual's understanding of his or her life.[21] Alternatively, the disclosure process may lead to a fundamental change in an individual's manner of living such that he or she copes differently with traumatic events in future, or no longer identifies particular events as such a danger or threat to his or her psychosocial self-construct. When these sorts of changes occur in the psychosocial domain, we would expect changes in the physiological domain to be coherent with them such that short-term changes related to emotional expression will be less relevant than more habitual changes in the manner of neuroimmune functioning. For example, changes in perceived controllability of stressful events should have immunomodulatory effects over and above those of the stressor *per se*,[22] or changes in the manner of coping with traumatic events might be reflected in a change in the balance of type 1 versus type 2 immune responses.[23] In the next section, we will explore some of the evidence suggesting that changes in the meaning and context of events at the psychosocial level lead to health-related changes in the physiological context of immune responses.

13.3 The empirical evidence: effects of emotional disclosure

13.3.1 Emotionally expressive writing in healthy volunteers

Following Pennebaker's initial explorations of emotionally expressive writing with first-year college students[1] (see section 13.1.1), subsequent studies by Pennebaker and colleagues revealed beneficial effects of emotionally expressive writing on grade averages of students,[24] absentee rates in university employees,[25] and re-employment rate following job loss.[26] Other researchers have found similar beneficial effects of emotionally expressive writing with student volunteers. These include a reduction in depressive symptoms and intrusive thoughts,[27,28] positive cognitive changes,[29] and improvements in upper respiratory illness symptoms following a relationship break-up relative to a control writing group.[30] Further, subjects who disclose more severe traumas report fewer physical symptoms over subsequent months than do low-severity trauma subjects, and, regardless of previous disclosure, health benefits occur when severe traumas are disclosed.[31] Only one published study, using a student population, has failed to find any subsequent physical health or psychological benefits in the emotional disclosure group,[32] but the reason for the discrepancy between this study and other research is not obvious.

Much of the research into emotional disclosure with healthy people has centred on college students or young people, but distress-driven symptoms are prevalent among older primary care patients and account for a large percentage of doctor visits and medical costs. Therefore does emotional self-disclosure have any benefits for elderly people in primary care settings? Klapow *et al.*[33] addressed this question in an elderly population without psychiatric symptoms by comparing the effects of three 20-min writing sessions focusing on either distressing experiences (intervention group) or health behaviours (control group). Although there was reduced use of out-patient services and associated costs in both groups, the reduction was twice as great in the intervention group than in the control group, indicating a clearly beneficial effect for elderly people.

With such impressive effects observable in experimental studies with healthy volunteers, it is natural to ask whether emotional disclosure has benefits for other groups. Over the last few years, several studies have reported effects in a variety of groups such as people who have undergone loss (e.g. bereavement) or trauma.

13.3.2 People who have undergone loss or trauma

Segal *et al.* [34] asked 30 bereaved older adults to disclose verbally their thoughts and feelings about the death of their spouses in four 20-min sessions. There were significant therapeutic effects, including a decrease in intrusive thoughts and distress, which were maintained for at least a year after the disclosure. In addition, higher levels of negative affect during disclosure sessions were associated with greater cognitive changes at 1 year. In other research,[35] talking to others about their loss was associated with better adjustment to the loss of a marital partner. Curiously, in a second randomized study by the same researchers, where recently bereaved individuals were assigned either to a Pennebaker-type emotional writing task or to a no-essay control condition, the writing task did not result in a reduction in distress or doctors' visits either immediately after the bereavement or at 6-month follow-up.

In an intriguing study of college women preselected for trauma experience, Greenberg *et al.*[36] examined whether disclosing emotions generated by imaginative immersion in a novel traumatic event would enhance health and adjustment similarly to emotional disclosure about real trauma. After being randomly assigned to write about real traumas, imaginary traumas, or trivial events, imaginary trauma participants were significantly less depressed than real trauma participants but they were similarly angry, fearful, and happy. Compared with control group participants, both trauma groups made significantly fewer illness visits at 1-month follow-up; however, real trauma participants reported more fatigue and avoidance than did the other groups. The authors suggested that the effects of disclosing imaginary trauma could reflect catharsis, emotional regulation, or construction of resilient possible selves.

With regard to trauma associated with sex offences, there appears to be a difference of outcome depending on whether the studies are conducted on victims or perpetrators. For example, when psychiatric prison inmates were randomly assigned to one of three conditions (trauma writing, trivial writing, or no-writing control), participants in the trauma condition relative to those in the other conditions reported experiencing more physical symptoms post-intervention. In contrast, sex offenders in the traumatic writing group decreased their post-writing infirmary visits.[37] Conversely, there were no significant symptom reductions in undergraduate women who acknowledged attempted or completed rape.[38] Similarly, no psychological or physical health benefits were observed in women who reported a history of child sexual abuse.[39]

13.4 Emotionally expressive writing in illness groups

It is clear from the studies outlined in the previous section that emotional disclosure has beneficial effects in a variety of healthy populations and can also benefit people following loss or trauma. However, it is not necessarily applicable or effective for all groups. For example, a Dutch study in a general practice setting[40] tested whether a disclosure intervention improved subjective health and medical care use in a group of somatizing patients. Three sessions of verbal emotional disclosure to general practitioners were compared with standard care, and although the intervention was well received by patients and doctors, disclosure had no effect on the health of the patients as assessed by medicine use, health care visits, sick leave, and subjective health rating. Other research has begun to explore the effects of emotional disclosure in clinical areas such as cancer, infections, and autoimmune illnesses.

13.4.1 Cancer survivors

Diagnosis of cancer can be a source of considerable stress, and cancer patients are often reticent about disclosing their experience of the condition. In a study of 300 women with breast cancer, Henderson et al.[41] assessed how much and with whom the women discussed their cancer in the month following diagnosis. Seven per cent reported little or no disclosure to anyone besides their spouse or doctor, while 20–30% reported little or no disclosure to entire subgroups of their social network (family, friends, and health professionals). Interestingly, greater disclosure about their disease was associated with younger participants, greater disease severity, optimism, and attitudes oriented towards disclosure.

Recent studies have addressed the effectiveness of emotional disclosure interventions in cancer patients. Forty-two terminally ill patients with metastatic renal cell carcinoma who were participating in a phase II clinical trial were randomly assigned to an expressive writing or neutral writing group.[42] While there were no group differences in symptoms of distress, perceived stress, or mood disturbance, patients in the expressive writing group reported significantly less sleep disturbance, better sleep quality and sleep duration, and less daytime dysfunction compared with those in the neutral writing group. In a pilot study, Rosenberg et al.[43] explored expressive disclosure in men with diagnosed prostate cancer. Compared with controls, patients in the expressive disclosure condition showed improvements in physical symptoms and health care utilization, but not in psychological variables or disease-relevant aspects of immuno-competence. Both studies suggest that actively expressing and processing emotions may be effective in dealing with distress and symptoms in at least some cancer patients.

Stanton et al.[44] explored this further in a cohort of breast cancer patients over a 3-month period following medical treatment. Women who, at study entry, coped through expressing emotions about cancer and their experience of it had enhanced physical health and vigour, decreased distress, and fewer medical appointments for cancer-related morbidities during the next 3 months compared with those women who were low in emotional expression. Expressive coping was also related to improved quality of life for those who perceived their social contexts as highly receptive. Subsequently, the same researchers extended this work by assessing the effects of emotional disclosure interventions on breast cancer patients.[45] Early-stage breast cancer patients were assigned randomly to write over four sessions about (1) their deepest thoughts and feelings regarding breast cancer, (2) positive thoughts and feelings regarding their experience with breast cancer, or (3) facts of their breast cancer experience, and then assessed 1 and 3 months later for distress, perceived somatic symptoms, and medical appointments for cancer-related morbidities. Emotionally expressive writing was relatively effective for women low in avoidance, while writing about positive thoughts and feelings was more useful for women high in avoidance. Compared with control writing participants, the emotional group reported significantly decreased physical symptoms, and both the emotional and positive writing participants had significantly fewer medical appointments for cancer-related morbidities.

13.4.2 People with HIV

People with HIV infection comprise a group in which relationships between emotional disclosure and immune function are perhaps most readily studied. This is because HIV infects helper (CD4) T lymphocytes, and the concentrations of circulating CD4 T lymphocytes and circulating HIV viral titres are the two most important prognostic indicators. Lutgendorf et al.[46] explored the effects of emotional disclosure in relation to notification of HIV status in men at risk of AIDS. In the weeks following HIV serostatus notification, increased avoidance of thinking about HIV positivity predicted poorer mitogen-induced T-lymphocyte proliferative responses as well as trends toward lower circulating CD4 (helper) T lymphocytes. These researchers suggested that increases in avoidant and intrusive thought processing may reflect difficulties in working through the trauma of seropositivity notification. Their results highlight the importance of cognitively processing stressful or emotional material for immune functioning in HIV+ individuals.

On theoretical grounds, the effectiveness of emotional disclosure should rest not with the degree of emotion expressed but with the manner in which understanding of the traumatic experiences is altered by cognitive processing and restructuring. In other words, effective emotional disclosure should involve people finding or changing the meaning of traumatic events in the context of their lives, rather than merely expressing emotion. Bower et al.[47] explored this concept in HIV-seropositive men who had recently experienced an AIDS-related bereavement. When interviews with these men were assessed for evidence of cognitive processing and finding meaning after the loss, it was found that men who engaged in cognitive processing were more likely to find meaning from the loss. More importantly, men who found meaning showed less rapid declines in CD4 T-lymphocyte levels and lower rates of AIDS-related mortality independent of health status at baseline, health behaviours, and other potential confounds.

The importance of cognitive processing, finding or reconstructing meaning, and working through, rather than simply releasing, emotion is also evident in three more recent studies with HIV+ subjects. In one study, subjects with the best immune status (i.e. highest circulating CD4 T-lymphocyte concentrations) were those with intermediate levels of expressed emotion and a high capacity for emotional processing.[48] In a second study,[49] coping interviews were used to assess HIV-specific emotional support and emotional expression and inhibition through an analysis of the percentage of positive/negative emotion words and inhibition words, respectively. After controlling for health behaviours and other variables, there was no relationship between availability of emotional support and CD4 T-lymphocyte levels, but a higher percentage of inhibition words were associated with lower CD4 T-lymphocyte levels. A third study of patients living with AIDS examined the relationship between long-term survival and emotional expression and depth of processing of trauma.[50] Subjects wrote essays describing their reactions to past traumas, and these were scored for emotional expression and depth of processing (positive cognitive appraisal change, experiential involvement, self-esteem enhancement, and adaptive coping strategies). A group of HIV+ people who had survived at least 4 years with an AIDS-defining symptom was compared with a group of HIV+ subjects who had comparably low CD4 T-lymphocyte numbers but no AIDS symptoms. The long-term survivor group scored significantly higher on emotional expression and depth processing. For women, depth of processing was positively related to CD4 T-lymphocyte numbers, while emotional expression was also significantly negatively related to viral load and positively related to CD4 T-lymphocyte numbers. These findings highlight the importance of depth of processing rather than just emotional expression of traumatic experiences for people living with HIV/AIDS.

Finally, the question of whether a standard 'Pennebaker-type' emotional disclosure study would result in health benefits for HIV+ subjects was recently investigated in our laboratory. In a pilot study, 37 HIV+ volunteers were randomly assigned to four daily sessions of emotionally expressive writing or descriptive writing, and viral load and CD4 T-lymphocyte levels were compared over the subsequent 6 months, controlling for prewriting levels.[51] Relative to the drop in viral load measure, CD4 T lymphocyte counts increased following the intervention for participants in the emotional writing condition compared with control writing participants, suggesting that emotionally expressive writing may well have therapeutic benefits in HIV-infected people.

13.4.3 People with other infectious diseases

Another immunological variable with potential health relevance is the response to Epstein–Barr virus (EBV). This is a latent virus that infects a high proportion of the population and spends much of the time hidden unexpressed in certain nerve cells. Under conditions of physical or psychological stress, EBV activates and this process is accompanied by an increase in circulating antibodies specific for the virus. Because effective control of EBV is mediated by T lymphocytes rather than antibodies, the appearance of high titres of EBV-specific antibodies is generally taken as an indication of ineffective immune control of the virus. Esterling et al.[52] investigated the effects of emotional disclosure on EBV+ volunteers by testing whether abstaining from disclosing emotional material would correlate with poor control of the virus. After the volunteers had written essays about stressful life events, the degree of emotional disclosure in the essays was correlated with EBV antibody titre. It was found that the less disclosure in the essays, the higher was the titre, indicating poorer immune control of the virus. Further, those subjects who had been characterized previously as having repressive interpersonal styles had high antibody titres irrespective of the level of disclosure, while those not characterized as repressors only had high titres if they did not disclose emotions in their essays.

In a subsequent study, these researchers compared written and spoken emotional expression with writing about superficial topics.[53] Subjects in both oral and written trauma expression groups had significantly lower EBV antibody titres after the intervention than did subjects in the control group. Content analysis indicated that the oral group achieved the greatest improvements in cognitive change, self-esteem, and adaptive coping strategies, although there were also some differences between written and oral groups in positive and negative emotional word use. Interestingly, individual differences in the ability of subjects to involve themselves in the disclosure process and abandon their avoidance of the stressful topic during the course of the study were predictive of lower anti-EBV antibody titres, and these associations were more pronounced for individuals who disclosed older and more troublesome events.[54]

13.4.4 Autoimmune disease

The behaviour of the immune system in autoimmune diseases is different from its behaviour during infections in that autoimmunity is characterized by inappropriately aggressive or inflammatory immune responsiveness towards some normal components of the body. It is as if the immune system has partially lost the ability to discriminate between 'physiological self' and non-self, and so treats some aspects of self as if they were foreign. Therefore effective treatment focuses on diminishing the anti-self responses or controlling the damaging effects of such aggression. Many patients with autoimmune diseases report that their disease activity fluctuates over time and is often worse at times of stress. Therefore whether emotional disclosure has any impact on the course of autoimmunity is a question that is beginning to be addressed experimentally.

One of the first studies to explore this was performed by Kelley *et al.*[55] who randomly assigned patients with rheumatoid arthritis either to talk privately about stressful events or to talk about trivial topics for four consecutive days. Two weeks later there were no differences between the groups on any health measure, but at 3 months the disclosure patients had less affective disturbance and better physical functioning in daily activities. As has been evident in all other emotional disclosure studies, participants found writing or talking about traumatic events to be an upsetting process and reported increased negative affect immediately after the experience. However, in the study by Kelley *et al.* those patients who experienced larger increases in negative affect immediately after emotional disclosure also demonstrated improvements in the condition of their joints.

A more recent study confirmed this effect with rheumatoid arthritis patients and also extended it to asthmatic patients.[56] Here, the health benefits were measured by clinically assessed disease activity in the case of rheumatoid arthritis and by objective lung function assessment for asthmatic patients. In the 2 weeks following emotionally expressive or trivial writing, patients in the emotional writing group had less positive affect, increased experience of stress, and more stressful thoughts.[57] However, 4 months after writing there were significant improvements in disease activity for both rheumatoid arthritis and asthma patients in the emotional writing group but no change in patients in the control group.[56] Moreover, these effects could not be accounted for by changes in activities, locations, or social contacts of the patients. To date, however, no studies have directly linked the beneficial effects of emotional disclosure in autoimmune patients with changes in immune function.

13.5 How does emotional disclosure lead to health benefits?

Various possibilities might account for the health and other benefits following emotional writing, the most obvious being a change in health-related behaviours such as diet, exercise, sleep patterns, alcohol consumption, or smoking. However, a meta-analysis of a number of emotional writing studies concluded that none of these health behaviour factors (with the possible exception of alcohol consumption in one study[26]) could account for the salutary effects of expressive writing.[58] The finding of de Moor et al.[42] (see section 13.4.1) that cancer patients in the expressive writing group reported significantly less sleep disturbance and better sleep quality and duration would seem to be at variance with the conclusions of Smyth's meta-analysis. However, de Moor et al. did not test sleep disturbance as a mediator of the effects of disclosure on health outcomes, and they were also studying emotional disclosure in terminally ill patients whose sleep requirements and behaviour might be different from less seriously ill patients. Therefore other possible explanations of the effects of emotional disclosure on health have focused on psychological changes or physiological effects. Moreover, in the light of the benefits beginning to be seen in groups of patients with cancer, HIV, other infections, and autoimmune illnesses, physiological effects involving immune mechanisms are particularly germane.

13.5.1 Psychological mechanisms to account for effects

With regard to psychological explanations, a 'behavioural inhibition' explanation was initially proposed to account for the effects of emotional disclosure on health.[59] This argues that our natural human response is to express emotions generated by trauma and, consequently, energy is required to suppress this emotional expression. Therefore the process of inhibition requires work which is taxing on the body and this constant necessity for inhibitory work affects the neuroimmune network to cause immunosuppression and adverse health outcomes. However, Littrell[60] contends that the link between suppression of emotion and the physiological–behavioural inhibition system is not well established, and so this hypothesis cannot provide a full explanation for the apparent beneficial effects of emotional expression. For example, according to inhibition theory, reporting about undisclosed traumas should produce greater health benefits. However, in a study in which healthy undergraduates wrote about undisclosed traumas, previously disclosed traumas, or trivial events, there were no significant between-group differences on longer-term health utilization or physical symptom measures.[31] Further, when college women were randomly assigned to write about real traumas, imaginary traumas, or trivial events, imaginary trauma participants were significantly less depressed than real trauma participants immediately after disclosure, but they were similar to real trauma participants in their experience of other emotions such as anger, fear, or happiness. Moreover, compared with control group participants, both the real and the imaginary trauma disclosure groups made significantly fewer illness visits over the subsequent month.

An alternative, and perhaps more tenable, explanation invokes self-regulation theory. This stems from observations that although there is generally dysphoria immediately after emotional disclosure, there is a change in the manner in which participants express themselves over time during successful emotional disclosure interventions. Rather than simply being a cathartic exercise or a release of inhibition, the process appears to involve some cognitive restructuring which is reflected in a change in the linguistic properties of expressive writing over time. For example, increasing use of insight and of causal and associated cognitive words over several days of writing has been linked to health improvements.[21] Thus the construction of a coherent story appears to work together with expression of negative emotions in therapeutic expressive disclosure. Building on this, Cameron and Nicholls[61] investigated the effectiveness of an expressive writing task designed to foster self-regulatory coping with stressful experiences. They asked student volunteers to express thoughts and feelings about a stressful experience and then to formulate coping plans (self-regulation task), and they compared this group with others who were instructed to express their thoughts and feelings only (disclosure task) or to write about trivial topics (control task). They found that relative to the control task, those participants who were high scorers on optimism scales in both the self-regulation task and the disclosure task groups reduced illness-related clinic visits during the subsequent month. However, only the self-regulation task reduced clinic visits among pessimists. A more recent study also found support for a self-regulatory component in expressive writing.[62] Here, emotional writing about a traumatic event was compared with writing about life goals in terms of the participant's best possible future self. As well as being less upsetting than writing about trauma, this was associated with an increase in subjective well-being and a comparable decrease in illness compared with a control group, suggesting that some form of cognitive restructuring may be an important facet of effective expressive writing.

13.5.2 Immunological mechanisms to account for effects

Emotional disclosure, either through writing or talking, is usually associated with immediate post-writing distress,[58] and this is reflected in changes in autonomic nervous system activity as indicated by skin conductance and heart rate measurements during the writing process.[63-65] There have also been reports of changes in immune measures immediately after or soon after emotional disclosure. These effects include proliferative responses in culture of mitogen-stimulated blood T lymphocytes,[66] changes in circulating T-lymphocyte numbers,[67] and changes in NK cell cytotoxicity.[68] Some or all of these effects are likely to be associated with the short-term emotional changes brought about by the disclosure process and may not necessarily be good predictors of longer-term health effects. Nevertheless, there are indications that some psychological processes, beyond the immediate dysphoric effects of the disclosure, may also be operating. For example, Petrie *et al.*[69] found that although emotional writing was associated with post-writing increases in circulating helper T-lymphocyte numbers, deliberate suppression of thoughts about the written events following writing decreased circulating T-cell numbers. Also, Christensen *et al.*[68] reported that subjects who scored high on a hostility scale exhibited a significantly greater increase in NK cell cytotoxicity following emotional writing than did low-hostility subjects.

However, as discussed earlier, it is likely that longer-term immune effects rather than short-term changes will be more directly responsible for the health benefits of emotional disclosure. Initial studies in this area focused on immune changes in healthy volunteers, although more recent work is beginning to reveal potentially salient effects in patient populations as well. A study of healthy medical students inoculated with hepatitis B vaccine following four daily sessions of writing emotionally about traumatic events or descriptively about mundane topics revealed small but significant differences in antibody response between the two groups at 4 and 6 months after writing.[65] The emotional disclosure group displayed higher antiviral antibody titres than the descriptive writing group, suggesting that the disclosure process was influencing the ability of B lymphocytes to generate a primary antibody response over a prolonged period.

13.6 Directions for future research

13.6.1 Generalizability of emotional disclosure

It is clear that written or verbal expression of emotion in relation to traumatic events, undertaken repeatedly over several days, can result in both health benefits and, in some cases, health-related immune changes. Also, although emotional expression is associated with transient autonomic, neuroendocrine, and immune changes, the venting of emotions *per se* does not appear to be associated with longer-term benefits. Rather, it is the increasing use of insight and of causal and associated cognitive words over several days of writing that is linked to health improvement.[21] Earlier in this chapter it is argued that, in an emotionally expressive context, it is the construction of a coherent story or the reshaping of previously disparate events to fit into an acceptable psychosocial 'self' framework that is relevant to therapeutic writing. In support of this, several studies have shown that finding meaning in adverse or traumatic events is a principal factor in the health and immune benefits of emotional disclosure. However, the situations in which this has been explored are relatively narrow and it may not necessarily be a general phenomenon. For example, a recent study with women who had lost a close relative to breast cancer[70] tested the hypothesis that cognitive processing about the bereavement would produce changes in goals and priorities indicative of finding positive meaning from the loss. The women were asked to write about the death (cognitive processing/disclosure group) or about non-emotional topics weekly for 4 weeks. Contrary to predictions, written disclosure did not induce changes in meaning-related goals or NK cell cytotoxicity. However, women in both groups who reported positive changes in meaning-related goals also showed increases in NK cell cytotoxicity. Thus, although prioritizing goals and striving for meaning in life may have positive physiological correlates, written disclosure may not be sufficient to induce changes in these goals in response to a past bereavement. Clearly, there is a need for future studies to explore the types of situation in which emotional disclosure is beneficial and what psychological and linguistic aspects of the process are required for effectiveness.

13.6.2 Neuroimmune effects of emotional disclosure

It has been argued that the immune system, in its sensory and effector integration with the nervous system, is part of 'physiological self' which acts in concert with a person's 'psychosocial self' with the purpose of maintaining a coherent and self-consistent relationship between the individual (self) and his or her context (non-self). Therefore a robust psychosocial self-construct might be expected to promote a robust physiology. In this regard, a sense of coherence has been found to be a strong predictor of health outcomes and life satisfaction, and has also been observed to buffer the adverse effects of stressful life transitions on NK cell activity in older adults.[71]

However, an effective or beneficial immune response in one situation may be inappropriate and adverse in another—for example, an excessive reaction to innocuous substances as seen in allergies, or a detrimental immune responsiveness towards self-components as seen in autoimmune conditions. Therefore would we expect emotional disclosure (or for that matter any psychosocial intervention) to have particular neuroimmune effects independent of context? Would we expect effective emotional disclosure to result in similarly increased helper T cell numbers in HIV-infected people and in people with autoimmune thyroiditis, for example? On theoretical grounds the answer is 'no', but experimentally we do not yet have sufficient evidence to judge. We have yet to distinguish experimentally between the compelling possibility that there is an 'intelligence' in the human body–mind that can tailor physiological effects to suit desired outcomes, and the more mundane explanation that emotional disclosure type interventions work through a generalized nervous-system-mediated enhancement or inhibition of immune activity.

If emotional disclosure interventions affect the immune system through effects on neuroimmune connections, it may be possible to identify long-term changes in stress reactivity as reflected in autonomic nervous system activity or the production of pituitary–adrenal hormones such as cortisol and catecholamines which influence T-lymphocyte responsiveness. This area has yet to be investigated systematically. Alternatively, health-related immune changes following emotional disclosure may be a consequence of alterations in inflammatory processes or in the balance of type 1 and type 2 helper cytokine production. Such effects could be explored by, for example, measuring pro-inflammatory and immunoregulatory cytokine concentrations following antigenic stimulation before and after effective emotional disclosure interventions. A further question concerns the extent of immune system involvement in the beneficial effects of emotional disclosure interventions in illness groups. The situation is reasonably straightforward with infectious diseases such as HIV because the blood-derived immune measure of circulating CD4 T-cell numbers is a strong predictor of disease activity. However, in many other conditions, such as cancer, asthma, rheumatoid arthritis, etc., there are few or no readily accessible blood-associated immune markers that correlate with the disease activity. Significant health benefits of emotional disclosure have been reported in many such conditions,[42–45,55–57] but in most cases no immune parameters were measured.

A final question concerns the type of immune effects expected in different clinical situations. For example, effective immune system involvement to deal with an infectious disease requires upregulation of specific responses against antigens of the infectious agent. In contrast, in an autoimmune disease the requirement is to downregulate responsiveness towards particular self-antigens. If emotional disclosure interventions are able to achieve both these feats, then the mechanism is clearly not straightforward and is unlikely to be reducible to simple neurologically mediated immune enhancement or suppression. Future research requires two steps. The first will be to demonstrate clear correlations between health benefits in illness groups and changes in relevant immune variables. The more challenging step with then be to make sense of the psychoneuroimmune mechanisms that account for such correlations.

13.6.3 Who benefits from emotional disclosure?

Whatever physiological pathways are eventually identified, a number of things are already clear about emotional disclosure: It can have health benefits and at least some of its effects are mediated through immune changes. It does not bring about health changes as a result of alterations in health-related behaviours (e.g. changes in exercise, smoking, or diet). It is generally more beneficial for men than for women, and for people with repressive, inhibited, or hostile coping styles. The question of psychological mechanisms responsible for the health benefits of emotional disclosure has been partially answered but further work is required. For example, as a broad generalization it seems less likely that behavioural inhibition and catharsis are primary factors and more likely that self-regulation and changes in attribution of meaning around traumatic events are influential. However, there may be different personality traits or coping styles that determine both the effectiveness and pathways to effectiveness of the disclosure process. Moreover, if some psychological characteristics (e.g. repressive personality, emotional inhibition, hostile coping style) predict beneficial effects from emotional disclosure interventions, are there also characteristics that might be associated with detrimental effects? Currently there is little information on this issue.

We also have to learn whether emotional disclosure is equally applicable to all cultures, ethnic groups, and ages. Much of the research published to date has drawn from populations of young adults, but there is some evidence of effectiveness in elderly groups.[33] With regard to ethnicity and culture, a comparison of emotionally expressive writing from students of three different ethnic groups at the University of Auckland revealed potentially important differences, not only in the types of events considered traumatic by the students, but also in their manner of writing about them (as assessed by categories of words used).[72] While most of the research to date indicates that multiple writing sessions (rather than a single session) are required for benefits, we can be less certain about whether directing people to generate goals or formulate coping plans, as in research based on self-regulation theory,[45,61] is more effective than simply asking them to explore their emotions in relation to traumatic events. Personality types, backgrounds, life histories, and illness experience all affect our perceptions and both our psychological and physiological responses to events in our lives. The extent to which these factors promote or mitigate against effective emotionally expressive therapeutic effects is largely unexplored. There is still much to learn about this fascinating area of psychoneuroimmunology.

References

1 **Pennebaker JW, Beall SK** (1986). Confronting a traumatic event: toward an understanding of inhibition and disease. *J Abnorm Psychol* **95**: 274–81.

2 **Labott SM, Ahleman S, Wolever ME, Martin RB** (1990). The physiological and psychological effects of the expression and inhibition of emotion. *Behav Med* **16**: 182–9.

3 **Martin RB, Guthrie CA, Pitts CG** (1993). Emotional crying, depressed mood, and secretory immunoglobulin A. *Behav Med* **19**: 111–14.

4 **Futterman AD, Kemeny ME, Shapiro D, Polonsky W, Fahey JL** (1992). Immunological variability associated with experimentally-induced positive and negative affective states. *Psychol Med* **22**: 231–8.

5 **Futterman AD, Kemeny ME, Shapiro D, Fahey JL** (1994). Immunological and physiological changes associated with induced positive and negative mood. *Psychosom Med* **56**: 499–511.

6 **Knapp PH, Levy EM, Giorgi RG, Black PH, Fox BH, Heeren TC** (1992). Short-term immunological effects of induced emotion. *Psychosom Med* **54**: 133–48.

7 Mittwoch-Jaffe T, Shalit F, Srendi B, Yehuda S (1995). Modification of cytokine secretion following mild emotional stimuli. *NeuroReport* **6**: 789–92.

8 Malarkey WB, Kiecolt-Glaser JK, Pearl D, Glaser R (1994). Hostile behavior during marital conflict alters pituitary and adrenal hormones. *Psychosom Med* **56**: 41–51.

9 Kiecolt-Glaser JK, Glaser R, Cacioppo JT, *et al.* (1997). Marital conflict in older adults: endocrinological and immunological correlates. *Psychosom Med* **59**: 339–49.

10 Kiecolt-Glaser JK, Malarkey WB, Chee M, *et al.* (1993). Negative behavior during marital conflict is associated with immunological down-regulation. *Psychosom Med* **55**: 395–409.

11 Miller GE, Dopp JM, Myers HF, Stevens SY, Fahey JL (1999). Psychosocial predictors of natural killer cell mobilization during marital conflict. *Health Psychol* **18**: 262–71.

12 Maier SF, Watkins LR (1998). Cytokines for psychologists: implications of bidirectional immune-to-brain communication for understanding behavior, mood, and cognition. *Psychol Rev* **105**: 83–107.

13 Kelley KW, Bluthe RM, Dantzer R, *et al.* (2003). Cytokine-induced sickness behavior. *Brain Behav Immun* **17**(Suppl 1): S112–18.

14 Matzinger P (1994). Tolerance, danger, and the extended family. *Annu Rev Immunol* **12**: 991–1045.

15 Booth RJ (2002). Psychospiritual healing and the immune system in cancer. In Lewis CE, O'Brien R, Barraclough J (eds) *The Psychoimmunology of Cancer* (2nd edn). Oxford: Oxford University Press, 164–81.

16 Marshall PS, O'Hara C, Steinberg P (2002). Effects of seasonal allergic rhinitis on fatigue levels and mood. *Psychosom Med* **64**: 684–91.

17 Pawlak CR, Jacobs R, Mikeska E, *et al.* (1999). Patients with systemic lupus erythematosus differ from healthy controls in their immunological response to acute psychological stress. *Brain Behav Immun* **13**: 287–302.

18 Booth RJ, Ashbridge KR (1992). Teleological coherence: exploring the dimensions of the immune system. *Scand J Immunol* **36**: 751–9.

19 Booth RJ, Ashbridge KR (1993). A fresh look at the relationship between the psyche and immune system: teleological coherence and harmony of purpose. *Adv Mind–Body Med* **9**: 4–23.

20 Aldridge D (1998). Life as jazz: Hope, meaning, and music therapy in the treatment of life-threatening illness. *Adv Mind–Body Med* **14**: 271–82.

21 Pennebaker JW (1993). Putting stress into words: health, linguistic, and therapeutic implications. *Behav Res Ther* **31**: 539–48.

22 Brosschot JF, Godaert GL, Benschop RJ, Olff M, Ballieux RE, Heijnen CJ (1998). Experimental stress and immunological reactivity: a closer look at perceived uncontrollability. *Psychosom Med* **60**: 359–61.

23 Marshall GD, Jr, Agarwal SK, Lloyd C, Cohen L, Henninger EM, Morris GJ (1998). Cytokine dysregulation associated with exam stress in healthy medical students. *Brain Behav Immun* **12**: 297–307.

24 Pennebaker JW, Colder M, Sharp LK (1990). Accelerating the coping process. *J Pers Soc Psychol* **58**: 528–37.

25 Francis ME, Pennebaker JW (1992). Putting stress into words: the impact of writing on physiological, absentee, and self-reported emotional well-being measures. *Am J Health Promot* **6**: 280–7.

26 Spera SP, Buhrfeind ED, Pennebaker JW (1994). Expressive writing and coping with job loss. *Acad Manage J* **37**: 722–33.

27 **Lepore SJ** (1997). Expressive writing moderates the relation between intrusive thoughts and depressive symptoms. *J Pers Soc Psychol* **73**: 1030–7.

28 **Schoutrop MJ, Lange A, Hanewald G, Davidovich U, Salomon H** (2002). Structured writing and processing major stressful events: a controlled trial. *Psychother Psychosom* **71**: 151–7.

29 **Murray EJ, Segal DL** (1994). Emotional processing in vocal and written expression of feelings about traumatic experiences. *J Trauma Stress* **7**: 391–405.

30 **Lepore SJ, Greenberg MA** (2002). Mending broken hearts: effects of expressive writing on mood, cognitive processing, social adjustment and health following a relationship breakup. *Psychol Health* **17**: 547–60.

31 **Greenberg MA, Stone AA** (1992). Emotional disclosure about traumas and its relation to health: effects of previous disclosure and trauma severity. *J Pers Soc Psychol* **63**: 75–84.

32 **Kloss JD, Lisman SA** (2002). An exposure-based examination of the effects of written emotional disclosure. *Br J Health Psychol* **7**: 31–46.

33 **Klapow JC, Schmidt SM, Taylor LAC, *et al.*** (2001). Symptom management in older primary care patients: feasibility of an experimental, written self-disclosure protocol. *Ann Intern Med* **134**: 905–11.

34 **Segal DL, Chatman C, Bogaards JA, Becker LA** (2001). One-year follow-up of an emotional expression intervention for bereaved older adults. *J Ment Health Aging* **7**: 465–72.

35 **Stroebe M, Stroebe W, Schut H, Zech E, van den Bout J** (2002). Does disclosure of emotions facilitate recovery from bereavement? Evidence from two prospective studies. *J Consult Clin Psychol* **70**: 169–78.

36 **Greenberg MA, Wortman CB, Stone AA** (1996). Emotional expression and physical health: revising traumatic memories or fostering self-regulation? *J Pers Soc Psychol* **71**: 588–602.

37 **Richards JM, Beal WE, Seagal JD, Pennebaker JW** (2000). Effects of disclosure of traumatic events on illness behavior among psychiatric prison inmates. *J Abnorm Psychol* **109**: 156–60.

38 **Brown EJ, Heimberg RG** (2001). Effects of writing about rape: evaluating Pennebaker's paradigm with a severe trauma. *J Trauma Stress* **14**: 781–90.

39 **Batten SV, Follette VM, Rasmussen Hall ML, Palm KM** (2002). Physical and psychological effects of written disclosure among sexual abuse survivors. *Behav Ther* **33**: 107–22.

40 **Schilte AF, Portegijs PJ, Blankenstein AH, *et al.*** (2001). Randomised controlled trial of disclosure of emotionally important events in somatisation in primary care. *BMJ* **323**: 86.

41 **Henderson BN, Davison KP, Pennebaker JW, Gatchel RJ, Baum A** (2002). Disease disclosure patterns among breast cancer patients. *Psychol Health* **17**: 51–62.

42 **de Moor C, Sterner J, Hall M, *et al.*** (2002). A pilot study of the effects of expressive writing on psychological and behavioral adjustment in patients enrolled in a phase II trial of vaccine therapy for metastatic renal cell carcinoma. *Health Psychol* **21**: 615–19.

43 **Rosenberg HJ, Rosenberg SD, Ernstoff MS, *et al.*** (2002). Expressive disclosure and health outcomes in a prostate cancer population. *Int J Psychiatry Med* **32**: 37–53.

44 **Stanton AL, Danoff-Burg S, Cameron CL, *et al.*** (2000). Emotionally expressive coping predicts psychological and physical adjustment to breast cancer. *J Consult Clin Psychol* **68**: 875–82.

45 **Stanton AL, Danoff-Burg S, Sworowski LA, *et al.*** (2002). Randomized, controlled trial of written emotional expression and benefit finding in breast cancer patients. *J Clin Oncol* **20**: 4160–8.

46 **Lutgendorf SK, Antoni MH, Ironson G, Klimas N, Fletcher MA, Schneiderman N** (1997). Cognitive processing style, mood, and immune function following hiv seropositivity notification. *Cogn Ther Res* **21**: 157–84.

47 **Bower JE, Kemeny ME, Taylor SE, Fahey JL** (1998). Cognitive processing, discovery of meaning, CD4 decline, and AIDS-related mortality among bereaved HIV-seropositive men. *J Consult Clin Psychol* **66**: 979–86.

48 Solano L, Montella F, Salvati S, *et al.* (2002). Expression and processing of emotions: relationships with CD4+ levels in 42 HIV-positive asymptomatic individuals. *Psychol Health* **16**: 689–98.

49 Eisenberger NI, Kemeny ME, Wyatt GE (2003). Psychological inhibition and CD4 T-cell levels in HIV-seropositive women. *J Psychosom Res* **54**: 213–24.

50 O'Cleirigh C, Ironson G, Antoni M, *et al.* (2003). Emotional expression and depth processing of trauma and their relation to long-term survival in patients with HIV/AIDS. *J Psychosom Res* **54**: 225–35.

51 Petrie KJ, Fonanilla I, Thomas MG, Booth RJ, Pennebaker JW (2004). Effect of written emotional expression on immune function in patients with human immunodeficiency virus infection: a randomized trial. *Psychosom Med* **66**: 272–5.

52 Esterling BA, Antoni MH, Kumar M, Schneiderman N (1990). Emotional repression, stress disclosure responses, and Epstein–Barr viral capsid antigen titers. *Psychosom Med* **52**: 397–410.

53 Esterling BA, Antoni MH, Fletcher MA, Margulies S, Schneiderman N (1994). Emotional disclosure through writing or speaking modulates latent Epstein–Barr virus antibody titers. *J Consult Clin Psychol* **62**: 130–40.

54 Lutgendorf SK, Antoni MH, Kumar M, Schneiderman N (1994). Changes in cognitive coping strategies predict EBV-antibody titre change following a stressor disclosure induction. *J Psychosom Res* **38**: 63–78.

55 Kelley JE, Lumley MA, Leisen JC (1997). Health effects of emotional disclosure in rheumatoid arthritis patients. *Health Psychol* **16**: 331–40.

56 Smyth JM, Stone AA, Hurewitz A, Kaell A (1999). Effects of writing about stressful experiences on symptom reduction in patients with asthma or rheumatoid arthritis: a randomized trial. *JAMA* **281**: 1304–9.

57 Smyth JM (1999). Written emotional disclosure: effects on symptoms, mood, and disease status in patients with asthma or rheumatoid arthritis. *Diss Abstr Int B Sci Eng* **59**(8B): 4543.

58 Smyth JM (1998). Written emotional expression: effect sizes, outcome types, and moderating variables. *J Consult Clin Psychol* **66**: 174–84.

59 Pennebaker JW (1989). Confession, inhibition, and disease. *Adv Exp Soc Psychol* **22**: 211–44.

60 Littrell J (1998). Is the reexperience of painful emotion therapeutic? *Clin Psychol Rev* **18**: 71–102.

61 Cameron LD, Nicholls G (1998). Expression of stressful experiences through writing: effects of a self- regulation manipulation for pessimists and optimists. *Health Psychol* **17**: 84–92.

62 King LA (2001). The health benefits of writing about life goals. *Pers Soc Psychol Bull* **27**: 798–807.

63 Berry DS, Pennebaker JW (1993). Nonverbal and verbal emotional expression and health. *Psychother Psychosom* **59**: 11–19.

64 Hughes CF, Uhlmann C, Pennebaker JW (1994). The body's response to processing emotional trauma: linking verbal text with autonomic activity. *J Pers* **62**: 565–85.

65 Petrie KJ, Booth RJ, Pennebaker JW, Davison KP, Thomas MG (1995). Disclosure of trauma and immune response to a hepatitis B vaccination program. *J Consult Clin Psychol* **63**: 787–92.

66 Pennebaker JW, Kiecolt-Glaser JK, Glaser R (1988). Disclosure of traumas and immune function: health implications for psychotherapy. *J Consult Clin Psychol* **56**: 239–45.

67 Booth RJ, Petrie KJ, Pennebaker JW (1997). Changes in circulating lymphocyte numbers following emotional disclosure: evidence of buffering? *Stress Med* **13**: 23–9.

68 Christensen AJ, Edwards DL, Wiebe JS, *et al.* (1996). Effect of verbal self-disclosure on natural killer cell activity: moderating influence of cynical hostility. *Psychosom Med* **58**: 150–5.

69 Petrie KJ, Booth RJ, Pennebaker JW (1998). The immunological effects of thought suppression. *J Pers Soc Psychol* **75**: 1264–72.

70 **Bower JE, Kemeny ME, Taylor SE, Fahey JL** (2003). Finding positive meaning and its association with natural killer cell cytotoxicity among participants in a bereavement-related disclosure intervention. *Ann Behav Med* **25**: 146–55.

71 **Lutgendorf SK, Vitaliano PP, Tripp-Reimer T, Harvey JH, Lubaroff DM** (1999). Sense of coherence moderates the relationship between life stress and natural killer cell activity in healthy older adults. *Psychol Aging* **14**: 552–63.

72 **Booth RJ, Davison KP** (2003). Relating to our worlds in a psychobiological context: the impact of disclosure on self-generation and immunity. In Wilce J (ed) *Social and Cultural Lives of Immune Systems*. London: Routledge, 36–48.

Integrative summary: on the clinical relevance of psychoneuroimmunology

Robert Ader

Introduction

Psychoneuroimmunology is concerned with the relationships among behaviour, neural and endocrine processes, and immune function. Research in the area has shown that immunoregulatory processes are part of a single complex network of adaptive responses. This new knowledge of interactions between the brain and the immune system holds considerable promise for expanding our understanding of the mechanisms underlying health and illness, and the role that emotions and 'stress' play in this equation. Thus, one focus of psychoneuroimmunological research—and the primary focus of this particular volume—concerns stress-related immune impairment in humans and the clinical significance of psychosocially induced changes in immune function.

Had I detected issues that provoked differences of opinion among the authors of these several chapters, I would have devoted this 'integrative summary' to just those issues. As it happened, however, the problems, needs, and solutions discussed were common to multiple content areas. With a minimum of references to specific chapters, it is some of these common themes that I will expand upon here.

With only slight variations in shading, the backdrop for these several chapters is similar. Affective responses to what are perceived to be stressful circumstances are accompanied by autonomic and neuroendocrine changes capable of influencing immune function and thus (increasing) susceptibility to a variety of diseases. Conversely, behavioural interventions that reduce anxiety or distress decrease the intensity or duration of autonomic and neuroendocrine responses, thereby effecting a change in immune function that promotes wellness and/or recovery from disease.

Depression, for example, has an impact on cardiovascular, infectious, and autoimmune diseases. Depression also alters autonomic and neuroendocrine activity which leads to changes in immune function. It is a reasonable hypothesis, but it remains to be established, that it is the alterations in immune function that mediate the effects of depression on the development or progression of a particular disease. Other emotions can also change immune function but, again, we do not know if these are responsible for the health-promoting aspects of emotional disclosure or any of the other behavioural interventions purported to reduce distress. Ascribing alterations in disease susceptibility to immune changes effected by acute or chronic stressful experiences or behavioural interventions is an experimental challenge. For example, immunopharmacological agents may be used to modify one or another aspect of immune function or as a targeted therapeutic intervention. Immunopharmacological agents also have neuroendocrine consequences. Therefore one cannot be certain whether the effects of an immunopharmacological manipulation are due to its actions on the immune system or its actions on the neuroendocrine system.

Are stress-induced changes in immune function clinically significant?

For the most part, the immunological effects of stressful life experiences have been 'small'—too small, it is argued, to be of clinical significance. However, given the complexity of the feedback and feedforward mechanisms within and between the immune and nervous systems, it is unreasonable to expect that psychosocial circumstances alone could perturb immune system defences to an extent that exceeded homeostatic limits. Therefore, when we speak of the role of stress in susceptibility to disease we are, in almost all cases, speaking of the effects of stress on the expression or progression of disease—not on the induction or cause of disease. The present authors presume that stress-induced neuroendocrine changes capable of altering immune processes involved in the pathogenesis of certain diseases can have clinical consequences and that such health effects are most likely the result of interactions among factors such as specific environmental pathogens, existing pathology, and/or an immune system compromised by endogenous or exogenously introduced circumstances.

The most direct way to investigate the effects of 'stress' on susceptibility to disease is in prospective studies—prospective with respect to stressful life experiences as well as disease processes. There is good evidence from animal studies that psychosocial factors can alter disease susceptibility via changes in immune function. However, the degree of control that can be exerted in studies with subhuman animals is not always feasible in studies of humans. Nevertheless, there are overlapping research strategies that have been adopted to address such questions. As discussed and illustrated by the present authors, these include the consideration and exploitation of several classes of variables such as 'vulnerable' or 'at-risk' populations, individual differences, qualitative and quantitative dimensions of stressful life experiences and immunogenic challenges, and, as a common denominator, outcome measures that are biologically relevant to specific disease processes.

Vulnerable populations

Penedo and Dahn, for example, ask if psychosocial factors such as stressful life experiences, coping skills, social support, and personality resources can exacerbate (or, presumably, attenuate) age-related decrements in immunocompetence. Ageing is accompanied by some changes in the immune system thought to reflect immunosenescence and by an altered susceptibility to disease. Thus the elderly may be considered a vulnerable population who may respond to stressful events with larger fluctuations of immune function and a greater propensity for the development or progression of disease than young or middle-aged people. Conversely, the elderly may display a greater 'gain' from certain behavioural interventions considering the reduced psychosocial resources that may be available in their current environment. Similar issues were raised regarding the interaction between psychosocial factors and other psychobiological vulnerabilities (e.g. depression) that are also characterized by alterations in immune function and increased susceptibility to or progression of disease. Vulnerable or immunocompromised individuals might also include patients taking certain prescribed medications or individuals who are abusing drugs.

Individuals with a genetic predisposition to particular diseases (e.g. autoimmune diseases, diabetes, some cancers) and individuals currently in remission from chronic disease also constitute 'vulnerable' or 'at-risk' populations in which one can investigate the effects of psychosocial factors on the progression, recurrence or exacerbation of existing disease rather than the development of new disease. By focusing on the reactivation of latent viruses (e.g. herpes, cytomegalovirus, Epstein–Barr virus) or bacteria (e.g. *Helicobacter pylori*), the majority of any adult population becomes, in that instance, a vulnerable population. And, of course, individuals at different stages of disease (e.g. HIV+ individuals and AIDS patients) are commonly selected to assess the effects of psychosocial factors on the progression or recovery from disease.

Experimentally induced immunogenic challenges

The most convincing evidence that stressful experiences heighten susceptibility to infectious disease in humans comes from studies that expose volunteer subjects to a controlled viral challenge. Miller and Cohen detail the advantages of such an experimental strategy, to which I would add the ability to systematically titrate the viral challenge. This would provide the latitude to observe psychosocial influences that might otherwise be masked by suprathreshold levels of immunogenic stimulation. Also, this strategy would further enable tracing the observed effects to immune function. The same strategy is exploited by studies measuring the effects of stress on the healing of experimentally induced wounds. Exposing volunteer participants to viral challenges and experimentally induced wounds has the additional potential for examining the psychobiological factors that might increase resistance to viral illness or accelerate wound healing, neither of which has yet been systematically addressed. These issues invariably direct attention to individual differences in the perception of and the psychobiological response to socioenvironmental circumstances.

Individual differences

One simple, universal observation underlies psychosomatic research . . . when a population of individuals is exposed to the same environmental pathogens only some individuals manifest disease. Despite the most sophisticated strategies designed to achieve uniformity, variability remains one of the most ubiquitous results of all natural and contrived biological experiments.[1]

As a subset of psychosomatic research, psychoneuroimmunology is challenged by the same observations—and the same opportunities. This, too, is a common theme throughout this volume. It is clear from the opening chapters that we know a great deal about how individual components of the immune system work and how individual components of the endocrine system respond to stress, yet we are only just beginning to understand how these systems interact in health and disease. Lewis Thomas expressed it most succinctly when he wrote: 'You'll never understand how bees make honey no matter how carefully you dissect a single bee'.

There are large individual differences in immunological reactivity, as there are in hormonal and autonomic responses, to stressful events. We are constantly reminded that the stress response is influenced by personality and dispositional factors that affect the individual's perception and appraisal of environmental circumstances, the individual and social resources available and required to cope effectively with the demands of the environment, and the biological substrate upon which the stressful stimuli are superimposed. The recognition and assessment of individual differences has been something of a problem in immunology. Investigators recognize genetically determined variability in lymphocyte activities and use inbred animals, conduct *in vitro* experiments, and pool blood samples from presumably identical individuals—techniques calculated to eliminate individual differences. Researchers in immunology are unaccustomed to dealing with the variability that typifies all biological phenomena. What one gains by ignoring variability is the 'illusion of simplicity'[2] that characterizes the traditional biomedical model of disease; however, the cost is a loss of generalizability.

In fact, host characteristics are not complications; they are opportunities. Individual differences in behaviour and in physiological, including immunological, function permit one to identify empirically derived factors that could mediate behaviourally induced changes in immune function and susceptibility to disease. Thus, rather than an intrusive manipulation that induces multiple physiological changes, often in a non-physiological manner, one can take advantage of the neuroendocrine and immunological differences between males and females, young and old people, and aggressive and non-aggressive individuals, or the difference in the pattern of cytokine responses that characterizes different strains of animals, for example, to explore potential mediating processes.

Clinical significance of behavioural interventions

Studying the effects of behavioural interventions has faced valid clinical implications. As a research strategy, interventions provide an alternative (the opposite side of the coin, if you will) to studies of chronic stress that can be difficult to implement in human subjects. However, the rationale for each is the same. Stressful experiences or behavioural interventions influence emotional, neural, and endocrine functions capable of altering immune responses that are generally viewed as negative, in the first instance, and positive in the second. This is an obvious oversimplification since physiological changes induced by either are neither negative nor positive except in relation to some specific outcome measure or disease process. Thus, the research strategies and variables that need to be considered in assessing the effects of behavioural interventions are essentially the same as those that apply to the effects of stressful life experiences.

Many different kinds of behavioural interventions are more or less effective in improving mood, quality of life, and health behaviours and in altering neuroendocrine and immune functions. However, the question remains as to whether these latter effects are sufficiently large or last long enough to contribute to one's health status or, to begin with, if they are even relevant to the development of a specific disease. Unfortunately, we have not yet reached the stage where the selection of a behavioural intervention is based on its ability to change those parameters of physiological function that are relevant to the progression of specific disease processes. In the same way that there is a behavioural target for change in the selection of a particular intervention, there needs to be a target for change in the neuroendocrine and immunological effects of therapeutic interventions.

The nature of potentially immunogenic stimuli

Finally, the qualitative and quantitative nature of stressful life experiences (and behavioural interventions) and immunogenic stimulation—methodological issues of strategic importance—should be emphasized. For example, the acute or chronic nature of a stressor and the disease process under study are factors that influence the health effects of stressful experiences and behavioural interventions. The findings described in previous chapters suggest that it is chronic ongoing stressful circumstances that have the greatest impact, especially, perhaps, in the case of acute disease. These are circumstances in which exposure to potentially pathogenic stimuli is superimposed on a neural, endocrine, and immunological milieu that has been altered in some way by chronic exposure to stressful conditions.

The health effects of acute exposure to a stressor are somewhat more complicated. Acute stressor effects superimposed on a *chronic* disease state (e.g. cardiovascular disease, cancer) do not appear to have consistent effects. Acute exposure to a stressor could also occur before or after *acute* exposure to a potential pathogen. In this case, the temporal relationship between exposure to the stressor and exposure to the potential pathogen becomes an additional variable that requires attention (e.g. where, in the cascade of immune responses to antigenic stimulation, are the neuroendocrine responses to a stressor exerting their effects?), emphasizing again the need for the repeated sampling of multiple measures of immune and neuroendocrine responses to the stressor.

Because the introduction of a defined viral or other antigenic challenge provides the greatest degree of experimental control, the magnitude of the immunogenic challenge is a critical variable. In keeping with the need to reduce variability, the use of an immunologically 'optimal' concentration of antigen is chosen to ensure a robust immune response. However, under the conditions that exist in the real world, as opposed to the laboratory, individuals are not generally exposed to pathogens in a dose or via a route that unconditionally elicits disease. Thus, the use of suprathreshold levels of stimulation provides little latitude for the expression of psychosocial factors that have the potential to contribute to the development or progression of disease as it naturally occurs. Therefore, it is not unlikely that the systematic variation of antigen dose would enable the observation of psychosocially based differences in immunological reactivity associated with increases and/or decreases in the development or progression of disease.

Some conclusions

'Stress' is supposed to be a constellation of non-specific responses to virtually any demand put upon one's body. Research on stress has, for the most part, concentrated on these non-specific responses as descriptors and as explanations of the effects of stressful life experiences. Indeed, there are neuroendocrine responses that are common to all stressors (e.g. adrenocortical responses), but different stressors also exert a variety of other stressor-specific responses. They must, because different stressors can have different effects on the same immune response or disease process—and the same stressor can have different effects on different disease processes. Thus, the common non-specific effects of stressful experiences cannot explain the myriad effects of stress on disease susceptibility. Several of these chapters more than hint at the simplicity and inadequacy of attempting to explain the effects of stress on immune function by invoking changes in circulating levels of adrenocortical steroids. Booth applies the same logic to an analysis of the mechanisms by which behavioural interventions might influence immune functions and susceptibility to different disease processes.

It is appropriate to recognize the need and attempt to document the clinical significance of behaviourally induced alterations in immune function, if only to parry the selectively applied criterion of 'practical application' to justify pursuing this integrative concept of adaptive processes. In a sense, though, the question is somewhat premature (as is the rush to influence disease susceptibility by applying behavioural interventions whose the immunological effects have not been adequately defined). We have more than enough data to feel confident of a robust relationship between the brain and the immune system that translates into questions of clinical relevance. More importantly, though, we recognize the basic information that is still missing. As we sharpen our tools and as the nature of the basic relationships among behavioural, neural and endocrine, and immune processes become clearer, questions about clinical relevance will be addressed with increasing sophistication. Indeed, as we learn more about how neural and endocrine states influence immunological-based diseases, and how immune processes affect behaviour and what are presumed to be endocrine or neurological disorders, there may be a need to redefine the nature of some diseases and the strategies for therapeutic interventions.[3] It is in this context that Heijnen and Kavelaars suggest that it might be worthwhile to consider using neuroendocrine mediators to enhance immunomodulatory therapies in some autoimmune diseases. This emerging view of immunoregulatory processes as the adaptive result of an integrated network of neural, endocrine, and immune responses promises a better understanding and a new appreciation of the multidetermined aetiology of pathophysiological states.

References

1 **Ader R** (1980). Presidential address: Psychosomatic and psychoimmunologic research. *Psychosom Med* **52**: 307–22.

2 **Weiner H** (1978). The illusion of simplicity: the medical model revisited. *Am J Psychiatry* **135**: 27–33.

3 **Ader R** (2001). Psychoneuroimmunology. *Curr Dir Psychol Sci* **10**: 94–8.

Index